NEW DEVELOPMENTS IN BIRTH DEFECTS RESEARCH

NEW DEVELOPMENTS IN BIRTH DEFECTS RESEARCH

NELSON A. GASLEM
EDITOR

Nova Biomedical Books
New York

For permission to use material from this book please contact us:
Telephone 631-231-7269; Fax 631-231-8175
Web Site: http://www.novapublishers.com

LIBRARY OF CONGRESS CATALOGING-IN-PUBLICATION DATA

New developments in birth defects research / Nelson A. Gaslem, editor.
p. ; cm.
Includes bibliographical references and index.
ISBN 13: 978-1-60021-400-4
ISBN 10: 1-60021-400-2
1. Abnormalities, Human--Research. I. Gaslem, Nelson A.
[DNLM: 1. Abnormalities. QS 675 N5323 2006]
RG6262.N3944 2006
616'.043--dc22 2006024936

Published by Nova Science Publishers, Inc. ✢ New York

CONTENTS

PREFACE

Birth defects are defined as abnormalities of structure, function, or body metabolism that are present at birth. These abnormalities lead to mental or physical disabilities or are fatal. There are more than 4,000 different known birth defects ranging from minor to serious, and although many of them can be treated or cured, they are the leading cause of death in the first year of life. This new book presents leading research in this field from around the world.

Chapter 1 - The lymphatic vascular system (LVS) is extended to almost every organ of the body and exists side by side to almost every tissue, in that way resembling the arterial and venous systems. We can trace its development as a separate entity in some regions of the body from the end of the fifth week of embryonic life. There is an obvious correlation between these sites and the appearance of some of the most common congenital lymphatic vessel malformations (LVM). They can cause minor or major health problems, affecting a large variety of organs and regions of the body. In this chapter we review varius aspects of the lymphatic system, both clinical and biological.

Lymphatic development is now being studied at the molecular level using lymphatic-specific markers. These methods revealed several mechanisms of regulation of lymphangiogenesis, involving glycoproteins, angiopoietines etc. The modulators that cause lymphatic malformations through their interaction with the endothelium (positive or negative) are not known yet exactly.

The spectrum of pathophysiologic perturbations caused by lymphatic defects, comprise derangements in fluid equilibrium, nutrient transport, leucocyte transport and anatomic relations. But the understanding of many basic aspects of lymphatic vessel function lags behind that of the blood vascular system, due mainly to the difficulty in working in small, thin-walled lymphatic vessels and the relative lack of lymphatic specific markers. Recent application of cellular and molecular techniques has produced some significant developments in lymphatic cell biology, mainly in our understanding of lymphatic muscle function, transport function and the regulation of an intrinsic lymph pump.

The variety of presentation of LVMs renders any attempt for a unified classification, at least in part, arbitrary, incomplete or useless. Classifications by clinical manifestation may easily overlap gross pathologic, histologic or cytochemical classification (and vice versa).

A classification of LVMs is proposed on the basis of the anatomical structures involved: lymph vessel-angiodysplasia, lymphadeno(nodal)-dysplasia and the coexistence of both (lymphangio-adenodysplasias). LVMs belong to the group of low-flow vascular lesions.

Among these lesions, we first discuss those that cause lymph accumulation in anatomic spaces. Some of these lesions have a congenital component and become symptomatic by the traumatic process of labour. Congenital chylothorax is the most interesting in this category.

Second, we discuss the lesions that develop on the LVS stroma, all of them with varying degree of adjacent tissue infiltration: from the lymphangioma circumscriptum to the diffuse lesion leading to macroglossia, or from the lymphatic obliteration lesions without other tissue involvement, to the complex Klippel-Trenaunay syndrome.

Diagnosis is based on clinical findings, imaging and histology. Several distinguishing characteristics must be looked for, mainly the presence of the lesion at birth, growth, involution, change in volume, pain, outflow.

Histology must distinguish between simple (capillary), cavernous, or cystic (hygroma) LVM, depending on the size of the lymphatic channels they contain.

Doppler ultrasound should be the initial imaging modality for recognizing vascular tumors from vascular malformations. It is also of special value for the fetal period.CT scan or MRI is best to evaluate the extent of the lesions prior to treatment. Lymphangioscintigraphy is a superb functional (but anatomically gross) exam.

In general, treatment is tailored according to pathology and age (fetus, newborn or older child). It may include dietary, pharmaceutical or surgical interventions more or less aggressive. The recently discovered inducers of lymphangiogenesis could, at least theoretically, constitute special targets for modifying lymphatic growth. This approach is mainly used for cancer treatment but may be promising for lympangioma treatment as well. On the other hand, stimulation of lymphangiogenesis might be a key for the treatment of lymphedema in the future.

Chapter 2 - Aim of the study: Follow-up of the development of children born with neural tube defect.

Material and method: We performed a follow-up study of 54 infants born with myelomeningocoele between 1991 and 2001 in the Department of Obstetrics of the Medical University of Gdansk.The selected group consisted of children that lived until the end of the observation period – till 28.02.2003. We analyzed: fetal age at diagnosis, the time of delivery, mode of delivery, the newborn`s Apgar score after birth, birth weight, the location of defect, mortality, the further development – sphincters function, motoric abilities.

Results: In the period between 1991 – 2001 22 534 births took place in the Department of Obstetrics of the Medical University of Gdansk. Most of the analyzed defects were diagnosed between 31st and 35th week pf pregnancy. Almost 54% of children were still born (13%) or died till the end of observation (40,1%). There was significant correlation between high level of spina bifida, presence of other malformations or late diagnosis and mortality. Most of the children had no ability of locomotion, some of them used wheelchairs or braces and only 3 of them needed no help in walking. Bladder and bowel problems were most common when spinal defect was localized in lumbo-sacral region.

Chapter 3 - Ostium Secundum Atrial Septal Defect (osASD) is a common, sometimes familial, form of congenital heart disease, accounting for approximately 10% of all congenital cardiac defects. Atrial septal defect is very well tolerated in most cases, and its diagnosis is often made during routine clinical evaluation in asymptomatic patients. In the last decade, percutaneous closure by device implantation has been proposed as the one-stop choice for ASD treatment. When compared to surgery, percutaneous approach is less invasive, does not require cardiopulmonary by-pass, preserves pericardial and atrial integrity, allows shorter admission time and faster reintegration to daily life and is less psychologically stressing for patients (especially in pediatric age). Mid-term follow-up studies underscore that percutaneous treatment is as effective as surgery in terms of ASD closure but is associated with less early and late complications (e.g. arrhythmias, unresolved right side dilation). Since percutaneous ASD closure has been routinely available for about 10 years, long term follow up studies are still warranted.

However, transcatheter option might be considered as an "unbiased" tool to study the impact of ASD closure on cardiac electro-geometric remodeling, allowing to differentiate the hemodynamic consequences of shunt disappearance from the artificial changes resulting from surgery. Indeed, improvements in cardiac electrical analysis (QT and PR dispersion, signal-averaged EKG, Monophasic Action Potential invasive recording) and imaging technologies (e.g. Doppler Tissue Imaging, Strain/Strain Rate, Integrated Backscatter, 3-D Echo, MRI) brought new insights both in patho-physiology of right ventricular volume overload and time-course of its normalization after percutaneous ASD closure. These data might help the clinical decision-making on timing for percutaneous ASD treatment in the era of device closure, In fact, while all symptomatic patients and asymptomatic adults should be treated as soon as ASD is diagnosed, the indication in asymptomatic children is usually given by subjective ultrasound or EKG signs of right heart suffering. In fact, it is unclear if all children significantly benefit from early treatment when benefits have to be weighed over risks related to dealing with growing hearts. Recent data show that in asymptomatic children, despite the general idea, ASD closure might be safely deferred to early adulthood with no difference in terms of cardiac remodeling and mid-term clinical endpoints. Indeed, it appears that traditional parameters do not select children who might most benefit from early treatment. In general, volume overload associated with ASD appears to be responsible for very mild, if any, impairment of cardiac function in childhood to early adulthood. In this age range, it appears that percutaneous ASD closure completely reverses to normal any adaptive cardiac remodeling. In conclusion, new advances in diagnostic technologies might help to better understand the patho-physiologic consequences of atrial shunt disappearance as well as to clarify the most appropriate timing for ASD closure in childhood.

Chapter 4 - Duplications of the alimentary tract make up a group of rare and interesting malformations that vary in size, location and presenting symptoms. Since 1733, when *Calder* published the first reported case of intestinal duplication, more than 500 cases have been published, to date. *Ladd,* in 1937, introduced the term "duplication" and described three features to define the same. Most duplications are possibly "enterogenous cysts" as the actual doubling of the alimentary tract is seen in only a few cases. The aetiology of duplications is still evolving with different theories suggesting different causes for this unusual condition.

Duplications are classified as either tubular or cystic and can occur anywhere along the alimentary tract with colonic mucosa being reported in cysts located in the tongue to gastric mucosa being identified in the rectum. Communication of these duplications with the normal intestinal tract may vary but are more frequently seen with the tubular type.

Clinical presentations of these uncommon anomalies depend upon the location and size of the duplication and some duplications can remain quiscent and persist into adulthood. Though excision remains the preferred treatment, it may not be always a possible option due to co-existing malformations in other organ systems. Further details are given in the discussion of the various types of duplications.

Chapter 5 - Cystic fibrosis (CF) is the most common autosomal recessively inherited disorders in Caucasian population. Prenatal diagnosis of CF is very frequently required and is performed by molecular analysis of the mutations that the fetus could have inherited of the parents. This procedure is carried out at 10-13 weeks of gestation using DNA from chorion villus sample (CVS) and includes 2% risk of abortion. During the last years, much attention has been paid to the possibility of developing non-invasive methods for prenatal diagnosis without any risk for the fetus. Recently, the discovery of fetal DNA in maternal plasma is offering a new strategy to study some conditions of the fetus in a safer way. Because of the presence of maternal DNA in plasma, these approaches are limited to paternally inherited disorders or present "de novo" in the fetus. Up to now, the studies carried out have mainly shown fetal sex detection, fetal RhD and quantitative variations in gestations at risk of pre-eclampsia or fetal chromosomal anomalies. As a prenatal diagnosis unit, these reports have prompted us to investigate the possibilities of using fetal DNA in maternal plasma as a possible alternative tool in the prenatal diagnosis routine.

We have evaluated our experience on the CF prenatal diagnosis field in 13 families. We have also tested the possibility of performing a prenatal diagnosis of a paternally inherited CF mutation using fetal DNA present in maternal plasma. Different diagnosis techniques and strategies were used depending on the mutation found in the families that participated in the present study. We show the results from parental and CVS DNA analyses and we comment the obtained results of these conventional CF prenatal diagnoses. On the other hand, we used maternal blood in order to detect and analyze fetal DNA in one of the families that participate in the study. This non-invasive diagnosis was performed at 13 weeks of gestation using DNA extracted from maternal plasma. We used a single PCR amplification of the paternal mutation (Q890X) and posterior restriction analysis of the PCR product. We successfully detected the presence of the mutation and thus, the fetal condition of being a carrier of the paternal mutation. We conclude that the use of fetal DNA for the diagnosis of cystic fibrosis could be a reliable technique that can substantially reduce invasive test.

Chapter 6 - Cystic fibrosis (CF) mutation analysis on 500 CF patients, characterized 83 different mutations (20 so far specific to our population) accounting for 92% of CF genes and generating 111 different genotypes. Seven mutations were common [p.F508del (54.5%), c.621+1G>T (6.3%), p.G542X (3.9%), p.N1303K (2.3%), c.2789+5G>A (2.0%), c.2183AA>G (1.5%), p.E822X (1.8%)], 16 showed frequencies between 0.4% and 1.1%, while the remaining (60) were very rare (1 to 3 alleles). Denaturing gradient gel electrophoresis (DGGE) screening of 15 exons (3, 4, 7, 9, 10, 11, 12, 13, 14b, 16, 17b, 19, 20, 21, and 23) detected 86% of CF alleles. Haplotypes for eight diallelic and three microsatellite markers have been characterized for the common, a few rare and novel Greek mutations. In order to test the contribution of the CFTR gene in male infertility, we carried out mutation testing on subjects suffering from the monosymptomatic form of CFTR. Mutation testing was carried out on 134 male infertility subjects including 88 suffering from azoospermia (Congenital bilateral absence of vas deferens-CBAVD and Obstructive azoospermia-OA) and 46 with severe oligospermia. The results showed that 56.2% of CBAVD males carried one mutation/variant in the CFTR gene while 27.1% were compound heterozygotes for one mild (belonging to class IV or V) and one severe mutation. Of the OA males, 27.5% had at least 1 CF allele while only 13% of the severe oligospermia males were carriers. Carrier screening was initiated, with emphasis on individuals and couples in high-risk groups –with a family history of CF, one partner with CF, and couples with male infertility seeking in vitro fertilization (IVF). Mutation analysis on 900 individuals (175 couples, 91 unaffected CF siblings, 285 CF family relatives and 174 general population subjects), identified a total of 188 heterozygotes the majority amongst siblings and relatives of index cases. Of the 175 couples, 23 had advanced ongoing pregnancies upon request for CF screening. In total six couples were found requiring prenatal diagnosis.

Results of 167 prenatal diagnoses (including 110 due to bowel echogenicity), testing a total of 57 different parental genotypes, are reported. One hundred and sixty-seven prenatal tests resulted in 41 affected, 80 heterozygous, 46 normal fetuses and one incomplete diagnosis. Of the echogenic bowel fetuses, 15 had one detectable mutation and in 4 cases homozygosity with severe mutations was detected.

Chapter 7 - Cystic fibrosis (CF) is a genetic disease at once tragic and theoretically puzzling. Predominantly found in Caucasian and Semitic populations, its incidence in the United States is 1 in approximately 3000 births. The global population of cystic fibrosis sufferers has been estimated to be about a quarter of a million persons, many of whom will never be accurately diagnosed during their lifetime. Average life expectancy in the United States has risen to about 32 years of age, but the median age at death for the most common mutation pair, delF508/delF508, remains about 23 years of age even with the most advanced care. The life expectancy of females with cystic fibrosis tends to be a few years shorter than the life expectancy of males. Proximate cause of death in about 95% of cases is respiratory failure [1].

In this essay, we will examine recent research findings and clinical trial results that offer a new specification of the linkage between genetics and disease in the case of CF: a linkage involving the transport of reduced glutathione (GSH).

Chapter 8 - Cystic fibrosis (CF), the most common severe autosomal recessive trait among Caucasians, is caused by molecular lesions in the cystic fibrosis transmembrane conductance regulator gene (*CFTR*). The course of the multi-organ disease CF is highly variable suggesting the influence of environmental factors and/or modulating genes other than *CFTR* on the disease phenotype.

The gene causing Cystic fibrosis (CF) was uncovered in 1989.[1] Within the cystic fibrosis transmembrane conductance regulator (*CFTR*) gene, more than 1300 variants have been described so far.[2] The allelic heterogeneity of the *CFTR* gene has instigated many genotype-phenotype studies [3-5] which all demonstrate that except for the pancreatic status, course and severity of the multi-organ CF cannot be predicted on the basis of the *CFTR* mutation genotype. Moreover, the variability of CF disease has also been observed among unrelated patients carrying the same *CFTR* mutation genotype [6,7] and within CF sib pairs.[8] These observations have been accepted by the CF community to indicate the role of other factors than the *CFTR* gene in shaping the disease phenotype, and several studies have been launched to study the role of inherited modulators in CF.

In 1994, the European CF twin and sibling study has been initiated during an EU BIOMED symposium. More than 500 CF twin and sibling pairs from 158 CF clinics of 14 European countries were enrolled in the study in 1995-1996. Out of these, less than 40 families with F508del homozygous twins or sibs were selected to study inherited modulators of CF disease based on their extreme clinical phenotype. This chapter describes the rationale for selecting these pairs [9] and summarizes the findings on the candidate gene region on 7q31.3-7qtel [10] among this set of highly informative CF siblings.

In: New Developments in Birth Defects Research
Editor: Nelson A. Gaslem, pp. 1-68

ISBN 1-60021-400-2

Chapter 1

BIRTH DEFECTS OF THE LYMPHATIC SYSTEM

Anastasios S. Petropoulos*, Dimitrios K. Sfougaris and Vassilios K. Mouravas

Aristotle University of Thessaloniki, Medical School –Clinic of Pediatric Surgery
General Hospital "Papageorgiou", Thessaloniki, Greece.

ABSTRACT

The lymphatic vascular system (LVS) is extended to almost every organ of the body and exists side by side to almost every tissue, in that way resembling the arterial and venous systems. We can trace its development as a separate entity in some regions of the body from the end of the fifth week of embryonic life. There is an obvious correlation between these sites and the appearance of some of the most common congenital lymphatic vessel malformations (LVM). They can cause minor or major health problems, affecting a large variety of organs and regions of the body. In this chapter we review varius aspects of the lymphatic system, both clinical and biological.

Lymphatic development is now being studied at the molecular level using lymphatic-specific markers. These methods revealed several mechanisms of regulation of lymphangiogenesis, involving glycoproteins, angiopoietines etc. The modulators that cause lymphatic malformations through their interaction with the endothelium (positive or negative) are not known yet exactly.

The spectrum of pathophysiologic perturbations caused by lymphatic defects, comprise derangements in fluid equilibrium, nutrient transport, leucocyte transport and anatomic relations. But the understanding of many basic aspects of lymphatic vessel function lags behind that of the blood vascular system, due mainly to the difficulty in working in small, thin-walled lymphatic vessels and the relative lack of lymphatic specific markers. Recent application of cellular and molecular techniques has produced some significant developments in lymphatic cell biology, mainly in our understanding of

* Correspondence concerning this article should be addressed to Prof. Anastasios S. Petropoulos Tel-Fax: 0030 2310 991.562; Tel: 0030 2310 693.818; e-mail: petrpesu@med.auth.gr. General Hospital "Papageorgiou", Ring Road, Nea Efkarpia, 56403 Thessaloniki, Greece.

lymphatic muscle function, transport function and the regulation of an intrinsic lymph pump.

The variety of presentation of LVMs renders any attempt for a unified classification, at least in part, arbitrary, incomplete or useless. Classifications by clinical manifestation may easily overlap gross pathologic, histologic or cytochemical classification (and vice versa).

A classification of LVMs is proposed on the basis of the anatomical structures involved: lymph vessel-angiodysplasia, lymphadeno(nodal)-dysplasia and the coexistence of both (lymphangio-adenodysplasias). LVMs belong to the group of low-flow vascular lesions.

Among these lesions, we first discuss those that cause lymph accumulation in anatomic spaces. Some of these lesions have a congenital component and become symptomatic by the traumatic process of labour. Congenital chylothorax is the most interesting in this category.

Second, we discuss the lesions that develop on the LVS stroma, all of them with varying degree of adjacent tissue infiltration: from the lymphangioma circumscriptum to the diffuse lesion leading to macroglossia, or from the lymphatic obliteration lesions without other tissue involvement, to the complex Klippel-Trenaunay syndrome.

Diagnosis is based on clinical findings, imaging and histology. Several distinguishing characteristics must be looked for, mainly the presence of the lesion at birth, growth, involution, change in volume, pain, outflow.

Histology must distinguish between simple (capillary), cavernous, or cystic (hygroma) LVM, depending on the size of the lymphatic channels they contain.

Doppler ultrasound should be the initial imaging modality for recognizing vascular tumors from vascular malformations. It is also of special value for the fetal period.CT scan or MRI is best to evaluate the extent of the lesions prior to treatment. Lymphangioscintigraphy is a superb functional (but anatomically gross) exam.

In general, treatment is tailored according to pathology and age (fetus, newborn or older child). It may include dietary, pharmaceutical or surgical interventions more or less aggressive. The recently discovered inducers of lymphangiogenesis could, at least theoretically, constitute special targets for modifying lymphatic growth. This approach is mainly used for cancer treatment but may be promising for lympangioma treatment as well. On the other hand, stimulation of lymphangiogenesis might be a key for the treatment of lymphedema in the future.

Keywords: Congenital Malformations, Lymphatic System, Vascular Dysplasias, Neonatal Chylous Efusions.

Historical Aspects

The presence of a 'clear' fluid in the organism was known from ancient times although its properties were not known. Ancient Greek writers refer to it as 'lemphos', which means 'clear' or 'shiny', in order to distinguish it from blood. This word was transformed as 'lymph' in English. Another well known English word derived from the same root is 'lamp'. Hippocrates (ca 400 BC) mentions lymph as a 'nutriment for vein and artery'. Aristotle, even more systematic, says that fibers of the body 'are supplied with fluid, the lymph'. His pupil Plato describes a kind of mystical anatomy considering lymph one of the basic fluid constituents of the body. Herophilus and Erasistratus in Alexandria (ca 300 BC) described vaguely the lacteals [1,2] that convey the white, milk-like fluid, which they called 'chylos (chyle)', which means the liquid inner part or the product after turning food into liquid. The best known word deriving from this root is "chemistry".

The famous physician, surgeon and animal dissector Galen from Pergamon (2nd century AD) gave the name 'chyle' to the product of digestion which is formed in the alimentary tract and brought via the portal vessel at the liver. He considered that the liver elaborated the chyle into venous blood [1].

Interest on the lymphatic system abated in the ensuing centuries along with the interest in science in general, only to regain a position as an object for research during the 17th century. The Italian Gasparo Aselli (Aselius) (1581-1626) was the first to describe and depict the lymphatic vessels of the mesentery and the mesenteric lymph nodes (pancreas of Aselli). His work was published posthumously in 1627 [1,3].

Pequet described in 1651 for the first time in detail the cisterna chyli and the thoracic duct. Olaus Rudbeck (1652) and Bartholinus (1653) made the point that the lymphatic vessels form a system separate from that of the blood vessels [1,4]. Bartolet in 1663 presented a case of chylothorax for the first time [5].

By 1700, the anatomy of the lymphatic system, its physiological role in the drainage of lymph from the various body parts and its delivery to the venous system was adequately described [6].

Baum, in 1918, described in detail the lymphatic system of the dog giving a big thrust to experimental work [7].

The first lymphangiography in animals was attempted by Carvalho, Rodrigues and Pereira in 1931 using a fluorine colloid [8]. The basic principles of direct lymphangiography with direct administration of lymphotropic contrast medium in the peripheral lymph vesels, were set by Kinmonth in 1952 [9]. But the tediousness of the method, its complications and lack of efficient therapy in many cases, led most physicians to abandon lymphatic imaging and to rely mainly on physical signs and patient history for diagnosis and therapy [10].

However, the introduction of computed tomography (CT) and magnetic resonance imaging (MRI) for examining lymph nodes quickly replaced conventional lymphography [11].

The diagnostic tool that has dramatically changed the diagnostic armamentarium is isotope lymphography (also known as lymphangioscintigraphy) capable for defining both anatomic and functional derangements [12].

Unfortunately, basic research on the lymphatic system was not so eminent past the 1980's partly because the conventional laboratory tools were exhausted. But this canged radically in the past few years, due mainly to molecular genetics, allowing the identification of lymph vessel with specific markers. This approach elucidated many dark areas and is promising for therapeutic applications in the future [13].

EMBRYOLOGY

Researchers had already accumulated a substantial amount of knowledge on the formation of the lymphatic vascular system (LVS) by the beginning of the 20th century. That is in spite of the difficulty inherent in working with the small and thin-walled lymphatic vessels of human and animal embryos. Later on, our knowledge on the LVS started lagging behind that of the blood vascular system. It was not until the last decade of the 20th c. that the application of cellular and molecular tools produced some significant development in the follow up of the differentiation and migration of lymphatic endothelial cells. The lymphatic system is formed through the development of 6 embryonic anlages which are called lymph sacs. These endothelial sacs are the following:

A) Two jugular sacs, each one siding the lower part of each jugular vein. B) A single retroperitoneal paraaortic lymph sac at the mesenteric root, between the adrenal glands. C) The cisterna chyli, which is also unpaired, situated anteriorly to the L3 and L4 vertebrae. D) The two posterior sacs also called tail or sciatic sacs, situated alongside the common sciatic veins (Figure 1) [1].

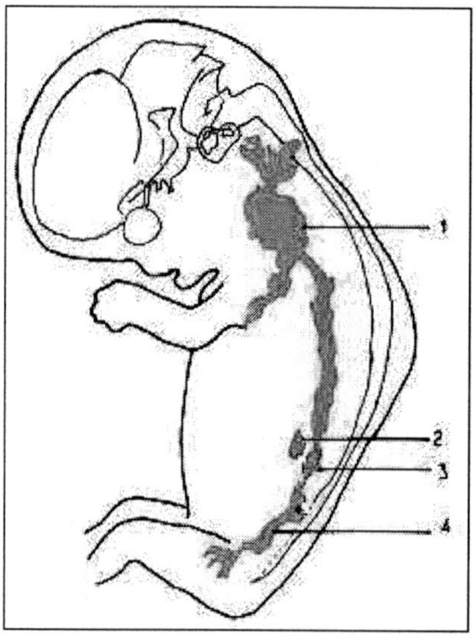

Figure 1. Development of the Lymphatic System in the Human Embryo at 8 Weeks, 30 mm. 1) Jugular Lymph Sac. 2) Retroperitoneal Lymph Sac, 3) Cisterna Chyli, 4) Posterior Lymph Sac (Petropoulos 1980).

The two jugular sacs appear by the 6th embryonic week at the angle forming between the internal jugular vein and the ipsilateral subclavian vein and they proliferate extending to the upper extremities. The unpaired retroperitoneal sac derives from a plexus of lymphatic capillaries at the root of the mesentery and is already formed by the end of the 8th embryonic weeek (e.w.). At the same time the cisterna chyli appears dorsaly to the aorta. Imediately afterwards the sciatic lymph sacs appear by the internal iliac and femoral veins. All the abovementioned lymph sacs are connected through a network of endothelial formations constituting the primordial lymph vessels which appear on the 9th e.w. [14].

The connection between the jugular sacs and the cisterna is established through two parallel lymph vessels (trunks) running alongside the spine and interconnected by anastomotic vessels crossing the midline. Gradually, parts of this network atrophy or are relatively less developed, leaving as most prominent parts, the left cranial trunk and right caudal trunk, interconnected with a diagonal anastomotic vessel. This structure constitutes the thoracic duct (TD).

Various theories on the origin of the lymphatic system saw the light since the discovery of the lymph sacs by Saxer in 1896 [15,16]. Initially it was widely accepted that the LS was formed by the developing vascular system, a theory advocated by William Hiss [17]. According to this theory, the two jugular sacs and the retroperitoneal sac are derived from the adjacent veins, while the lymphatic vessels are formed by endothelial ingrowths to the surrounding mesenchyme. Lewis' observations [18] that the lymph sacs separate from the venous system when the embryo is 16-20 mm long and subsequently reunite when the embryo is 30 mm long, added to this theory which is known as the centrifugal theory. Sabin in 1902 studied ink-injected chick embryos and concluded that the earliest primitive lymphatics arise as a result of endothelial cell sprouting from the cardinal veins. Subsequently, these cells proliferate and migrate toward the internal organs and the skin of the embryo forming the lymphatic system.

In contrast, Huntington and McClure advocated the centripedal theory in 1910 [19]. According to this, the lymph vessels are formed initially in the mesenchyme and only later do they converge and form a union with the venous system.

Kampmeier supports the theory according to which the lymph vessels form within the mesenchyme from the lymphatic stem cells (lymphangioblasts), in the perivascular space of the primordial venous vessels which later on atrophy. These cells invade the mesenchyme in order to form primitive lymphatic sacs [20].

As for the origin of the lymph nodes, Sabin supported that they initially appear in the cervical region on the 9th e.w. as an agglomeration of connective tissue in the small lymph sacs [21]. Subsequently these spaces are colonized by lymphocytes. Later on, lymph vessels and lymph nodules are formed at these same sites and develop into lymph nodes.

Recent work with the chick embryo limb buds has shown that the lymphatic vessels can be derived both by sprouting of vessels from the cardinal vein and by mesodermal lymphangioblasts [22,23]

The earliest expressed marker for developing lymphatic endothelial cells is the homeobox transcription factor Prox-1 which first becomes expressed in the vascular system in the lateral aspect of the posterior cardinal vein in mice, shortly before the onset of sprouting of lymphatic endothelial cells from this vein. After specification of lymphatic endothelial cells has occurred, these cells normally migrate to form the first embryonic lymph sacs. Migration of the lymphatic endothelial cells towards the lymph sacs depends critically on the presence of the growth factor VEGF-C [24] (Figure 2). There are also investigational results which strongly suggest that the superficial lymphatics develop independently from the deep ones, and are derived from mesenchymal lymphangioblasts rather than veins [25].

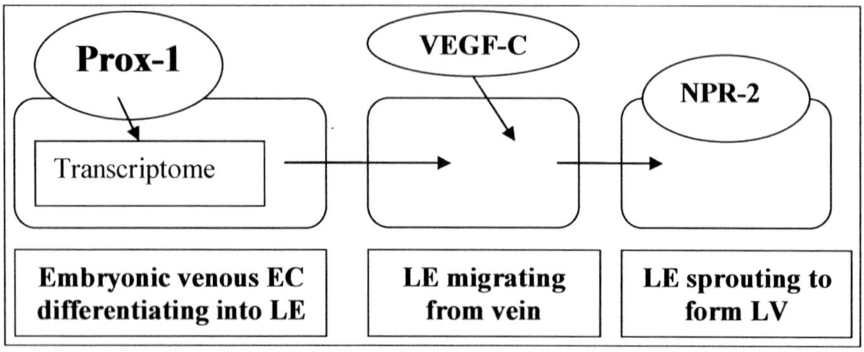

Figure. 2. Lymphangiogenesis in embryonic life. Endothelial cells (EC) differentiating into lymphatic endothelium (LE) and formation of lymphatic vessels (LV).

In a mouse model of skin regeneration, it has been shown that interstitial fluid channels form before the lymphatic endothelial cells organize. Lymphatic cell migration, vascular endothelial growth factor (VEGF)-C expression, and lymphatic capillary network organization are initiated primarily in the direction of lymph flow, suggesting that interstitial fluid channeling precedes and may even direct lymphangiogenesis [26]

We may say that to this time the embryogenesis and development of the LS is not totally understood and described. But the use of modern molecular tools in lymphatics is very recent and has a long way to go.

Anatomy and Histology

The lymphatic system consists of the *lymphatic vessels* (lymphatics) and lymphoid tissue, which is either aggregated in several organs or circulates being carried by the blood and lymph.

Lymphatic vessels originate as capillaries side by side with the blood capillaries. In general they are very difficult to recognize in sections because they do not contain erythrocytes. They resemble large-diameter capillaries in which erythrocytes are absent in the section.

On their peripheral extreme they have blind endings and form sacculations of 40-60 μm. They continue centrally as lymphatic capillaries 5-50 μm wide with anastomosing tubes, and they form plexuses in the tissue spaces (much wider meshes than those of the adjacent blood capillaries). Lymphatic capillaries are absent from the CNS, bone marrow, eye, and parts of the spleen. Those located in the villi of the small intestine are called lacteals because the lymph fluid within them is milky in appearance due to absorbed triglycerides [3].

Studies of the gross anatomy of the lymphatic system are few and difficult to perform. Of considerable help is to demonstrate the lymphatic vessels radiographically using a lead oxide suspension prior to dissecting them out in adult human cadavers [27] or in the anesthesized animal in experimental settings.

Lymphatic capillaries merge into larger lymph collector vessels which have very thin walls of endothelium, basal lamina and collagen, and numerous valves formed by endothelial foldings. These gradually form the afferent lymph vessels of the lymph nodes which are arranged largely in regional groups. The flow continues through the efferent vessel of the lymph nodes to larger lymph vessels, the lymphatic channels and to the major lymphatic channels (Figure 3, Figure 4) [28].

Modern tissue histochemistry has permitted to distinguish lymphatic from blood vascular endothelium and to study it separately [1]. The lymph capillaries, like blood capillaries, are lined with a continuous endothelium, but are irregular in diameter and wider than blood capillaries. In electron microscopy it is shown that their basal lamina is discontinuous or absent. The endothelial cells have fine anchoring fibrils to the extracellular matrix and between them. These junctions attach to all parts of the endothelial cells except to the part of the endothelial cell that is redundant to the inside of the lumen i.e. where there is an overlap with its adjacent cell, forming the flap valve. This structure is actually a one-way valve that allows fluid to enter the lymphatic capillary whenever the pressure differences are permissive (Figure 5).

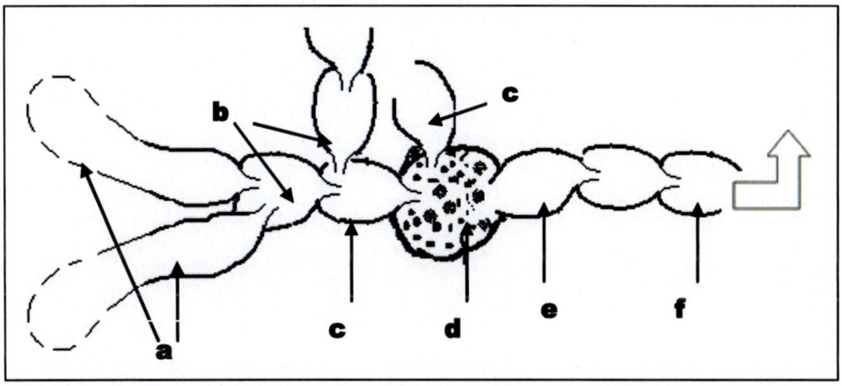

Figure 3. Schematic representation of the lymphatic vessel tree: a)Lymphatic capillaries with sacculations b) collector vessels c) afferent vessels d) lymph node e) efferent vessel f) lymphatic channel, leading to major lymphatic channel.

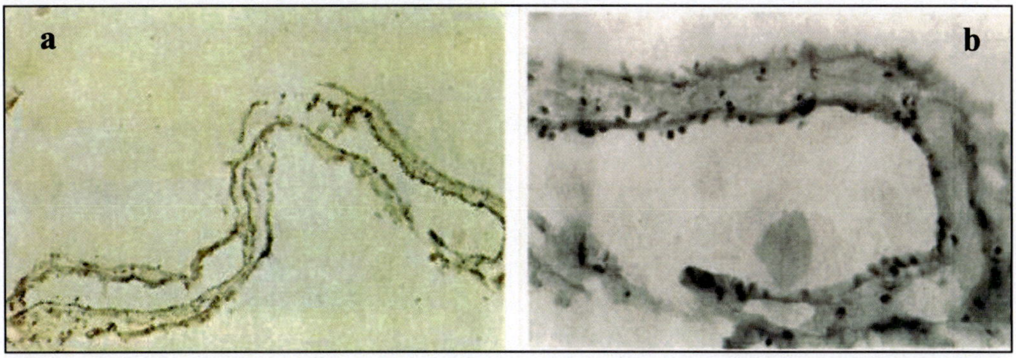

Figure 4. Two fixed histological specimens of the thoracic duct of a dog. Eosin –Hematoxyline, Longitudinal section 63X. a) Transverse section 252X b) The vessel is thin walled consisting of of a layer of loose connective tissue lined by endothelium. It is partly surrounded by adipose tissue. Only lymph cells and no red blood cells are observed in the lumen (Petropoulos 1980).

The most important major lymphatic channels are the thoracic duct (TD), that will be described in the section on chylothorax, and the Right Lymphatic duct. They contain valves consisted of two semilunar cusps. The TD was found to contain on the average 14.7 valves in man. Most of these valves were found in the upper third of the thoracic duct, and the fewer in its middle part [29].

The Right Lymphatic duct drains into the junction of the right internal jugular and right subclavian veins. It is formed by the confluence of the right jugular, the subclavicular and bronchomediastinal trunks. It is about 2 cm in length and there are several anatomic variations, the most common being the non union of the bronchomediastinal trunk that drains directly to the subclavian vein. The right jugular trunk drains the right side of the neck and head. The bronchomediastinal trunk drains the right hemithorax and lung, most of the heart and some of the right lobe of the liver. The subclavicular trunk drains the right upper limb.

PHYSIOLOGY

Our understanding of many aspects of lymphatic physiology is by far behind our knowledge on the blood vascular system. This is in part due to the less rewarding therapeutics for lymphatic vascular diseases (less funding), the inherent difficulty in working with small, thin-walled, clear lymph vessels and the lack, for many years, of specific molecular/cellular markers. The application of cellular and molecular tools to the field of lymphatic biology has recently produced some significant developments in lymphatic endothelial cell biology and the understanding of lymphatic physiology [30].

Lymph vessels and lymph nodes function as a tissue drainage and as an "immunoexposing" system. That is, returning to circulation the fluid that leaks out of the blood capillaries to the interstitium. This fluid contains plasma protein in excess, that cannot be reabsorbed directly back into the circulation. They also perform a special kind of drainage of nutrients from the intestines. Their other major function is to expose pathogens and antigens to the immuno-reacting and filtering lymph nodes.

The Functions of the lymphatic system can be summarized as follows:

1. Transport of tissue fluid formed in the capillary bed;
2. Removal of cell debris and foreign matter (e.g. bacteria) by mononuclear phagocytic series cells and prevention of bacteria and foreign material from entering the blood stream;
3. Production of lymphocytes and control of the immune responses.
4. Adds to the blood substances and cells such as: proteins that leaked from blood capillaries, new and recirculated lymphocytes, antibodies, fat droplets (chylomicrons), etc.
5. Fat is collected from the gut in blind lymphatic capillaries lying centrally in intestinal villi. The fat-whitened lymph (chyle) gives these vessels a milky colour, hence their name 'lacteals'.

However, we have not yet established a unified picture of the regulating mechanisms of lymph formation and transport in physiological and pathological conditions [31].

The terminal vessels of the lymphatic system, the lymphatic capillaries, have the characteristics that make them highly permeable to macromolecules, pathogens and migrating cells. The basis for the mechanical function of the capillary pump at this level is directly related to its ultrastructure. The wall of lymph capillaries is endothelium; this endothelium is generally more permeable to various molecules and cells than that of blood capillaries.

The mechanism for interstitial fluid uptake into the lymphatics is not fully understood [32]. Whenever pressure outside the capillary is greater than the pressure inside, the flap valve (described in the section on Histology) is pushed inside the lumen leaving an open space between the endothelial cells, allowing fluid to enter the lymphatic capillary (Figure 5). Whenever the pressure inside the capillary becomes greater than that outside, the endothelial flap closes over the space between the endothelial cells, and the fluid can not escape. Any compression or relaxation of the tissues, or of the lymphatic capillaries themselves will create alternating pressure differences across the capillary membrane and eventually suction the interstitial fluid.

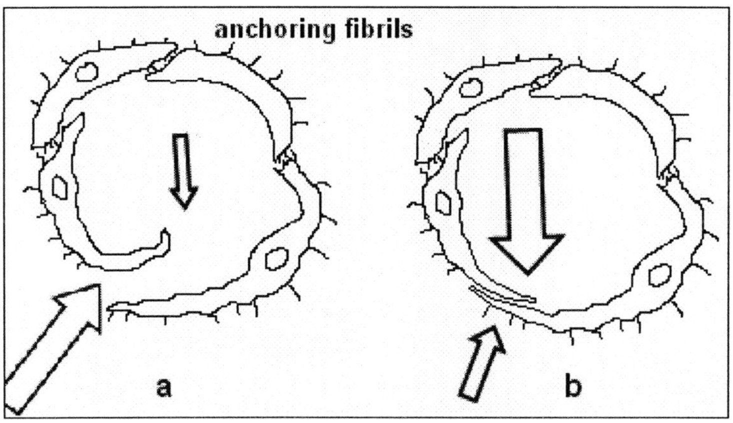

Figure 5. Schematic representation of the flap valves at the lymphatic capillaries: a) valves open when intracapillary pressure is less than the interstitial fluid pressure. b) valves close when intracapillary pressure exceeds that of the interstitium.

There exists a system of intralymphatic valves that prevent backflow along the length of the lymphatic channels. The contraction of the muscles surrounding the lymphatics compress their lumen and propulse the lymph towards one direction, the other direction not being allowed because of the intraluminal valves which function permissively only towards the larger more central lymph vessels and upper trunk veins. Intrathoracic pressure fluctuations, during the respiratory cycle, functions in a similar way. Lymphatics have a two-valve system: a (primary) valve system in addition to the classical (secondary). The primary valves at the level of the capillary endothelium, in conjunction with the secondary intralymphatic valves, provide a mechanism that facilitates the unidirectional flow during periodic compression and expansion of the lymphatics.

It has been shown that lymphatic capillary endothelial cells themselves have an ability to contract. Their cytoplasm contains actinomyosin. In horses it has been shown that myofibroblasts may act as pacemaker cells for the contraction of smooth muscle cells [33].

The resting membrane potential sometimes shows rhythmic fluctuations or slow waves that resemble those in visceral smooth muscle [34]. The minimum depolarization necessary for inducing the spontaneous contraction is about 6 mV in the lymphatic smooth muscle cells [35].

The use of some molecular marker techniques in lymphatic muscle biology has somewhat lagged behind those in the endothelium, but recent developments in lymphatic muscle contractile and electrical physiology have led to advances in our understanding of lymphatic transport function, particularly in the regulation of the intrinsic lymph pump [30]. In some animals and in humans it has been shown that the larger collecting lymph vessels develop spontaneous rhythmic contractions [36,37,38]. This rhythmical activity, aided by the presence of valves inside these vessels, can create pumping pressures as great as 20–30 mm Hg [39].

The frequency of contractions seems to be determined mainly by the amount of fluid in the lymph vessel. When a segment of vessel immediately below a valve becomes distended, it contracts, and the fluid is pushed forward beyond the valve. But there are also other conditions that affect the contractile ability and consequently the lymphatic circulation, especially in localized parts of the body.

The lymphatic endothelial cells seem to function physiologicaly only under lower oxygen tension in lymph (8–35 mm Hg) and so does their rhythmic pump activity (20–35 mm Hg). In addition, endogenous NO as well as activation of K-ATP channels play important roles in the regulation of the lymphatic pump activity. All of these factors inhibit lymph transport, contributing in the formation of edema. We may suppose that the purpose of all these non selectively acting factors is to act rapidly aiming to dilute the toxic and irritating substances released from pathogens. Excitatory substances that could induce lymph formation and transport, have not been identified yet. These could play a role against the formation of tissue edema.

VEGFs and their receptors (VEGFR) on the endothelial cells as well as specific hyaluronan (HA) receptors have been implicated in some functions of the lymphatic endothelium. VEGF was originally described as a permeability factor, as it increases permeability of the endothelium through the formation of intercellular gaps, vesico-vascular organelles, vacuoles and fenestrations. VEGF also causes vasodilatation through the induction of the endothelial nitric oxide synthetase (eNOS) and the subsequent increase in nitric oxide production [40].

Immediately after birth the lymph is clear and hey-colored. After feeding the baby with milk the lymph obtains its characteristic whitish color due to the presence of chylomicrons. Depending on the quantity and quality of ingested milk its lipid load ranges from 0.4 to 4 gr/100ml [41].

The lymph is rich in T lemphocytes and its concentration in electrolytes is similar to that of plasma.

The daily production of lymph exceeds 1.7 times the baby's total blood volume, causing serious repercussions if lymph is lost in the third space, such as hypovolemia, hyponatremia, hypoproteinemia, metabolic acidosis and leucopenia.

GENETICS AND MOLECULAR BIOLOGY

The study of the genetic basis of lymphatic disease with the help of molecular biology is expected to elucidate the pathogenesis of this wide group of diseases. In addition it is expected to help in the development of targeted molecular therapies for the treatment of both primary and secondary forms of lymphatic pathology. We are now able to study lymphatics because we can locate the Vascular Endothelial Growth Factors (VEGF) and their Receptors (VEGFR) on the endothelial cells.

Several changes to the expression of genes result in creating anomalous lymphatics. These changes are produced in a number of ways, either naturally or experimentally: ethylnitrosourea-induced mutagenesis, missense mutations in the VEGFR-3 gene, mutations of transcription factors, functional blockade of endogenous VEGF-C and VEGF-D signalling, targeted deletions of genes etc. Even the experimental application of several factors for therapeutic purposes such as VEGF-C-expressing adenovirus or administration of recombinant VEGF-C had analogous results.

Ligands and Receptors

The VEGF family of secreted glycoproteins and their receptors are very important in the development of the vascular and the lymphatic vascular system. Later in life, these molecules are required for processes involving tissue repair. There are receptors that are expressed on both lymphatic and blood vessels and some that are found exclusively on lymphatics and there are substances identified that bind on these receptors and promote lymphangiogenesis and many other functions of the lymphatics [42,43] (Figure 6).

Prox1 is a homeodomain protein that specifies lymphatic cell fate by directly reprogramming the transcriptome of embryonic venous endothelial cells. Lack or inactivation of Prox1 in mice leads to embryonic death or (in cases of heterozygotes) to chylous ascites [43].

VEGFR-2, is a receptor for VEGF-A, VEGF-C, and VEGF-D, and is expressed by blood vascular and lymphatic endothelial cells. There are clues indicating the importance of VEGFR-2 for repair-associated lymphangiogenesis [44,45]

VEGFR-3, was the first gene whose expression was shown to be specific for lymphatic endothelial cells [43]. It serves as a signaling receptor for the lymphatic-specific growth factors VEGF-C and VEGF-D. Missense mutations in VEGFR-3 have been linked to hereditary lymphedema in humans and also to a similar condition in a mouse model of lymphedema [46].

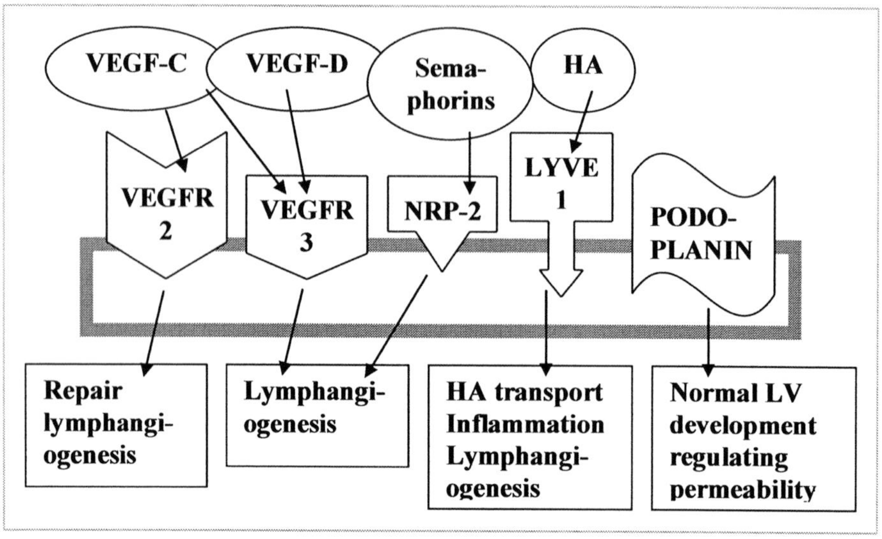

Figure 6. Receptors on the lymphatic endothelium, their ligands and the functions that they promote.

VEGF-C and VEGF-D were originally cloned as ligands for VEGFR-3. VEGF-C plays an essential role during embryonic lymphangiogenesis, as revealed by the phenotype of VEGF-C-deficient mice. During development, VEGF-C is expressed along with its receptor VEGFR-3 predominantly in regions where lymphatic vessels develop around embryonic veins and including mesenchymal cells [47]. The expression then decreases in most tissues, remaining high in the lymph nodes. VEGF-C induces selective lymphangiogenesis without accompanying angiogenesis [48]. The VEGF-C signaling through VEGFR-3 can also induce lymphangiogenesis in adult tissues.

LYVE-1 has been identified as a Lymphatic Vascular Endothelium-specific Hyaluronan (HA) receptor. During tissue injury or in other pathological situations, HA turnover increases and HA breakdown products serve as inducers of inflammatory responses, leading to angiogenesis and lymphangiogenesis, enhanced production of chemokines, and recruitment of dendritic cells [49].

Podoplanin is a mucin-type transmembrane glycoprotein that is expressed by lymphatic, but not by blood vascular endothelial cells. Podoplanin-deficient mice die at birth exhibiting lung failure. Neonatal mutant mice display cutaneous lymphedema associated with impaired lymphatic transport [50].

Neuropilin-2 (NRP-2) is a nonkinase transmembrane protein that serves as a receptor for class III semaphorins and for several VEGF family ligands, including VEGF-A_{165}, PlGF-2, and VEGF-C. It is expressed mainly in visceral lymphatic vessels, and less in the cutaneous lymphatics [48]. NRP-2-deficient mice show a severe reduction of small lymphatic vessels during development [51].

Mutations

Milroy disease, a primary lymphedema present at birth [52], has been linked to missense mutations of the VEGFR-3 locus on distal chromosome 5q. The function of this receptor is inhibited with resulting lymphedema [48]. Hereditary early onset lymphedema may also exhibit VEGFR-3 locus mutation.

Lymphedema-distichiasis has been linked to the FOXC2 gene, encoding a transcription factor, involved in diverse developmental pathways [53].

Hypotrichosis-lymphedema-telangiectasia syndrome is connected with a mutation on the SOX18 gene on chromosome 20q13.

Lymphedema also has been detected in several genetic mouse models originally generated by ethylnitrosourea-induced mutagenesis and the phenotype recently has been linked to an amino acid substitution mutation in the highly conserved VEGFR-3 tyrosine kinase domain [54]. Mouse embryos with targeted deletion of the Net gene, an Ets ternary complex transcription factor, develop chylothorax and dilated lymphatic vessels [55].

Targeted Molecular Therapies

To date, VEGFs are the best manipulated inducers of angiogenesis and lymphangiogenesis. The first VEGF inhibitor has recently entered the clinic for treatment of cancer.

VEGF-C proteins are being considered for stimulation of angiogenesis in the context of ischemic disease and also as the most promising molecular tool for the treatment of both primary and secondary lymphedema in animal models [56].

Application of a VEGF-C-expressing adenovirus promoted lymphangiogenesis and resulted in the generation of functional new lymphatic vessels in the Chy mutant mice [54]. When human recombinant VEGF-C was applied to rabbit ears (in which lymphatics were surgically ablated) lymphangiogenesis increased.

Although many parameters of the VEGF-C therapy remain to be studied, this treatment strategy remains as a potentially developing for the benefit of lymphedema patients.

Perspectives

As it was emphasized before, the slow progress in our understanding of the development of the lymphatic vascular system, largely due to the lack of reliable molecular tools, was followed by an acceleration phase. We can say that there has been a "quantum leap" in lymphatic research over the past several years. Nonetheless, lymphatic research is still allmost at the beginning. It will be of particular importance to identify the ultimate signaling mechanisms that initiate lymphatic endothelial cell differentiation during embryogenesis, and to further elucidate the molecular interactions between blood and lymphatic vessels. These are interesting and promising fields of research for the development of new therapeutics for lymphedema and related disorders.

Congenital Chylothorax

Chylothorax (Ch) is the accumulation of lymph or chyle in the pleural cavity. The term congenital chylothorax (CCh) has been used to describe chylothorax in infants of less than three months old [57]. We must acknowledge that this terminology is somehow misleading because the underlying pathology is not, necessarily, a congenital dysplasia of the lymphatics. On the other hand, chylothorax occurring at this age may be managed by neonatologists and pediatric surgeons using a single diagnostic-therapeutic algorythm. Therefore, adopting this terminology is not completely unjustified.

In cases where no external influence (e.g. trauma) justifies the chylothorax we refer to it as spontaneous chylothorax [58]. If, after the proper diagnostic evaluation, no cause is recognized we refer to it as idiopathic chylothorax. When ch is attributed to a primary cause other than malformation of lymphatics, we refer to it as secondary ch (Table 1).

Lymph or chyle is the most common kind of liquid intrapleural collection during the neonatal and fetal periods [59]. Therapy is usually conservative, aiming at the evacuation of the pleural space, reduction of chyle production, control of nutritional, metabolic and immunological repercussions and maintenance of respiratory function. In many cases surgical intervention might be necessary if the conservative measures fail and the life of the young patient is endangered.

Prompt diagnosis and early start of supportive therapy together with the surgical options available nowdays have lowered the mortality rate for this disease from 50% in 1950 to 10-20% today [1] which is still a very high proportion.

Table 1. Types of Congenital Chylothorax and its onomatology

Spontaneous	Idiopathic	(Diagnosis of exclusion)	***Primary***
	Birth defect of lymphatics	(Not easy to demonstrate)	
	Birth defect of other system	Usually cardiac	***Secondary***
	Part of a syndrome	Trisomy 21, Noonan etc	
Following disease other than birth defect		Venous thrombosis, neuroblastoma	
Traumatic	Birth trauma	(History)	
	Postoperative complication	Usually PDA	

Anatomy

The largest lymph vessel in the human body is the thoracic duct (TD). In grown ups its length is 38-45 cm and its diameter 12-15 mm (Figure 7) [1,60]. It originates from the cisterna chyli and ends at the left jugular vein at its junction with the left subclavian vein.

The cisterna chili is actually a spindle shaped aneurysm of the of the lymphatic system situated retroperitoneally, in front of the vertebrae T12, L1 and L2. It forms at the confluence of three important lymphatic vessels: the right and left lumbar and the intestinal. These three vessels drain the lymph from the inferior limbs and the abdominal viscera. The course of the TD from the cisterna upwards is, initially at the right of the midline, in front of the vertebral column. It enters the thoracic cage from the abdomen through the aortic foramen of the diaphragm and continues its upward course, initially coursing between the azygos and the aorta receiving paired intercostal tributaries. It gradually passes to the left of the midline at the level of T4-T6 vertebrae and to the left of the esophagus. At the level of C7 it quits its contact to the vertebral column, and turns laterally (left), anterior to the vertebral vessels, the phrenic nerve and the anterior scalene, posterior to the carotid sheath structures, to reach the veins of the thoracic outlet. There are several anatomical variants of the TD at this junction point. It joins the venous system either as a single vessel, either bifurcated, even as multiple branches. It may enter the jugular vein, the subclavian or their junction or even the anonymous vein [61].There might even exist a cystic dilatation of the trunk at that region, a remnant of the jugular sac. The TD rarely reaches the veins at the right side of the body, when it comes with an anomalous retroesophageal right subclavian artery.

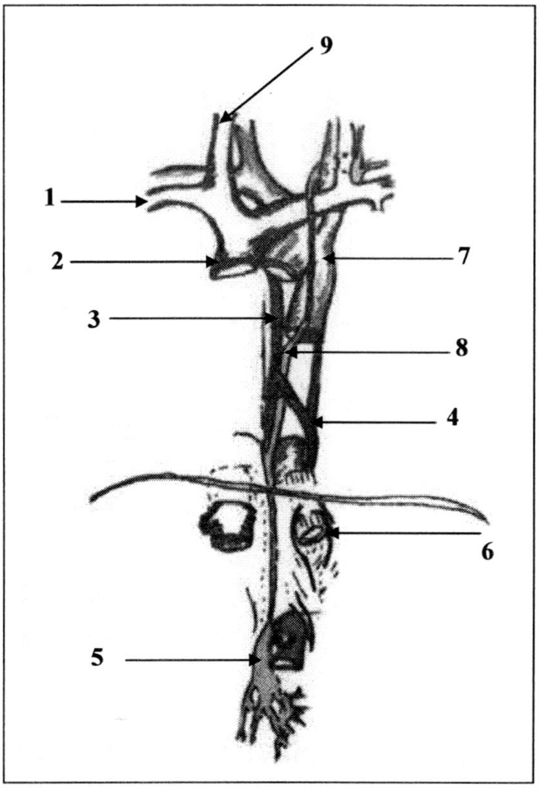

Figure+ 7. Anatomic relations of the TD 1)Subclavian vein 2)Superior vena cava 3)Azygos vein 4)Hemiazygos vein 5)Inferior vena cava 5)Cisterna chyli 6) Esophagus 7)Aorta 8)TD 9)Internal jugular vein (Petropoulos 1980).

The course of the TD in the abdomen and thorax, as described above, is observed in more than 60% of the population. In 38.7% of cases two or more TDs are found [61,62].

The usual course of the TD, shows why leakage of lymph from the inferior part of the trunk causes a right chylothorax and leakage from the superior part a left sided chylothorax. The good knowledge of the TD anatomy is very helpful in the interpretation of the imaging examinations and the surgical treatment of these lesions.

Etiology

The causes of CCh include trauma, malformations of the lymphatic system, acquired or congenital neonatal pathology, or it may occure with no evident cause at all. Underlying pathology, as well as patient history, distinguish Ch as 'spontaneous', 'primary', 'idiopathic' etc (Table 1).

Birth trauma is considered as the major cause when no other etiology is evident, especially when delivery was troublesome. The mechanism of injury is considered, most often, to be hyperextension of the cervical and thoracic spine. Another mechanism may be the increasing pressure in the venous and lymphatic system during delivery. The thin walled lymphatics are prone to be disrupted and release lymph in the thoracic cavity [63]. Untill several years ago most neonatal chylothoraces were considered either traumatic or idiopathic [64]

Chylothoraces are increasingly recognized in the fetal period on routine ultrasound at about the 29th week of gestation. One cannot resist to assume that several years ago some of these cases would have been considered as secondary to birth trauma. The U/S findings are liquid accumulation in one or both thoracic cavities. There may be associated findings of nonimmune hydrops fetalis (generalized and placental edema), thyrotoxicosis (with tachycardia) or congenital cardiac defects [65,66,67].

Table 2. Congenital defects of the major lymphatic vessels.

Congenital defecs of the lymphatics
1. Complete agenesis of the TD
2. TD atresia
3. Non communication between peripheral lymph vessels with those situated more centrally with the result of congestion and leaking of those peripheraly situated.
4. Multiple fistulas between the TD and the pleural cavity originating from non union between different embryonic parts of the TD

Congenital lymphatic disorders are being increasingly recognized in the pediatric and adult population. The pathology, obviously, is present before birth, rendering the lymphatics vulnerable to disruption but not always symptomatic in the neonatal period (Table 2). These LVDs have various localizations and clinical manifestations such as generalized lymphangiomatosis [68], congenital pulmonary lymphangiectasia [69,70], Gorham's disease (one or more bones are substituted by lymphatic tissue) [71.72], distichiasis-lymphedema syndrome [73]. Congenital pulmonary lymphangiectasia (PL) is recognised today as a separate entity that may or may not have a syndromic appearance and may exhibit ch (see section on PL).

In recent years the coexistence of CCh and several rare diseases such as mediastinal neuroblastoma [74] and neonatal thyreotoxicosis [67] has been described.

CCh can accompany a number of genetic defects. CCh has been described in children with Turner's and Noonan's syndrome [75,76], trisomy 21 [77],cardio-facio-cutaneous syndrome [78] or may appear in siblings [79].

Venous thrombosis may cause increasing pressure in the venous and lymphatic system and produce CCh. There have been reported cases of congenital superior vena cava obstruction [80], and left subclavian vein thrombosis [81]. Venous thrombosis may be secondary to catheterization, a practice much more common today in the neonatal ICU with more babies of low birth weight surviving. Superior vena cava syndrome secondary to central intravenous nutrition has been reported to cause CCh [64].

Another category is that of Ch complicating neonatal thoracic surgery [64]. To accept the term CCh in these cases is a matter of convention. Many kinds of thoracic operations in neonates have been implicated, such as those for correction of patent ductus arteriosus [82,83], cardiac anomalies, congenital cystic adenomatoid malformation of the lung [84] congenital diaphragmatic hernia [85].

The incidence of CCh following thoracic surgery is estimated between 0.25 and 0.9% [86]. We could not establish, even in approximation, the relative frequency of each etiologic factor. Medical literature is not unanimous on this question. Some investigators conclude that Ch occurs in newborn and pediatric patients most commonly as a complication of thoracic and cardiac surgery [87], while others consider idiopathic CCh as the most commonly occurring [64]. But in absolute numbers, the congenital idiopathic form is rare (1/15000 births) [88].

Some reasons for this descrepancy in statistics are the pool of patients of each institution and the thoroughness of patient evaluation.

Clinical Presentation and Diagnosis

CCh is the most common cause of intrapleural liquid accumulation in the neonatal period. It affects boys twice as common as girls and in 60% of cases occurs on the right side. In half of the cases it appears just after birth or within the first week of life. It may accompany a major congenital syndrome such as Noonan's, Turner's, Down's or cardio-facio-cutaneous syndrome. Intrapleural liquid accumulation found in prenatal diagnosis is most likely to be lymph.

In prenatal ultrasound the presence of pleural effusion, hydrops fetalis or associated lymphatic malformation is highly suggestive of CCh. Polyhydramnios may be present.

Signaling symptoms of CCh are those of shortness of breath i.e. tachypnea, dyspnea, retraction of intercostal spaces and cyanosis. Clinical examination reveals dullness of the ipsilateral hemithorax, reduced respiratory sounds and shift of the heart and great vessels towards the contralateral side.

The appearance of these symptoms depend on the time and rate of collection of chyle and whether it is uni- or bilateral. If CCh was present before birth, the symptoms are apparent immediately after birth. If chyle accumulation begins after birth, as is following birth injury, it may be initially insidious and symptoms may not be apparent until the first or second week of age.

If the rate of accumulation is slow and the child is in an intensive care unit, the radiograph (babygram) may be the first to reveal it.

A case of CCh can come into the physician's notice under the following settings:

- Antenatal u/s of the fetus with uni- or bilateral pleural effusion
- Pleural effusion in a newborn following a traumatic delivery
- Pleural effusion in a newborn (or child) with no apparent reason, without coexistent (or suspected) anomaly
- Pleural effusion in a newborn with a coexistent anomaly
- Pleural effusion in a newborn or infant after catheterization or surgery
- Pleural effusion in a newborn, infant or child with another lymphatic vascular disorder.

Therefore, a history of pathological findings on antenatal ultrasound, of traumatic labour or surgical manipulation may be very helpful. Attention must be given to recognize any genetic syndrome that may appear with CCh. The presence of CCh in the neonatal period without apparent defects of other body systems is indicative of either trauma during delivery (most often hyperextension of the cervical spine) or congenital defects of the TD and the lymphatics. In cases of defects of other organ systems, CCh may be the first sign [89].

The most important step in diagnosis is the characterization of the pleural cavity content. The sample is taken by thoracentesis, it is analysed chemically and a cell count is obtained. The color and consistency of the aspirate depends on the quality and quantity of consumed nutrients. The newborns that are not yet fed, or those who receive a formula with high concentration of medium chain triglycerides (MCT), have a clear, straw colored chyle. After they are fed with milk their chyle becomes thicker and whitish. A pleural collection resembling chyle can be due to tubrculosis, filariasis, rheumatoid arthritis, and other inflammatory conditions,. In these cases the effusion conteins large quantities of cholesterol and not triglycerides. It is known as pseudochylothorax.

The milky aspect of the effusion can only serve as a hint for further investigations; it is not a proof that the effusion is chylous. Coloring with Sudan III reveals the presence of lipids whose concentration, as well as that of the proteins is depended on the diet.

Pleural effusion in children is chyle when it contains > 1.1 mmol/L triglycerides (with oral fat intake) and has a total cell count ≥1,000 cells/μL, with a lymphocyte fraction > 80% [87].

It has been suggested, though, that pleural fluid lymphocyte counts alone are not reliable in establishing the cause of hydrothorax before birth [90].

An additional challenge is to recognize a possible underlying cause before considering CCh as 'idiopathic' or 'traumatic'. Congenital lymphatic disorders are being increasingly recognized in association with CCh. The spectrum of thoracic manifestations of lymphatic disorders ranges from incidental radiographic findings to diffuse lymphatic disease with respiratory failure [91].

Antenatal diagnosis is feasible today with the use of ultrasound and MRI that seems to be particularly useful for the investigation of thoracic lesions that are atypical or complicated by multiple abnormalities. [92,93].

After birth, a simple X-ray of the thorax may show unilateral thoracic opacification, with contralateral mediastinal shift. In premature babies there might be difficulty in radiograph interpretation because of possible underlying pulmonary pathology. In these cases ultrasound examination is helpful. Children with lymphatic malformations are at increased risk in developing Ch.

In cases of lymphangiomatosis the X ray shows a characteristic picture of multiple linear densities on the lung fields. Biopsy of the lung and the pleura shows dilated lymphatic vessels [94]. The immunohistochemical study of the specimens show the presence of endothelial cells reacting positively with the factor VIII-related antigen.

Conventional lymphangiography with contrast media is practically impossible to perform on neonates and difficult for infants. Even for older children it is cumbersome and has largely been superseded or used in combination with CT or MRI. For the imaging of the TD lymphoscintigraphy is very useful in showing the course of the TD but not accurate in revealing the site of lymph leakage [95,96,97,98].

Immunity

It is well documented that several parameters of immunity are compromised as a consequence of loss of immunity factors in the pleural cavity [99]. These patients are hypogammaglobulinemic. Mean IgG levels are below the 5th percentile for age. On the contrary, IgM and IgA levels are within normal ranges. The preservation of protective levels of tetanus-specific antibody and lack of infectious complications attributable to hypogammaglobulinemia or cellular immunodeficiency suggest that there is no clinical immunodeficiency associated with CCh in the vast majority of cases. Furthermore, some hallmark infections of hypogammaglobulinemia were not commonly found. These results demonstrate that hypogammaglobulinemia in patients with CCh does not necessarily indicate inadequate protection afforded by specific antibody induced by previous immunization. The lack of other infections typical in hypogammaglobulinemia may be a feature of the quality of the immunoglobulin retained in the circulation. In infants, this may represent the function of maternal IgG, and in older patients, the continued or increased production of pathogen-specific IgG. Immunoglobulin replacement has not been of clinical benefit, and CCh without evidence of immune dysfunction should not be considered an indication for such therapy.

Although total peripheral blood leukocyte counts are above 2500 cells/mm^3 and the mean of 8235±4326 cells/mm^3 is within normal limits, the absolute lymphocyte counts of CD3$^+$, CD4$^+$, and CD8$^+$ T cells is consistently below the 5th percentile for age. These subsets are found in increased numbers in the pleural chyle. Altogether, these data strongly suggest that the depletion of lymphocytes in children losing chylous fluid is selective for T cells (especially CD4$^+$ T cells) with a concomitant relative increase in the proportion of Natural

Killer cells in the blood [100]. Loss of lymphocytes theoretically increases the risk of infections. This risk is considered high by some investigators and not significant by others. No correlation between infectious complications and lymphocyte count could be demonstrated by several authors [86]. It is notable that despite extreme lymphopenia and T-cell depletion, a large series [100] failed to observe infections characteristic of T-cell immunodeficiency in patients studied. There are, however, isolated case reports of infections characteristic of T cell deficiency in acute chylothorax, including disseminated candidiasis or other fungal infection [101] and cytomegalovirus. In one study, cutaneous delayed-type hypersensitivity was also depressed.

Infection of the chyle in CCh is thought not to occur because chyle is inherently bacteriostatic. A case has nevertheless been reported in an immunocompromised patient with pneumonia [102].

The duration of these disturbances is significantly correlated with the duration of lymph accumulation or drainage.

Treatment

Antenatal

Thoracocentesis can be performed in the operating theatre under ultrasound guidance prior to Caesarean delivery. Gestational age at the time of diagnosis ranged between 26-34 weeks and that of thoracocentesis between 31-34 weeks. Intrapartum thoracocentesis is considered a relatively simple procedure and allows these babys, immediately postpartum, to breathe spontaneously or be more easily ventilated. This in turn, reduces the need to introduce chest tubes in an emergency situation [103].

The prognosis of a fetus with hydrothorax at mid-trimester is extremely poor. A fetus who developed bilateral chylothoraces at 23 weeks of gestation had bilateral pleuroamniotic shunts with double-basket catheters successfully installed as early as the 25th week of gestation. Hydrothorax did not recur in this fetus. After the shunting, however, polyhydroamnios, fetal hypoproteinemia, and placental edema developed, and the hydrops worsened [104].

The follow-up results indicate that pleural drainage in utero and prevention of premature delivery should be proposed to improve the outcome of non immune hydrops fetalis (NIHF) patients [65].

We should bear in mind though, that the presence of prenatal pericardial and pleural effusion or congenital anomalies carries a very poor prognosis in patients with NIHF [105].

Maternal dietary therapy has been tried with the hope to influence the fetus. Despite some early improvement the effusion recurs and the overall result is not encouraging [106].

Postnatal

As already mentioned CCh can accompany a number of congenital defects which might need to be treated, sometimes urgently. Children with Turner's syndrome may suffer from aortic malformations (aortic coarctation, aortic stenosis, bicuspid aorta) and from anomalous pulmonary venous drainage [107]. Children with Noonan's syndrome may also have heart disease, most commonly pulmonary stenosis (39%), hypertrophic cardiomyopathy (10%) and atrial septal defect (8%) [108]. They may also have bleeding diathesis. In those children the presence of other lymphatic malformations such as cystic hygroma is possible which, if extensive, may compromise the airway. In children with trisomy 21, ventricular septal defect, was found in 49% and common atrioventricular canal, was found in 15% [109].

Conservative Treatment

As for the treatment of CCh per se, it is generally accepted that a diagnostic evacuating pleural paracentesis should be performed at the start. This will offer an immediate relief from the pressure effect and relief from respiratory distress if no other underlying reason exists. In cases of persistence of symptoms and reaccumulation of fluid after 2-3 evacuations, a thoracic drain should be inserted and mechanical ventilation should be used.

Conservative treatment is successful in some patients but should be abandoned if the fluid loss exceeds 1.5 l/day for more than 5-7 days in an adult or more than 100 ml/day in a child. Danger due to malnutrition is added a few days after. The above mentioned losses cause hypovolemia, hyponatremia, hypoalbuminemia, important immune deficiency and weight loss. Lymphocyte count may be less than 1000/mm3.

Spontaneous cessation and cure occurs in more than 70% of patients after an average drainage duration of less than two weeks (of less than a month at maximum). The patients designated for surgical therapy drained for an average of a month (25 to 40 days). The amount of drainage per day may not be significantly different between patients treated operatively and those treated nonoperatively. Failure of nonoperative management was associated with venous hypertension from increased right-sided cardiac pressures or central venous thrombosis [101]. The most serious complications during this period are undernutrition and immunological disturbances. The duration of conservative treatment should not exceed four weeks.

At the same time a supportive treatment should be instituted to avoid malnutrition, metabolic and immunological disturbances.

In the cases where the baby can be orally fed we consider the administration of formula with large concentration of MCT. In persistent cases the patient receives TPN [110]. With these measures we usually observe an improvement in symptoms and a reduction of chylothorax. Both total parenteral nutrition and MCT-enriched enteral regimens provide adequate nutritional support in children [86].

There are recent reports that the administration of somatostatin or its analogue octreotide might accelerate the resolution of chylothorax. It has been used with success in a number of idiopathic, postoperative and iatrogenic chylothoraces [111] Reported effective doses of intravenous somatostatin range from 3.5-12 mcg/kg/h. Care must be taken to watch for side effects of somatostatin therapy, including diarrhea, hypoglycemia, and hypotension and necrotizing enterocolitis [112,113,114].

Nitric oxide has been used for the treatment of postoperative Ch in neonates with pulmonary hypertension [115]. This has not been used for idiopathic CCh.

Surgical management is considered in cases that do not improve with conservative measures because of the high mortality of the long lasting disease [116,117]. We also consider surgical management in cases of CCh accompanied by SVC thrombosis and increases CVP [116].

Surgical Therapy

There are various surgical options: Ligation of the TD, pleuroperitoneal or pleurovascular drainage, pleurodesis and pulmonary decortication. An open or a thoracoscopic approach can be used.

TD ligation used to be the only possible intervention for the treatment of CCh in the past. An impotant disadvantage of this method is that it involves a major operation on a baby already in suboptimal, if not in precarious, condition. It still remains as an acceptable option in cases where Ch persists even after drainage operations [118,119,120,121].

The ligation usually takes place at the right mediastinum between the the 5th and the 8th thoracic vertebrae, through a retrolateral thoracotomy at the 7th or 8th intercostal space. The dilated duct is recognized coursing on the anterior surface of the vertebrae. It is ligated on both sides of the leaking point with non absorbable sutures. A meal containing fat, administered an hour before the operation facilitates the localization of the this point. We must not forget that identifying an isolated chylous leak in the chest is difficult and many times impossible [122].

Pleuroperitoneal shunt was first described by Azizkhan in 1983 [123].The aim was to divert the lymph towards the peritoneal cavity and its resorpion by the peritoneum. That way the possibility of malnutrition is diminished and time is given for new lymph vessels to be formed in the thoracic cavity. The draining system consists of a one-way valve permitting flow from the pleural cavity (with lower mean pressure) to the peritoneal cavity (with higher mean pressure) [124]. It also consists of a pumping chamber that can deal with high viscosity fluids such as lymph which is placed subcutaneously, over a rib. The system allows the pumping of lymph with periodic pump pressing. This allows the child to leave the hospital for home care under parental surveillance. The valves mostly in use today are the ventriculoperitoneal low pressure Hakim valves.

In order to avoid the frequent applications of pressure on the valve from over the skin, a new kind of large flow valve has been recently designed which is connected to the draining tubes but is not implanted [125].

This method is applied mainly for the treatment of congenital hydrothorax in patients younger than 4 months of age and smaller than 8 kg weight. If the resorptive capacity of the peritoneum is diminished for reasons such as right cardiac failure and venous congestion, the method will not be successful.

Lymph drainage in the systematic circulation was first advocated by Kirkland in 1965 [61]. It was initially applied in cases where the peritoneal cavity couldn't accept lymph for drainage. We have applied this method in our clinic through a Holter or a Hakim low pressure valve. During the decade of 1980 one of us (A.S. Petropoulos) performed experimental imaging studies of the TD (ductography) in dogs after injection of contrast medium in mesenteric lymph nodes (Figure 8). Following that, chylothorax was created by obliteration of the TD with various techniques (Figure 9) [94,95,96,97] and was successfully drained into the circulation through the IVC with the use of Holter valve (Figure 10).

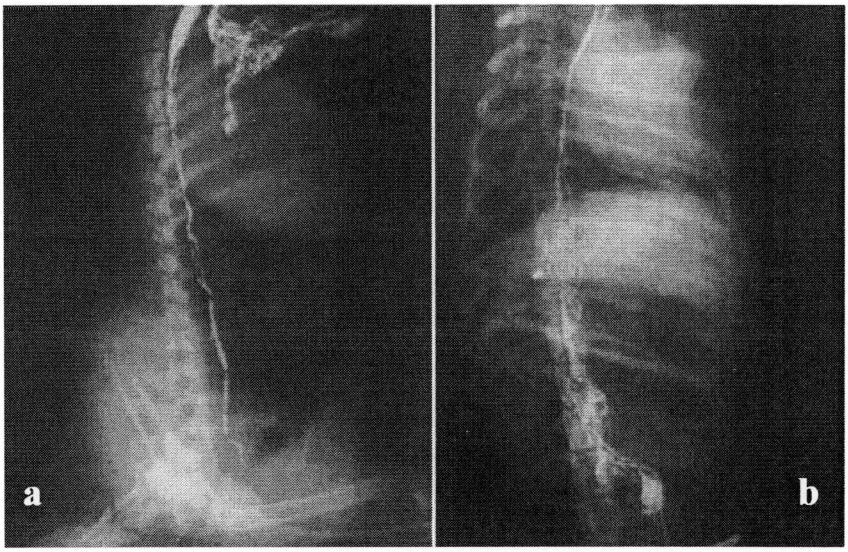

Figure 8. Imaging of a normal TD of a dog after injection of contrast medium in a mesenteric lymph node a) Front b) lateral view.

Following that, we applied this method to a series of 4 patients, all of them boys. One was a newborn and the others 16-25 months of age. Two of them had bilateral CCh, one had right sided, one left sided and one of them had chyloperitoneum as well.

One of these (the neonate), with bilateral CCh and severe circulatory decompensation, succumbed 3 months after bilateral drainage to the IVC, with two Holter valves.

The other 3 are being followed up for 21, 10 and 5 years after their initial operation. They have alltogether 5 valves, two for the bilateral CCh (one of them draining to the SVC), 2 for the CCh with chyloperitoneum, and one for the unilateral. All of them drain to the IVC, either directly or through the Iliac vein. One is draining the cisterna chyli to the IVC. (Figures11, 12, 13, 14, 15) [117,118,119,120].

During the followup years we had to do two revisions of the valves, with substitution, because of obliteration of the draining lumen and valve.

One of these patients has difuse lymphangiomatosis, with huge retroperitoneal lymphangioma and severe limb involvement.

The advantage is that the operation is well tolerated, there are no operative complications, convalescence is quick and the replacement of an obstructed catheter is easy. The disadvantage of the method is that the long catheters needed increase the possibility of obstruction or displacement.

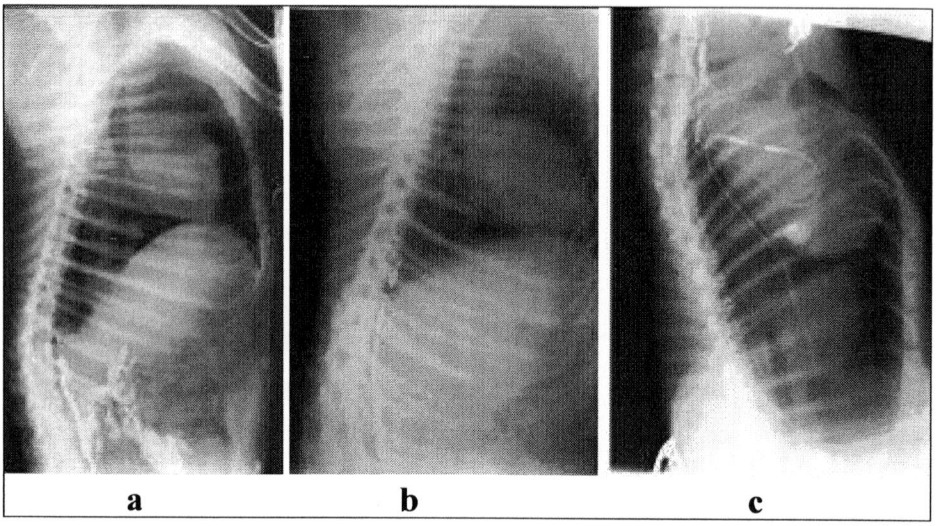

Figure 9. a) Transection of the TD at the level of the cisterna chyli. b) Partial recanalization of the TD after 4 weeks c) drainage of experimental chylothorax to the IVC through a Holter valve.

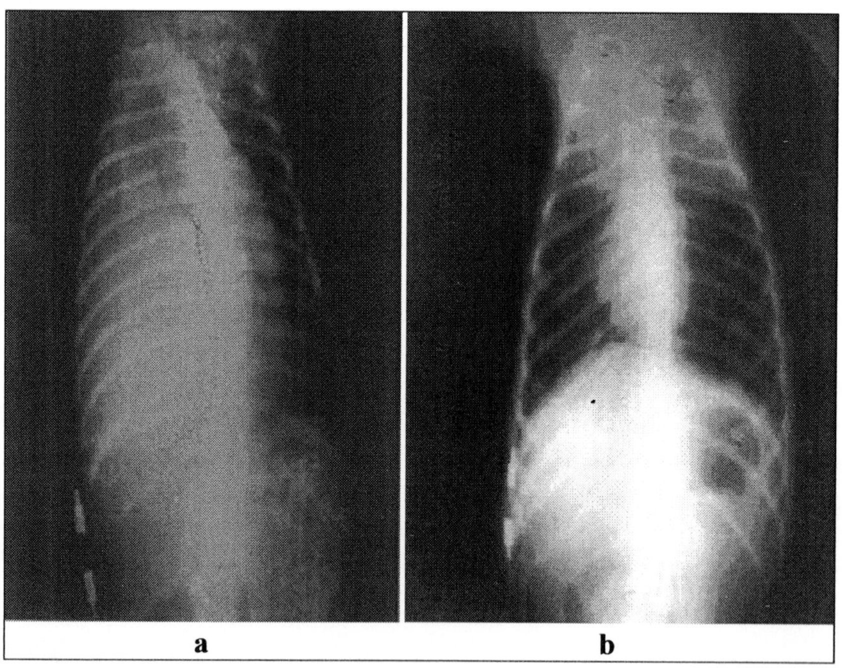

Figure 10. a) Radiograph of the thorax of the dog immediately after the insertion of the valve and draning of the lymph from the thoracic cavity to IVC. b) the same case 4 weeks later: complete drainage of the lymph

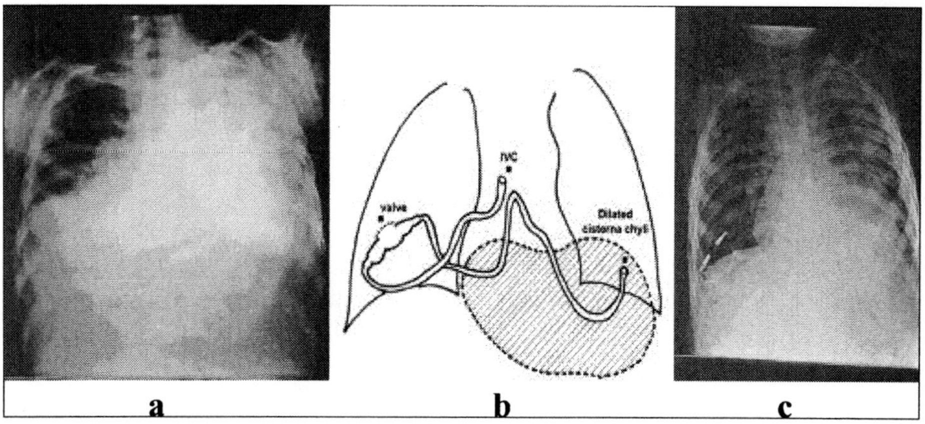

Figure 11. a) Bilateral chylothorax b)Schematic representation of the valve placement in the cisterna chyli and drainage to the IVC c) Six months later: Expansion of the lungs.

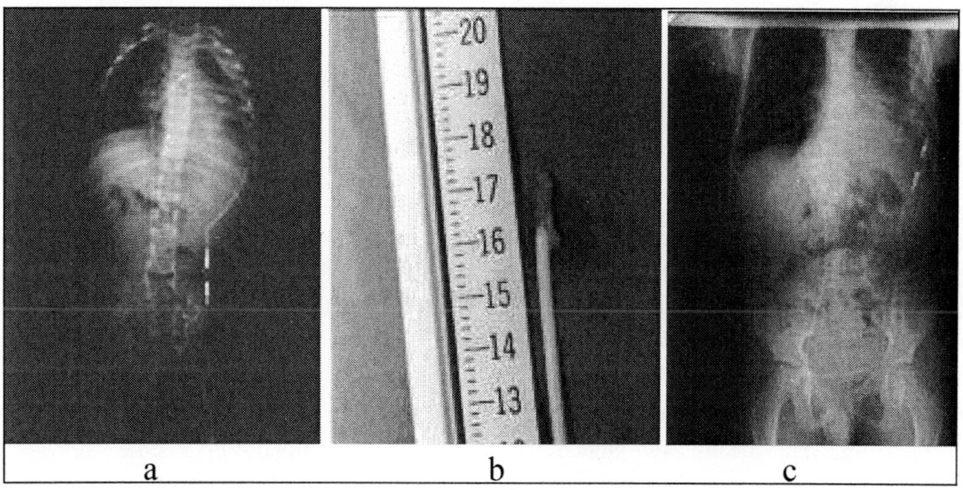

Figure 12. a) drainage of chylothorax with a Holter valve through the left iliac vein to the right atrium b)obstruction of the distal part of the catheter two years after c) replacement of the catheter.

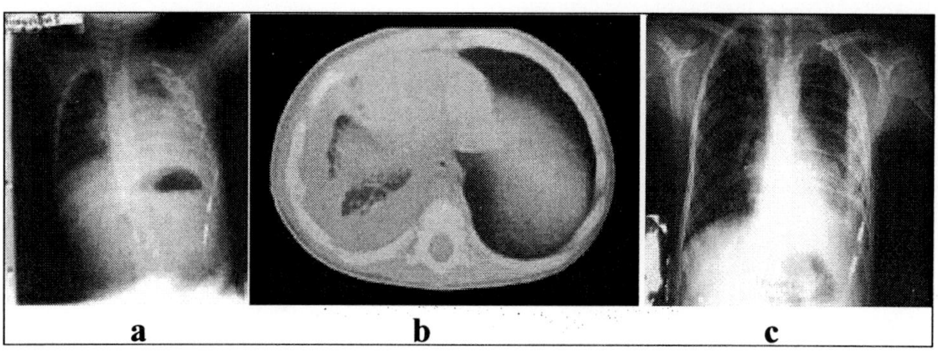

Figure 13. a) Left side chylothorax – drainage through the left iliac vein to the circulation b) CAT of left side chylothorax c) Same patient one year after, satisfactory lymph drainage, expansion of ipsilateral lung and small degree of pachypleuritis.

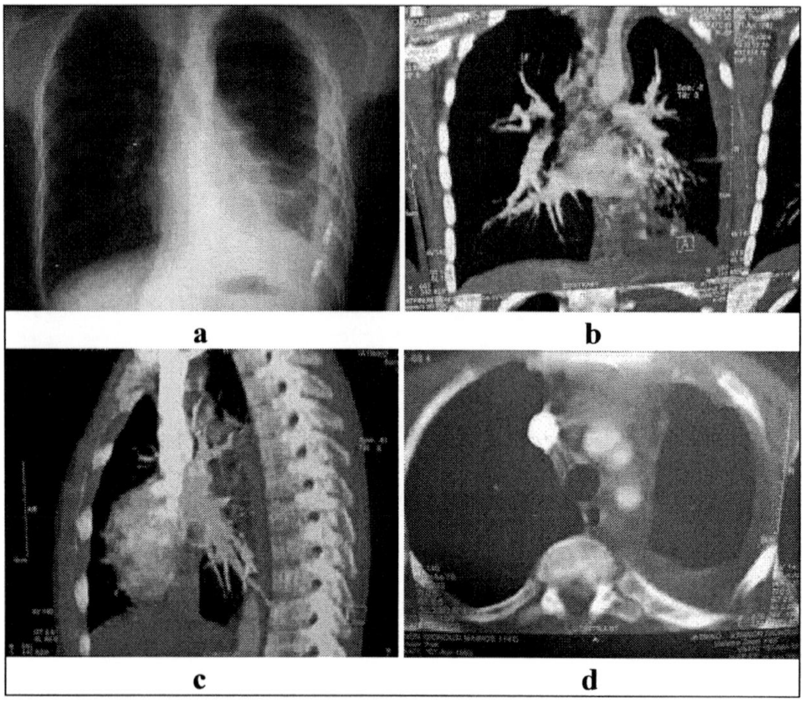

Figure 14. a) Radiography 8 years after drainage of chylothorax with small degree of pachypleuritis. b) and c) MRI d) CAT of the above patient.

Pleurodesis. This method aims at the formation of adhesions in the pleural cavity that will obstruct the leakage of lymph. Several agents have been used for this purpose as antineoplastic drugs, antimalarial drugs, antibiotics, talc powder, microbial immuroreactive products as OK-432 , fibrin glue and povidone-iodine.

Bleomycine has been used successfully in ch. Unfortunately, it was sometimes accompanied by toxic systematic effects because it was absorbed and reached the circulation. Quinacrine was also used for both pneumothorax and ch.

Fibrin glue has been used even in premature babies for CCh. Its application must be directly over the leaking point and has very good results especially if used in conjunction with pleurodesis or other surgical intervention [126].

Lastly, OK-432 was used which induces fibrin clots in the pleural cavity [127].

Pulmonary decortication is applied where other measures have failed [128]. In the course of the operation an attempt is made to find and close the leaking point.

Parietal pleurectomy can be a successful treatment when no distinct chylous leak can be identified [122].

Video assisted thoracoscopy. This method has the advantage of viewing the whole of the thoracic cavity and the mediastinal structures. It allows the positioning of clips to the TD at the level of the aortic foramen or at the leaking point [129]. Ultrasonic coagulating shears can be used to seal the TD. As a disantvantage we might mention the difficulty of finding the leaking point , the restrictions due to the small size of the patient and the fact that many had undergone thoracotomies before.

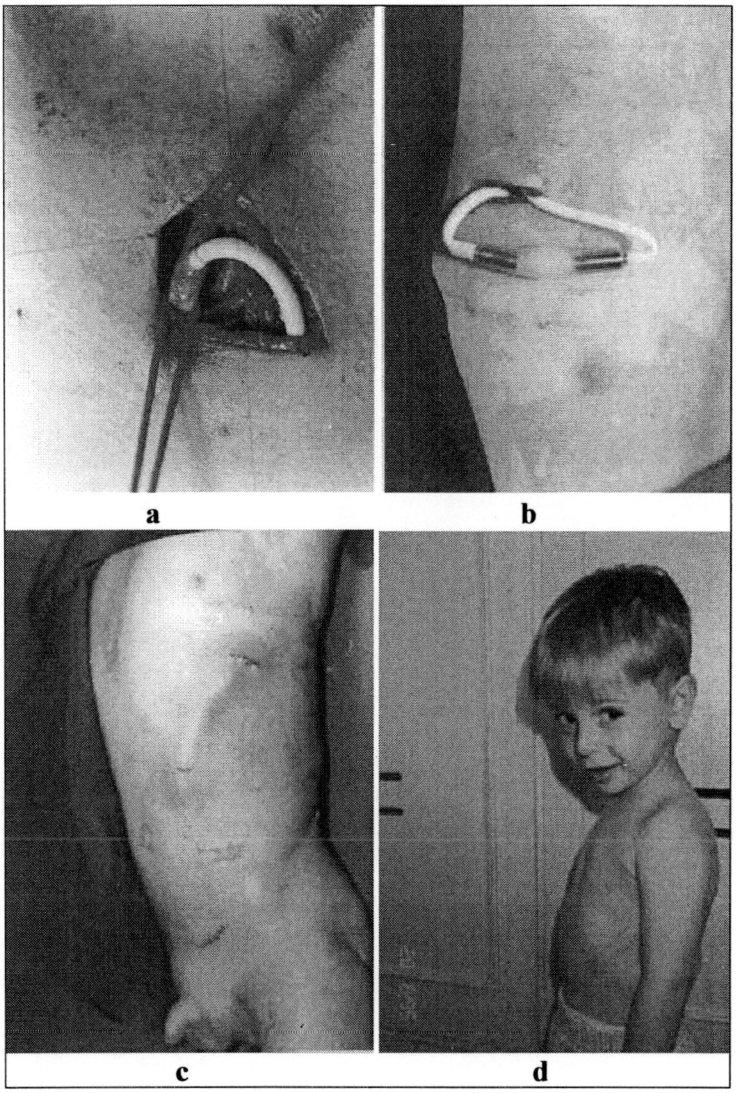

Figure 15. a) Cutdown and insertion of draining catheter to the external iliac vein b) Placement of Holter valve to the thoracic wall) drained lymph is shown c) The patient immediately after the operation d) The same patient two years later.

CONGENITAL CHYLOUS ASCITES

Chylous ascites (ChA) is the excessive collection of lymph in the peritoneal cavity. As an uncommon disorder, ChA has a reported incidence of 1 in 56,000 to 177,000 hospital admissions [130]. The most common cause (in 43% to 70% of cases) in infants and children is congenital malformation of the lymphatic channels [131]. Lymphangiography-documented lymphatic abnormalities leading to ChA include 1) atresia or stenosis of the major lacteals at the base of the mesentery or the cisterna chyli 2) mesenteric cysts, and 3) generalized lymphangiomatosis [132].

Congenital chylous ascitis is more common in patients with other forms of congenital lymphatic abnormalities. Primary lymphatic hypoplasia is a condition seen in childhood and characterized by lymphedema, chylothorax, and/or ChA [133]. Klippel-Trenaunay syndrome is sometimes accompanied with ChA [134]. The Yellow-Nail syndrome is a disorder of unclear etiology seen in childhood. Patients have hypoplastic lymphatics leading to chylous effusions. This condition exhibits the characteristic triad of lymphedema, pleural effusion and/or ChA and yellow discoloration together with dystrophy of the nails [135]. Primary lymphatic hyperplasia has also been recognized as a cause of chylous ascitec [136]. There are two forms: "bilateral hyperplasia" in which the lymphatics are not severely dilated and contain valves, and lymphangiectasia (megalymphatics) in which lymphatics are dilated and lack valves.

Other causes of ChA are external compression with obstruction of the lymphatics (25%-30%) because of intussusception, malrotation, incarcerated hernia, metastatic cancer, and inflamatory lesions causing lymph node enlargement Traumatic injury of the lymphatics is responsible for about 15% of cases.

Clinical Presentation

Most pediatric cases described were in males and were diagnosed in the 1st year of life [133]. ChA frequently appear as painless abdominal distention. As in other types of ascites, respiratory embarrassment is a common feature. A delay in diagnosis may result in weight loss, inanition, and ultimately death. Vomiting and scrotal edema (patent processus vaginalis) are more common in children. Anorexia and weakness are inevitable signs. Most patients present with a slowly increasing abdominal girth, although approximately 20% present themselves with an acute form characterized by rapid development of abdominal distention and signs of peritonitis, which is called the "acute chylous peritonitis". In the latter situation the pain is severe, and a physical examination may demonstrate well localized tenderness or rigidity. In these instances, the diagnosis is almost always established at laparotomy. Free chyle in the peritoneal cavity does not cause pain by itself, but pain results from stretching of the retroperitoneum and mesenteric serosa or from infection [137].

Diagnosis

Sampling peritoneal fluid by paracentesis is critical to diagnosing ChA. Chyle is the only body fluid with a fat content greater than plasma. Its protein content is approximately one half that of the plasma, and the electrolyte composition is nearly the same. The criteria commonly used to define chyle are not rigid because the chemical composition of chylous fluid is known to vary greatly from one individual to the other. Total fat and protein have been shown to vary along with diet [138]. Jahsman's [139] chief characteristics of chylous effusions, which still stands today, include milky appearance, separation into a creamy layer on standing, lacking an odor, alkaline chemical properties, specific gravity greater than 1.012, bacteriostatic properties, 3% total protein, staining of fat globules with Sudan Red stain, fat content of 0.4% to 4%, and total solids greater than 4%. The cell differential is 70% to 90% lymphocytes. With the advancement of molecular biology and accurate measurability of triglyceride levels, this value has become an important diagnostic tool. Triglyceride values are typically 2 to 8 times that of plasma [140]. Some authors have set arbitrary values for ascitic fluid triglycerides to define chyle. Staats stated that a triglyceride level greater than 110mg/dl was highly suggestive of chylous effusions [141]. For equivocal values (50-100), lipoprotein analysis could be obtained, which in chyle shows predominantly chylomicrons. True ChA must be distinguished from "chyliform" and "pseudochylous" effusions, in which the turbid appearance is due to cellular degeneration from bacterial peritonitis or neoplasm.

Determining the cause of congenital ChA can be a challenge. In abdominal tomography, the chyle has a low attenuation and can be readily distinguished. Another useful radiological study is lymphoscintigraphy. This technique involves injection of technitium Tc 99m-labeled sulfur colloid and dextran into intergigital web spaces. Lymphoscintigraphy allows for the functional assesment of lymphatic transport. In the setting of congenital chyloperitoneum, leakage of chyle is visualized. Proponents argue that this more physiologic technique is less invasive and should be used, especially when lymphangiography is contraindicated. A high quality image can be obtained, altough this may be technically difficult. Recently, there have been multiple reports of succesful identification of lymphatic leaks in congenital ChA through lymphoscintigraphy [142,143]. Postrepair evaluation has also been used to document the resolution of the leak. Advantages over lymphangiography include 1) no adverse effects 2) no contraindications 3) the ability to perform repetitive studies.

Although its use is declining with present-day noninvasive imaging, lymphangiography remains the gold standart in defining cases of lymphatic obstruction. The lymphangiogram is abnormal in almost every case of ChA. The identification of the site of extravasation is of primary importance when celiotomy is planned. Bipedal lymphangiography has been used successfully to evaluate the retroperitoneal lymphatics and / or lymphoperitoneal fistula. Complications are proportional to the volume of contrast used and the rate of infusion. Several larger series have demonstrated a 1,2% incidence of serious side effects due to the dye. Over 50% of these represent pulmonary sequelae of oil emboli. The mortality rate is 0,2%. Transient lympedema, including exacerbation of chyloperitoneum after lymphangiography, occurs in 4% of patients. Good results for lymphangiography have been reported when the patient is given a lipophilic dye orally with milk or creamy food before surgery.

Recently, laparoscopy has been mentioned more frequently as a diagnostic and potentially therapeutic modality [136,144]. Laparoscopy is a very accurate method to diagnose and identify the area of chylous leakage. Its therapeutic use is, however, limited by the difficulty of identification, ligation, and repair of retroperitoneal cisterna chyli or other lymphatic structures.

Treatment

Goals of nonoperative therapy for chylous ascites include 1) maintaining or improving nutririon 2) decreasing the rate of chyle formation and 3) correcting the underlying disorder.

Considerable controversy existed regarding the effectiveness of a high-protein, low fat diet with medium chain triglycerides. Most chylous effusions respond to an initial approach with a high -protein, low fat diet with MCT. Dietary restriction of long-chain triglycerides avoids the conversion of these into monoglycerides and free fatty acids, which are transported as chylomicrons to the intestinal lymph ducts. In contrast, MCT are absorbed directly into intestinal cells and transported as free fatty acids and glycerol directly to the liver via portal vein. The use of low fat diet with medium chain triglycerides supplementation therefore reduces the production and flow of chyle.

Patients who do not respond to the above measures should be fasted to reduce lymph flow and started on long-term total parenteral nutrition. This regimen, which can be administered at home [145], provides proper nutrition, reduces the rate of chyle flow, and is superior to medium chain triglycerides diet. However, its major drawbacks are the risks associated with use of central venous lines. The duration of TPN may be up to 10 weeks [146]. A minimum of 4 weeks for the effectiveness has been proposed [147]. Complementary with TPN, parecentesis of chylous ascites can relief dyspnea and abdominal discomfort. Patients who undergo multiple paracentesis are at risk for developing hypoproteinemia, malnutrition, and peritonitis.

In some recent studies [148,149], the use of somatostatine or ocreotide is associated with complete resolution of chylous ascites.

Surgical treatment should be considered in cases resistant to conservative therapy for over a month, and for those patients who have shown a temporary initial response with decrease of ascites, but are ultimately not cured by conservative therapy for more than 2 months [150].

During surgical exploration, the duodenum and the head of the pancreas should be mobilized (Kocher maneuver) to expose the root of the mesentery and the origin of the superior mesenteric vessels. The operative resolution of chyloperitoneum is achieved most commonly when a discrete leak of chyle can be identified in this region and repair with fine nonabsorbable ligatures is feasible. Chylous cysts should be excised. Adjunctive sclerotherapy with tetracycline, or topical application of fibrin glue is done [151]. Occasionaly, bowel resection is performed if large mesenteric lymphatics are localized to one segment. Preoperative nodal lymphangiography, or preoperative administration of lipophylic dye via oral or subcutaneous routes, may be helpful.

In patients with recurrence of chylous ascites after operation, or generalized lymphangiomatosis the use of peritoneovenous shunt is a reasonable therapeutic option (Fig.16). Initial success rates as high as 75% have been reported [152]. Unfortunately their use is associated with possible multiple complications. The high viscosity of chyle has rendered shunt patency in jeopardy. other potential serious problems are sepsis, fever, disseminated intravascular coagulopathy, hypokaliemia, pulmonary edema, and risk for air embolism. Advocates for peritoneovenous shunting state thet long-term patency have been improved with repeated manual valve compressions. A successful alternative approach to simple shunting has been described in a pediatric patient. Chylous fluid was reinfused into the venous circulation through a "peritoneal fluid filtration circuit". This technique uses a peritoneal dialysis catheter to drain the chylous fluid. A hemofilter is then used to remove water and electrolytes while reinfusing protein, fat, white cells, and other formed elements [153].

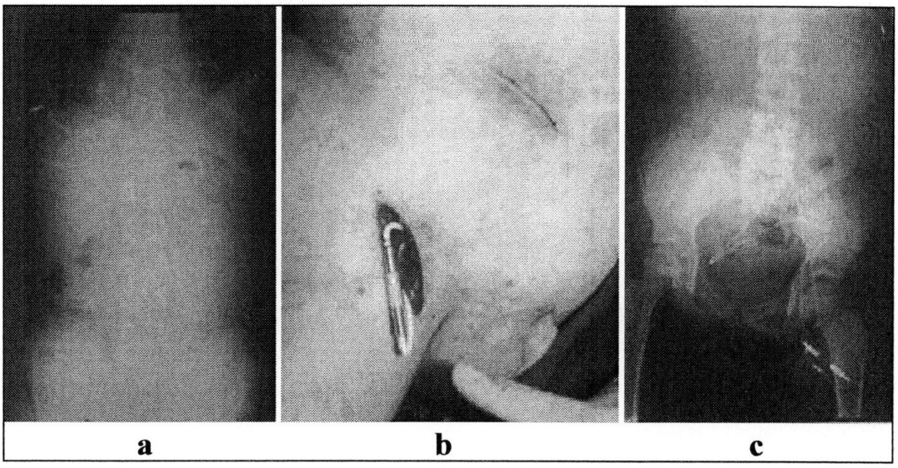

Figure 16. a) Chyloperitoneum b) Placement of Holter valve c) Postoperative picture of the patient with clinical improvement.

PULMONARY LYMPHANGIECTASIA

Pulmonary lymphangiectasia (PL) was first described by Virchow in 1856. It is a rare congenital disorder involving mainly the lungs. It is mostly sporadic, although some familial cases have been described with postulated modes of inheritance being either autosomal recessive or dominant inheritance with variable penetrance. Patients with primary PL have a developmental defect characterized by abnormal lymphatics mainly in the pulmonary connective tissue. The pulmonary septal, perivascular, peribronchial and subpleural spaces are dilated. The lymphatics in other organs may be defective as well.

Noonan [154] identified three pathologic types that are referred as:

a) primary pulmonary involvement,
b) PL secondary to pulmonary venous obstruction due either to venous or cardiac morphological abnormalities,
c) generalized lymphatic abnormality [155].

Wagenaar's classification, modified by Esther and Barker [155,156], distinguishes the forms of the disease as follows:

a) primary: (1) limited to the lungs, (2) with pulmonary and mediastinal involvement, (3) generalized (4) syndromic form
b) secondary, due to obstruction of the pulmonary venous outflow.

The incidence of the disease is not well established but necropsy studies suggest that approximately 0.5–1% of stillborns or infants who die in the neonatal period have pulmonary lymphangiectasia [157,158].Aborted fetuses with PL usually have additional congenital malformations detected on prenatal ultrasound scan such as trisomy 21, anencephaly, spinal dysraphism, Arnold-Chiari and other multiple malformations. They may present with in utero chylothorax causing pulmonary hypoplasia or hydrops fetalis [159,160,161].

The generalized form involves lymphangiectatic changes in many organ systems including the subcutaneous tissue, intestine, and lung. PL can be associated with multiple congenital anomaly syndromes such as Noonan, Ulrich-Turner, and Down' syndrome [161]. Secondary PL is due to severe cardiac malformations causing obstruction of the pulmonary venous outflow [162].

There is a male preponderance, and the child that is born alive typically suffers from respiratory distress with a mortality rate close to 100%. There are only sporadic cases of survivors or cases presenting later in life [155,163]. In those cases, the diagnosis of PL is usually made by the 3rd month of age. In one series only 5 out of 11 liveborn with PL survived infancy. Those that died suffered mainly by secondary PL to cardiac anomalies [161].

If the malformation is limited to the lungs and it may be localized to one or both lungs, in one or two lobes. The most common presenting symptoms are some degree of respiratory distress, chronic productive cough, recurrent pneumonia, bronchial asthma, choking and chylothorax. Chest x-ray findings of surviving children include generalized hyperinflation, pleural effusion, perihilar interstitial infiltrate, pneumothorax [164]. It may be difficult to distinguish PL from pulmonary interstitial emphysema or chronic lung disease on a radiological basis in older children.

Lung biopsy on these sick children is required to exclude or confirm this diagnosis. In rare circumstances of localized disease, surgical resection can be curative. Pulmonary lymphangiectasia should thus be included in the differential diagnosis of pulmonary cystic lesions, bilateral obstructive emphysema, and in cases of chronic pneumonia and asthma. Most patients die shortly after birth, but survival has been sporadically reported.

The generalized form involves lymphangiectatic changes in many organ systems including the subcutaneous tissue, intestine, and lung. The major symptoms include generalized edema and protein loss from intestinal lymphangiectasia. Hemihypertrophy may be present [165]. Pulmonary involvement in patients with generalized disease is typically less severe, and survival is reported to be better than with other forms of PL.

Assisted ventilation and thoracic drainage may be necessary for infants with PL. The children that survive beyond infancy tend to improve over time. Apart from lung biopsy, segmentectomy or lobectomy may be performed for localized lung involvement.

PRIMARY LYMPHEDEMA

Lympedema is the general term for a set of pathologic conditions in which there is excessive regional interstitial accumulation of protein-rich fluid. It can be either a primary or aquired (secondary) condition. Both forms share a common pathophysiology which is inadequate clearance of lymph fluid. Lymphedema usually involves abnormalities in the regional lymphatic drainage of the extremities, although visceral lymphatic abnormalities can also occur. Generalized developmental insufficiency of the lymphatic circulation is not compatible with life [166].

In addition to the chronic changes in the size and structure of the subcutaneous and integumentary structures, lympedema may have a substantial effect on quality of life and perception of well-being. Patients commonly present with painless swelling of an extremity. The swelling decreases with bed rest but does not disappear. Fifteen percent of patients have accompanying hemangiomas, lymphangiomas, double row of eyelashes, and yellow toenails and fingernails. In this chapter we are going to refer to primary lymphedema.

Pathophysiology

In contrast with venous edema, in which enhanced capillary pressure can indirectly stimulate lymph production, lymphedema is caused by a reduction in lymphatic transport. Several anatomic problems can lead to primary lymphedema including lymphatic hypoplasia and functional insufficiency or absent of lymphatic valves. Some patients may have an impairment of intrinsic contractility of the lymphatic vessel [167]. Much of the current understanding of the pathophysiology of lympedema derives from the experimental work of Olszewski in dogs [168]. In his and in other more recent experimental models [98], mechanical interruption of lymph vessels of the limb was sufficient produce lympedema after a period of months to years. Before overt edema occurred, marked lymphangiographic changes were observed in the absence of detectable accumulation of interstitial fluid. Eventually, lymph collectors became fibrotic and lost their normal permeability. In addition, electron micrographs of skin lymph capillaries disclosed permanent incompetence of the interendothelial junctions. In contrast, the pattern observed in edematous states and chronic limb lymphedema secondary to venous hypertension, such as congestive heart failure and thrombotic venous disorders, is one that is not accompanied by lymphatic hypertension that might otherwise have been theoretically prediced.

The most common cause of primary lymphedema is hypoplasia of the lymphatics in the subcutaneous tissue [169]. Most but not all authors [170,171] believe that the lymphatic system has a valveless superficial component and a valved deep one. In cases of lymphedema, the fluid is accumulated in the (superficial) system of the subcutaneous tissue. The deep system of lymphatics beneath the fascia and the muscles is separate and unaffected. The universal observation that the muscles and their deep lymphatics are competent in all cases of lymphedema has been the key consideration in the design of procedures that attempt to divert lymph into the valved deep systems so that the fluid can move upward.

Once established, lymphatic stasis fosters the accumulation of protein and cellular metabolites, such as macromolecular protein and hyaluronin within the extracellular space. Impaired lymphatic transport produces accumulation of both macromolecular protein and hyaluronin [172]. This is followed by an increase in the tissue colloid osmotic pressure, which leads to water accumulation and increased interstitial hydraulic pressure.

Chronic lymphedematic stasis often produces an increase in the number of fibroblasts, adipocytes, and keratinocytes in the edematous tissues. Mononuclear cells, like macrophages, often demarcate the chronic inflammatory response [173]. In most patients, there is an increase in collagen deposition, with adipose and connective tissue overgrowth in the edematous skin and subcutaneous tissues [174]. Histopathologic findings in chronic lymphedema include thickening of the basement membrane of lymphatic vessels, fragmentation and degeneration of elastic fibers, increased numbers of fibroblasts and inflammatory cells, and increased amounts of ground substance and pathological collagen fibers [175]. Ultimately, these processes lead to progressive fibrosis.

Classification

The simplest classification of primary lymphedema is according to the age at which the edema first appears. 1) congenital lymphedema or Milroy's disease is apparent at birth or become recognized within the first 2 years of life. 2) Meige's disease or lymphedema praecox typically occurs peripubertally or in association with pregnancy, but may appear as late as the third decade of life. 3) Lymphedema tarda develops after the age of 35 years. Some traits that occur in association with hereditary lymphedema include hypoparathyroidism, microcephaly, intestinal lymphangiectasia, ptosis, yellow nails and pleural effusions, cerebral arteriovenous anomalies, distichiasis and congenital heart defects, and webbing of the neck in Noonan syndrome [176]. Two genes mutated in hereditary lymphedema have been identified. Linkage of hereditary lymphedema to chromosome 5q34-q35 was first esdtablished in 1998, and unique causative mutations in FLT4, coding for vascular endothelial growth factor receptor-3, were subsequently identified in several families with Milroy congenital lymphedema [46]. Lymphedema-distichiasis syndrome is linked to 16q24.3, and unique mutations in FOXC2 have been identified as the cause of lymphedema-distichiasis syndrome in multiple families with pubertal or early adult onset lymphedema [177]. These two genes account for only a fraction of families with lymphedema.

When cases of congenital lymphedema cluster in families, an autosomal dominant pattern of transmission is most frequently described. However, isolated cases are much more common. There is a strong association between intrauterine and congenital lymphatic dysfunction and several heritable chromosomal abnormalities [178].

Clinical Presentation and Development

In congenital lymphedema, the swelling can involve only a single lower extremity, but edema of multiple limbs, the genitalia, and even the face can be seen. Bilateral leg swelling and involvement of the entire lower extremity is more likely in congenital cases than in other forms of primary lymphedema [179].

Lymphedema praecox, the most common form of primary lympedema, is responsible for as many as 94% of the cases in large series. The estimated 20:1 ratio of females to males suggests that estrogenic hormones are involved [180]. Edema is usually unilateral and is limited to the foot and calf in the majority of patients.

Lymphedema tarda is relatively uncommon, and accounts for fewer than 10% of cases of primary lymphedema.

An alternative classification of primary lymphedema relies upon morphologic characteristics [179]. Distal hypoplasia of the lymphatics is typically associated with bilateral peripheral edema of the lower extremities. There is usually a family history of similar symptoms, a female predominance, and a tendency for indolent progression. When isolated proximal obstructive hypoplasia is observed, clinical involvement of the entire limb is more likely, usually accompanied by relentless worsening of the edema. Patients who have unilateral edema involving the entire lower extremity are likely to have lymphatic hyperplasia with megalymphatics, although this syndrome is uncommon.

The time of the initial onset of lymhedema is uncertain, particularly as it may be asymptomatic. In many forms of primary lymphedema, there may be a protracted phase of apparently normal lymphatic function, despite an inherited anatomic or functional disturbance of this microcirculation. This latent phase of lymphedema may represent a balance between the existing increased lymph load and the reduced outflow capacity. Lymphedema may become manifest when compensatory mechanisms, which may include lymphatic regeneration, become inadequate to compensate for lymphatic flow.

The precipitating factors for overt lymphedema are not known [181]. At the onset of clinical lymphedema, swelling of the involved extremity is typically desdcribed as puffy, and the disturbance may be intermittent (Figure 17) [119]. With chronicity, the involved structures develop the chracteristic feature of induration and fibrosis.

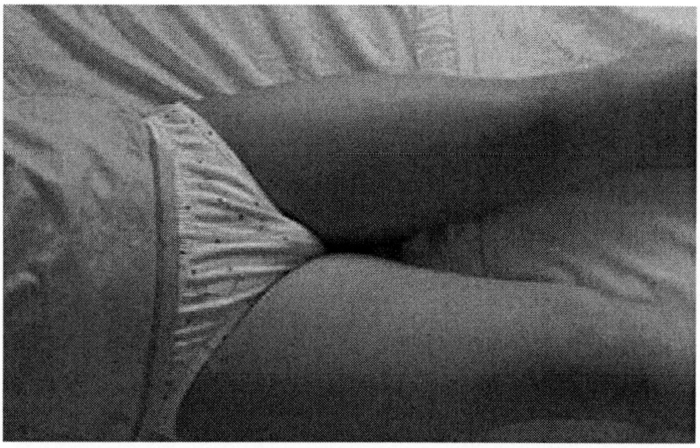

Figure 17. a) Primary lymphedema of right lower limb in a 13 year old patient.

In many patients, the maximal increase in girth of the involved limb is determined within the first year after onset, unless there are supervening complications like recurrent cellulitis. The propensity to recurrent cellulitis is one of the most troublesome aspects of long-standing lymphedema. Microbial growth is encouraged by the surplus of fluid and accumulated proteins. Lymphatic dysfunction also impairs local immune responses [182]. With recurrent infections, there is progressive damage of lymphatic capillaries.

The clinical presentation of soft-tissue infection in lymphedema can be variable, from very subtle exacerbations of lymphedema characterized by skin changes without fever, to rapidly progressive soft tissue infection with high fever and systemic toxicity. Recurrent attacks of cellulitis further damage the cutaneous lymphatics, worsen the skin quality, and aggravate the edema.

In very rare cases chronic lymphedema may be complicated by the local development of malignant tumors such as lymphangiosarcoma, which can present either as sclerotic plaques or multicentric lesions with blue-tinged nodules or bullous changes. Other cutaneous malignancies that have been observed in association with chronic lymphedema include lymphoma, melanoma, squamous cell carcinoma, and Kaposi's sarcoma [183].

Diagnosis

The diagnosis of primary lymphedema is best established by a thorough clinical history and physical examination. Localized edema may be due to inflammation caused by infection or allergic reaction, obstruction or compression of the venous system, or obstruction or compression of the lymphatic vessels. The presence of localized edema of a limb at birth suggests a congenital obstruction of the lymph vessels. A history of a major trauma, surgical intervention or radiation therapy is mainly indicative of lymph injury. Fever, local signs of inflammation, lymphadenitis and increased size of regional lymph nodes suggest venous thrombosis, microbial infection or cat scratch disease. Malignancies must always be taken into account, especially when patients report sudden onset, rapid progression or associated pain. Exposure to environmental factors, such as insect stings or bites, burns, or freezing should also be considered. Filariasis is a common cause of lymphedema in tropical climates. IgA nephritis, xanthomatosis, reflex sympathetic dystrophy, connective tissue disease, and Aagenaes syndrome (cholestasis-lymphedema syndrome) are other rare conditions that may cause secondary lymphedema [184,185].

Several physical features distinguish lympedema from other causes of chronic edema of the extremities. Among these are the classic changes of cutaneous and subcutaneous fibrosis (peau d' orange), and the Stemmer sign, which is an inability to tent the skin on the dorsum of the digits of the feet. Although the Stemmer sign has not been validated, it was initially reported to discriminate patients with lymphedema [186]. Lymphedema in the legs often produces preferential swelling of the dorsum of the foot, as well as the characteristic blunt, "squared-off" appearance of the digits in the involved extremity.

When the physical examination does not conlcusively support the diagnosis of lymphedema, additional evidence may be necessary to confirm impaired lymphatic function. Available tests include isotopic lymphoscintigraphy, indirect and direct lymphography, lymphatic capillaroscopy, magnetic reasonance imaging (MRI), axial tomography, and ultrasonography. Direct lymphangiography is generelly limited to the evaluation of canditates for lymphatic surgery. Isotopic lymphoscintigraphy is the most commonly used test and is generally considered to be the gold standart for the diagnosis of lymphedema. A radiolabeled macromolecular tracer is administer into the subdermal, interdigital region of the affected limb. The lymphatic transport of the radiolabeled macromolecule can be monitored in a semiquantitative fashion with gamma camera. Major lymphatic trunks and lymph nodes can be visualized. Useful diagnostic criteria are: i) absent or delayed radiotracer transport after injection ii)absence or paucity of lymphatic collectors iii) dermal diffusion of radiotracer (dermal backflow) iv) poorly visualized or absent regional lymph nodes (Fig 18) [187].

Magnetic resonance imaging and computerized tomographic imaging allow the objective documentation of structural changes attributable to lymphedema [188,189].

The characteristic absence of edema within the muscular compartment helps to differentiate lymphedema from other forms of edema. Characteristic of lymphedema is the honeycomb distribution in the epifascial plane, along with the thickening of the skin.

Other techniques such as tissue tonometry and bioelectrical impedance analysis allow detection of small changes in tissue turgor in subclinical states of lymphatic impairment and in the in the assesmant of response to treatrment [190].

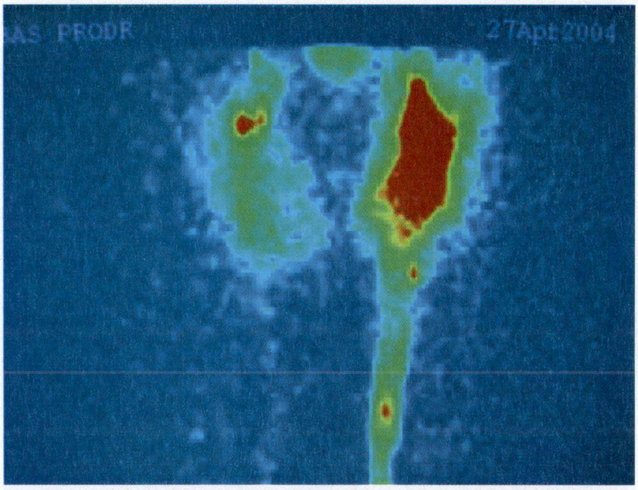

Figure 18. Radioscintigraphy of the patient on fig. 17: delayed transfer of tracer in the right limb and absence of visualization of lymphatic vessels until the right midthigh.

Treatment

Most patients with lymphedema respond to conservative treatment. Surgical interventions is seldom indicated except in difficult cases with extreme disabilities or recurrent complications.

Medical Therapy: Elevation of the extremity can be useful in some patients but this form of therapy is difficult to enforce in an active child. Supportive stockings, in the form of compressive garments, is a necessary adjunct to all other kinds of therapy. Relatively inelastic sleeves and underwear that transmit compression will prevent reaccumulation of fluid after successful decongestive treatment. These stockings are especially effective when combined with intermittent pneumatic compression. The intermittent pneumatic compression is best used overnight and the elastic garment during the day. Rapid reduction of the size is usually obtained, but the decrease is difficult to maintain due to lack of patients compliance.

The specialized massage technique for these patients is intended to enhance lymphatic contractility and to augment and redirect lymph flow through the nonobstructed cutaneous lymphatics. Manual lymphatic drainage should not be confused with other forms of therapeutic massage that have no effect on lymphatic contractility. The mild tissue compression during manual lymphatic drainage produces better filling of the initial lymphatics and enhances transport capacity, through the cutaneous lymphatic dilation and development of accessory lymph collectors [191].

Skin care is extremely important to prevent breakdown and infection. Infection should be treated promtly with antibiotics and bed rest. Diuretics, anticoagulants and other pharmacologic agents have limited value in the treatment of children with lymphedema.

Other treatments are under investigation. Some promising responses have been reported after local hyperthermia [192] and intraarterial injection of autologous lymphocytes [193].

As far as pharmacotherapy, the reported benefit of coumarin (5,6-benzo-[a]-pyrone) in lymphedema is ascribed to its stimulatory effect upon cutaneous macrophages and, thereby, upon local proteolysis [194]. Coumarin also stimulates other cellular elements of the immune system and may promote protein reabsorption. However, coumarin administered orally may cause idiosyncratic hepatitis. Also there are some data concerning the therapeutic benefit of augmenting dietary flavenoids and that dietary restriction of long-chain triglycerides provides some relief of edema in these patients [195].

Surgical Treatment: Many surgical techniques have been attempted in the treatment of lymphedema. The two basic goals have been to encourage lymph drainage and to remove lymphedematous tissue [196]. Ideally, appropriate lymphatic flow is reestablished. Implants of different material, such as silk, nylon, fascia, and rubber, have generally failed to provide long term relief of the lymphedema. Omental flaps have not produced good results, despite early successful reports. Pedicle flaps and myocutaneous flaps have failed to provide consistently good results.

A variety of lymphatic anastomoses have been tried, including lymph node-to-venous anastomosis, lymph vessel-to-vein anastomosis, and lymphatico-lymphatic anastomosis. Some of these techniques are theoretically attractive but require microsurgical expertise.

Excision techniques can produce good results in some patients. Split and full thickness skin grafts have some drawbacks, such as hypertrophic scarring, sensory loss in the skin, graft loss, scar contracture, keratoses, ulcerations, and aggravation of edema in the feet. Staged excision of sucutaneous tissue and skin may produce reasonably good results in selected patients. Staged excision has less risk of complications than does grafting, but necrosis of the flaps, sensory difficulty, and inadequate reduction in the size of the limb can occur. Surgery for cosmetic reasons alone is contraindicated because disproportion persists along with scars from the procedure. Function takes priority over cosmesis. Emotional support to patient and family is extremely important.

Lymphatic Vascular Dysplasias

Lymphatic vascular dysplasias (LVD), also known as cystic hygromas (CH) or lymphangiomas, are a group of lesions originating from errors in vascular formation during embryonic life. They do not proliferate but they gradually enlarge. They are usually apparent from the neonatal period but they can appear in the first or the second decade of life [197].

Lymphangiomas vary greatly in their size, site, and tissue infiltration, affecting the surrounding tissues in variable ways, transforming the anatomic relations and impairing the function the adjacent organs. Consequently, they may present clinically in a variety of ways. Their localization varies according to various authors, a combined estimate being approximately as follows: head and neck 48-75%, trunk and limbs 20-42%, internal organs 10% (Figure 19, 20) [198,199].

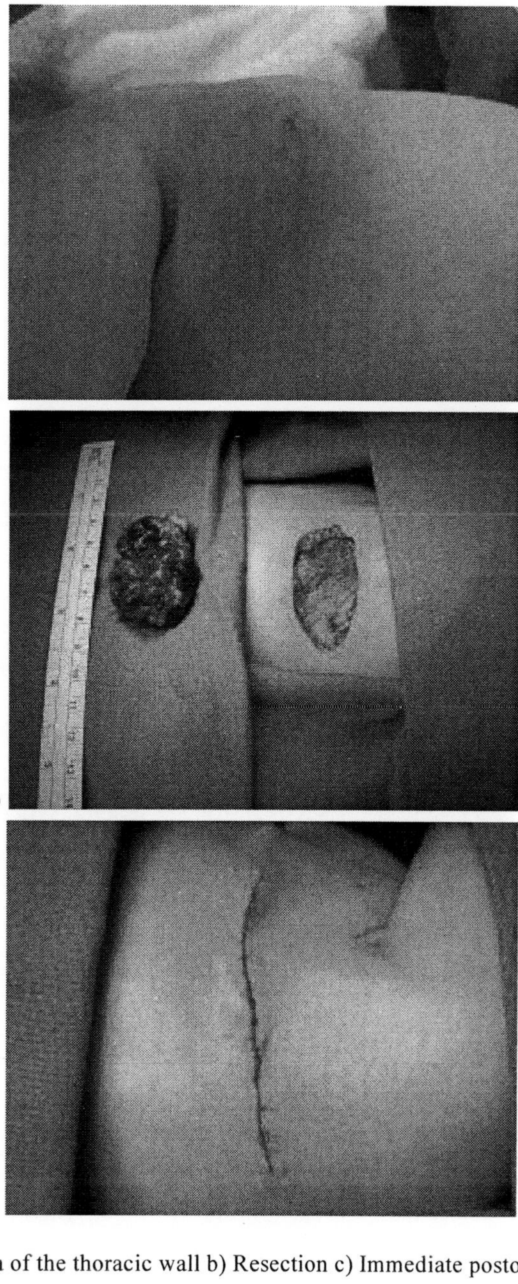

a b c

Figure 19. a) Lymphangioma of the thoracic wall b) Resection c) Immediate postoperative images.

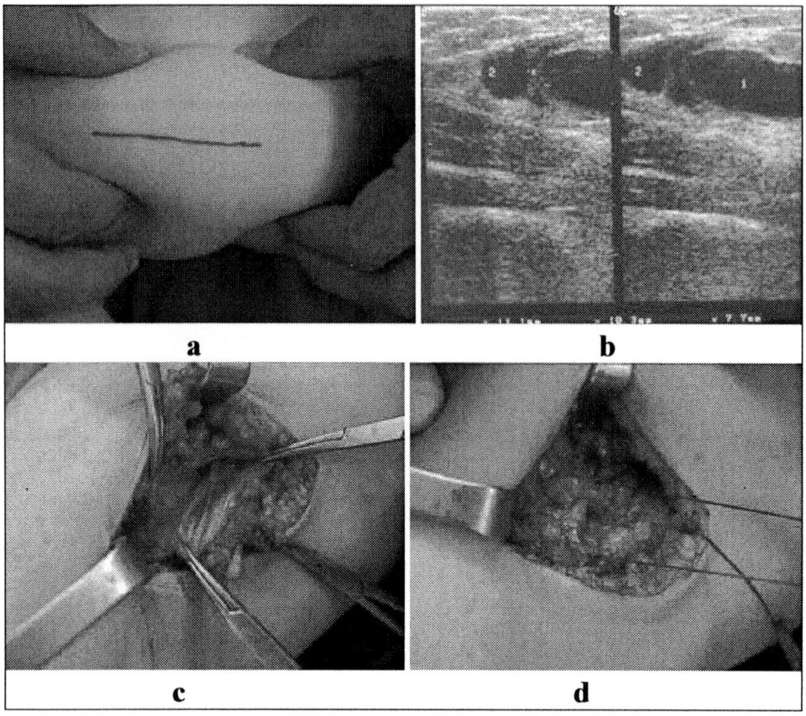

Figure 20. 16 a) Lymphangioma of the thigh b) Ultrasound c) Operative view d)Ligation of two aberrant lymphatic vessels in the above patient.

These apparent and sometimes impressive lesions are well known from the antiquity. At middle ages, together with the blood vessel dysplasias, they were simply classified either as signs of God or stains of Satan, according to the collective fears of the society or the interests of the authorities.

The classifications of vascular lesions by Jaccoud, Virchow and Wegener in the 19th c. and the terminology that they used were quite confusing [200]. Mulliken and Glowacki in1982 [201] proposed a classification based on the endothelial characteristics of vascular lesions. This classification has been adopted by the International Society for the Study of Vascular Anomalies (ISSVA) [202]. They identified two major types of vascular lesions:

a) hemangiomas: with rapid neonatal growth and hypercellularity with increased thymidine uptake during that period, and slow involution characterized by fibrosis and diminishing cellularity
b) vascular malformations: being present at birth and growing with a normal rate of endothelial cell turnover.

The group of malformations was further subdivided by Burrows et al. into low- and high-flow malformations (LFM and HFM) [203]. HFMs are connected to the arterial or capillary system, and therefore exhibit arterial flow. LFMs have a connection with the venous or the lymphatic system. Lymphatic malformations result from abnormal development of lymphatic vessels, and consist of fluid-filled lymphatic spaces that are either microcystic or macrocystic. In 70–80%, they are located in the head–neck region.

The more recent classifications such as the "Hamburg Classification", based on the work of Degni and Malan [204] deal mainly with venous malformations or are orientated to be used for therapy planning [205].

Pathology

Lymphatic vascular dysplasias are vascular malformations of the low flow type. They represent cystic cavities lined with endothelium and filled with clear or straw – colored fluid. They grow slowly, often surround and may even infiltrate adjacent structures.

Multiple histologic staging systems have been developed for LVDs. Traditionally, three categories are recognized, although they represent a clinicopathologic continuum:

1) Lymphangioma simplex, composed of small capillary-sized lymphatic channels (as in the common form of lymphangioma circumscriptum),

2) Cavernous lymphangioma, consisting of dilated lymphatic channels, often with fibrous covering and

3) Cystic lymphangioma or hygroma, with larger cavities than the categories above.

All three kinds of lymphangiomas can coexist in the same lesion. These histologic categories do not correlate with clinical behavior and therapeutic response. For that reason, the newer histologic patterns categorize lymphangiomas as macrocystic (previously termed cystic hygromas), microcystic (previously termed lymphangiomas) and mixed type [206], based on the size of the lymph lumens and response to sclerotherapy [207].

Another classification frequently used divides these lesions into two groups based on the depth and the size of the lesion. The superficial vescicles represent the lesion known as lymphangioma circumscriptum. The more deep situated lesions comprise the cavernous lymphangioma and the cystic hygroma. Many consider cystic hygroma as a type of cavernous lymphangioma.

The lesions of the mixed type have venous and lymphatic parts and it is relatively difficult to distinguish them from each other. Extensive LVDs may involve the whole limb. These lesions might be mislabelled as Klippel–Trenaunay, Parkes–Weber or Servelle–Martorell syndrome [208].

The cysts are lined by endothelium and they contain fluid which is often identical with lymph. The endothelium of lymphatic vessels and malformations express a specific receptor subtype, the vascular endothelial growth factor receptor 3 (VEGFR-3), which is essential for the lymphangiogenesis [24,209,210]. The visualization of the VEGFR-3 by means of specific stain techniques is used for histopathological diagnostic purposes. Also podoplanin and M2A oncofetal antigen have been reported to be specific for lymphatic endothelium [211].

Etiology

The reason for transforming of the lymphatic vessels into cystic hygromas is uncertain. Several mechanisms have been postulated for the formation of lymphatic malformations which include failure of the lymphatic system to connect with or to separate from venous system, abnormal budding of lymphatic structures from the cardinal vein, abnormal sequestration of lymphatic tissue in early embryogenesis, and acquired processes such as infection of the malformation, chronic inflammation, lymphatic obstruction or hemorrhage into it [212]. It has been suggested that lymphatic malformations are true neoplasms with potential for rapid growth and development. But there is no unanimity about the precise embryonic origin of the LVDs.

Cystic hygromas are thought to originate in the lymphatic sacs, from a specific deviation in the lymphatics development, resulting from a "pinching off or sequestration" of tissue in the sacs. LVDs may therefore form through sequestration of a sac or part of a sac, failure of fusion with venous system [213], or secondary obstruction of lymphatic drainage [214].

It has been suggested that abnormalities of the extracellular matrix and the neural crest migration during early embryonic development might be a cause, since there are recognized associations of LVDs with cardiovascular and venous malformations. Of course there may not be a one and only mechanism which may result in an LVD.

Molecular Pathology

Recent study of lymphatic endothelium has shed light on how the lymphatic system is formed and grows. In the future this will form the basis for new LM treatment options.

Lymphatic endothelial cells and blood vascular endothelial cells maintain distinct expression of lineage-specific genes (see Genetics and molecular biology) including Prox-1, lymphatic vessel endothelial hyaluronan receptor-1, vascular endothelial growth factor (VEGF) receptor 3, podoplanin, and CCL21 in the lymphatic system, and that VEGF-C and VEGF-D Huang et al [215] characterized the expression of VEGF and VEGF receptors in 29 LVDs using RNA in situ hybridization and found that endothelial cells in LVDs express transcripts of VEGF-C, VEGFR-3, and VEGFR-2 that are not expressed in the surrounding tissues, normal lynphatic tissue, or other vascular malformations. This suggests that VEGF-C and its receptors may play an important role in the formation of LVMs.

Further identification of genes only expressed by lymphatic endothelium should facilitate identification of usable markers that can enable analysis of the underlying biology, physiology, pathology, and treatment of lymphatic system and its malformations.

The distinction between lymphatic and other vascular vessels on microscopic sections is challenging. The antibody D2-40, , has been reported to be selective for lymphatic endothelium with a tendency of more consistent D2-40 staining of small versus large lymphatic channels [216].

Prenatal Diagnosis

Lymphatic malformations are often diagnosed sonographically before birth [217]. Sonographic examination of an LVD generally shows a cystic, anechoic mass that may be uni- or multiloculated with thin septae. Hemaorrhagic areas within LVD may be detected as hyperechoic foci within mass. The differential diagnosis of a cervical mass include cystic teratoma, thymic cyst, and congenital fibrosarcoma. A clear distinction should be made between posterior nuchal translucency, seen during the first and early second trimester, and cervicofacial LVD diagnosed during the second and third trimesters. Posterior nuchal translucency is associated with increased risk of aneuploidy [218,219]. In the presence of a normal karyotype, a fetus with a first trimester nuchal translucency has an equivocal prognosis with a normal outcome expected in 80% of pregnancies carried to the third trimaster. Dysmorphic features are noted in 20% of liveborn infants, but do not include LVDs. Normal outcome is highest when the fetal translucency resolves spontaneously, typically before 20 weeks gestation [220]. In contrast, an LVD is typically noted at a later gestational age, is generally anterior or lateral, and may be unilateral or bilateral.

Once the lesion is detected, antenatal MRI provides a detailed evaluation of the airway anatomy and is helpful in determining whether airway obstruction is likely to occure at birth [221].

Most infants with prenatal diagnosis of airway compromise and planned for the ex utero intrapartum treatment procedure (EXIT), can survive [222]. A two team approach is required for the procedure, with one team performing the caesarian section and another team managing neonatal airway. Maintaining maternal-fetal circulation via delaying placental separation and promoting fetal circulation pattern is the key to succesful management of neonates with airway obstruction. Techniques to secure the airway include direct laryngoscopy or beonchoscopy followed by intubation and/or tracheostomy.

Clinical Presentation and Diagnosis

The majority of lymphatic malformations occur in the head and neck, axilla and retroperitoneum (Figure 21, 22, 23). Involvement of the mediastinum, groin, extremities or face are less common. Approximately 80% are diagnosed before the patient is 5 years old, and over half present in the newborn period. The diagnosis of lymphangioma, whether cutaneous or cystic below the level of the skin, is generaly evident on clinical examination because these lesions are quite characteristic. They present as a soft, fluctuant swellings in the lateral or anterior neck, which may or may not increase in size with age and are often asymptomatic. Occasionally, huge malformations involving the floor of the mouth or the larynx will present at birth in a newborn with airway obstruction. Small or subtle lesions may not be apparent on initial neonatal physical examination and may be brought to medical attention only when infection or hemorrhage produces symptoms or rapid enlargement.

Ultrasonography may be used to confirm the diagnosis. If the extension of a cystic lesion into deeper structures of the body is uncertain, computer tomography (CT) with intravenous contrast enhancement can accurately show the full extent of the mass. An alternate approach is magnetic resonance imaging (MRI). Magnetic resonance imaging is an excellent technique for determining anatomic location in complicating cases, and is superior to CT in illustrating the relationship of the lesion to vital neurovascular structures such as carotid artery and branchial plexus [223]. The new generation of ultrafast MRI scanners has permitted this technique to be used more frequently in small infants, and even in affected fetuses [224]. Newer modalities such as magnetic resonance angiography and lymphatic MRI, may give us the opportunity to combine the inspection of the two circulation systems. The collected data may further be analyzed to reconstruct the 3D images [188].

Lymphoscintigraphy is able to define the lymphatic supply of a large lymphatic malformation, and this technique may be useful for planning a surgical approach or for identifying the source of a persistent lymphatic leak [225]. Often, a combination of techniques must be used to completely define the anatomic relationships of a large or complicated lesion.

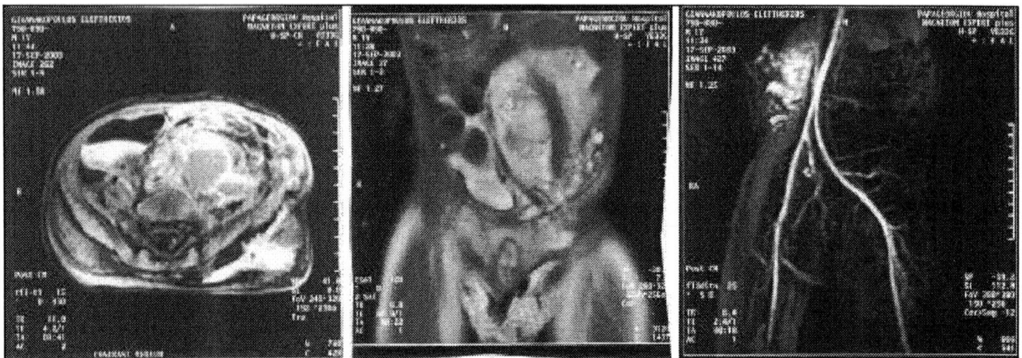

a b c

Figure 21. a) MRI of a large retroperitoneal lymphangioma displacing adjacent structures b) Coronal view c) MRA showing the relations to the great vessels.

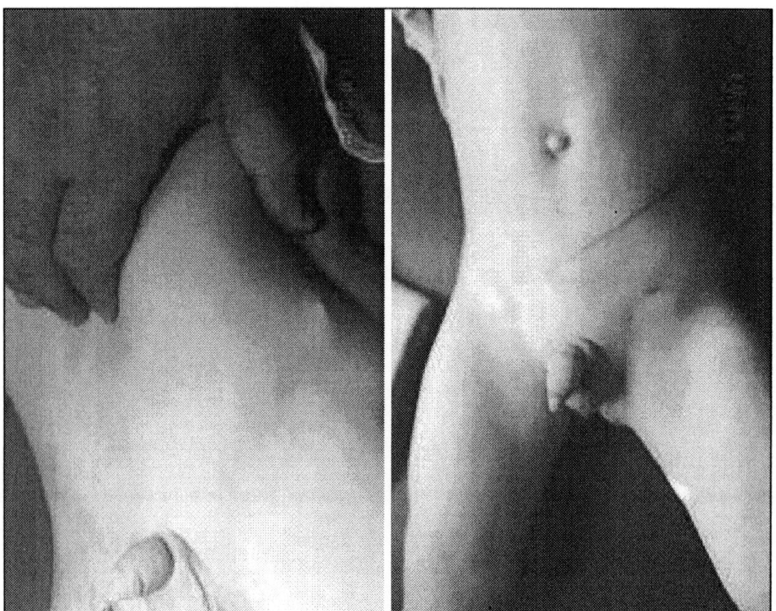

a b

Figure 22. a) Preoperative and b) Postoperative view of the previous patient.

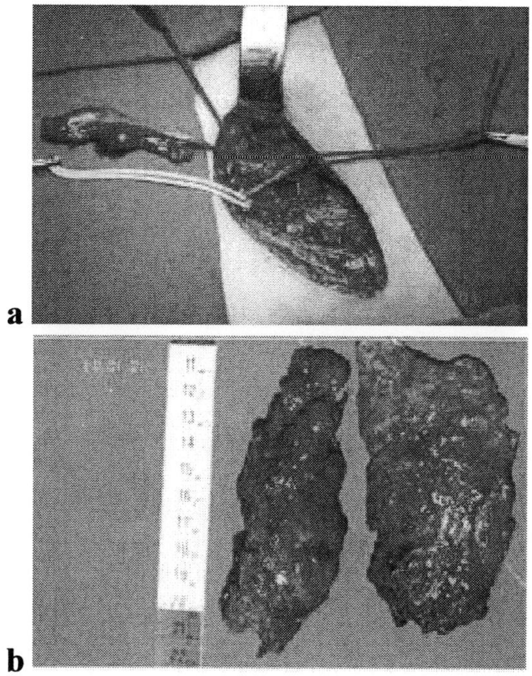

Figure 23. a) Operative view, b) Surgical specimen.

Treatment

Nonoperative Treatment

Surgical excision of localized lymphangiomas is the treatment of choice, but surgeons often worry about the infiltrative nature of some lesions and the difficulty in achieving complete resection. Spontaneous regression of these lesions after birth is thought to be rare [198]. In the past, the high mortality rate associated with resection stimulated the development of nonsurgical techniques using iradiation, incision and drainage, or injection of sclerosing agents.

Aspiration is not a definitive treatment but may be useful for emergency decompression. Radiation treatment has not been of benefit in the treatment of LVDs. Argon beam ablation and laser technology have been reported to be effective in the treatment of lymphangiomas, especially of complex type [226].

Percutaneous sclerotherapy involves the injection of sclerosing substances intravascularly in order to eliminate abnormal cystic cavities and vessels. It is important to maximize contact of the sclerosing agent with the lymphatic endothelium while avoiding extravasation into the surrounding tissues. During the past few years, varius sclerosant agents and techniques have been developed for use on LVDs. Sclerosants commonly used for this purpose include pure ethanol and OK-432.

Recently, a simple technique has developed aiming to inject and drain ethanol in the vascular malformation using a double needle. The flow of ethanol is controled locally by fluoroscopic visualization of a contrast material mixed with the a ethanol injected with one needle. Ethanol is drained through the second needle located in a distal section of the malformation. Fifteen pediatric patients with LVDs have been reported as succesfully treated without extravasation of ethanol or other complications [227].

OK-432 is a lyophilized incubation mixture of group A streptococcus pyogenes of human origin treated with benzylpenicillin potassium. Several recent reports have described success with few complications using OK-432 to treat LVDs [228,229]. A recent multiinstitutional, prospective, randomized trial and parallel case series [230] reported that 19 of 22 patients (86%) with predominantly macrocystic LVDs had complete or substantial (>60%) response to a four-dose injection series of OK-432 scheduled 6 to 8 weeks apart. The five patients with microcystic disease failed to show any response to OK-432 therapy. Minor adverse effects, including erythema, swelling, pain, and fever, were reported by most patients. Three major adverse effects were reported: left side proptosis after intracystic hemorrhage four weeks after therapy of an LVD adjacent to the left orbit, cervical cellulitis 4 weeks after therapy that required intravenous antibiotics, and respiratory compromise requiring emergent tracheostomy immediately after treatment of a large cervical LVD with intrathoracic extension. In another study sclerotherapy with OK-432 is recommended in patients with one to four large LVD cysts as first-line therapy [231]. Hall et al [232] found that lesions larger than 5 cm and outside the head and neck region did not respond well to OK-432 therapy. Additional concerns applicable to sclerotherapy include the need for multiple treatments, the risks associated with the associated postinjectional swelling, and the lack of long-term outcome data.

Fujino et al [233] prospectively evaluated the changes in cytokine levels in patients with LVDs for several weeks after OK-432 therapy in order to understand better the process of tumor regression. They found marked elevation of interleukin-8, VEGF, and transforming growth factor-β1 levels for several weeks after injection of OK-432. No significant elevation in interleukin-12, tumor necrosis factor-α, and interferon-γ was seen 1 week after injection of OK-432. These elevations may be nonspecific indicators of inflammation and may not be unique to OK-432. Fujino suggest that a cytotoxic action against endothelial cells in the LMs is an inadequete explanation for the mechanism of action of OK-432, and that fibrotic changes related to cytokine action also play a role.

Other types of sclerosants have been described in small case series such as bleomycin [234], cyclophosphamide [235], and fibrin sealant [236]. The concern with bleomycin is pulmonary toxicity with a total dose excceding 500 mg.

Surgical Treatment

Complete excision of all gross tumor tissue without the sacrifice of important normal adjacent structures remains the goal for the surgical treatment of children with lymphangiomas. For the usual well localized unilateral mediastinal lesion, this can best be achieved through a standart lateral thoracotomy. For the more common extensive midline or bilateral cervicomediastinal cystic hygroma, a one-stage procedure utilizing a median srernotomy with a transverse cervical extension is recommended. Because of the diffuse, frequently infiltrative nature of these lesions, the phrenic, vagus, and recurrent laryngeal nerves may be encased by adherent hygroma tissue, and temporaray or permanent nerve damage is a well-known complication of hygroma resection. Tracheal and esophageal perforations have also been reported. All important normal structures must be precisely identified intraoperatively, and carefully separated from the surrounding hygroma tissue. At times it may be necessary to leave behind small portions of the cyst wall if a complete resection cannot be achived safely. Chylothorax is another reasonably frequent postoperative complication. Although most chylothoraces resolve spontaneously with parenteral nutrition and effective drainage of the pleural space, TD ligation may be necessary.

Lymphatic malformations of the neck can usually be approached through a transverse cervical incision under general intratracheal anesthesia (Figure 24). After division of the platysma muscle, the mass is carefully dissected from all surrounding structures. The large cystic malformations are usually well-encapsulated, and every attempt should be made not to rupture the cysts. The fluid within the cyst aids the surgeon in defining the cyst wall, and therefore in finding the correct plane in which to dissect. Particular care must be taken to avoid injury to the carotid artery and its branches, or to the internal jugular vein. Preservation of other large venous channels if possible may also be beneficial in promoting regional drainade. A number of nerves are often closely associated with the lesion, including the facial nerve, spinal accessory nerve, vagus nerve, and brachial plexus. Although pathological studies have shown that microscopic tumor is often left behind [237], recurrence is rare when all gross tumor is removed. Once the malformation has been removed and, if possible, the lymphatic supply to the malformation ligated, a closed suction drain should be left in the tumor bed to prevent early accumulation of fluid. Dietary restriction of long-chain triglycerides in the postoperative period may be of some benefit in reducing the amount of chylous lymph production.

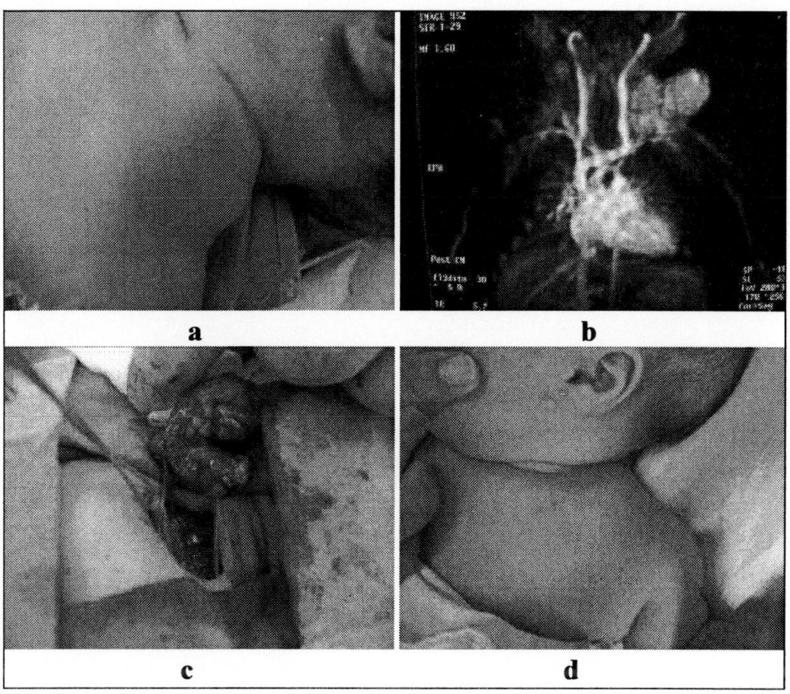

Figure 24. a) Cystic hygroma of the neck b) MRA of the patient c) Operative view d)Postoperative view.

KLIPPEL-TRENAUNAY SYNDROME

In 1900, French physicians Klippel and Trenaunay described a rare syndrome, which comprised capillary malformations, varicose veins or varicose malformations, with soft and bony hypertrophy of the extremity [238].

The syndrome is characterised by the following 3 features: 1) cuteneous capillary malformation sometimes associated with angiokeratomas usually affecting one limb, 2) soft tissue or bony hypertrophy of the affected extremity, and 3) abnormal development of the deep and superficial veins resulting in varicose veins, persistent lateral embryonic veins, deep venous malformations and lymhatic malformations (Fig 25). Currently, Klippel-Trenaunay syndrome (KTS) can be diagnosed on the basis of any two of these features [239].

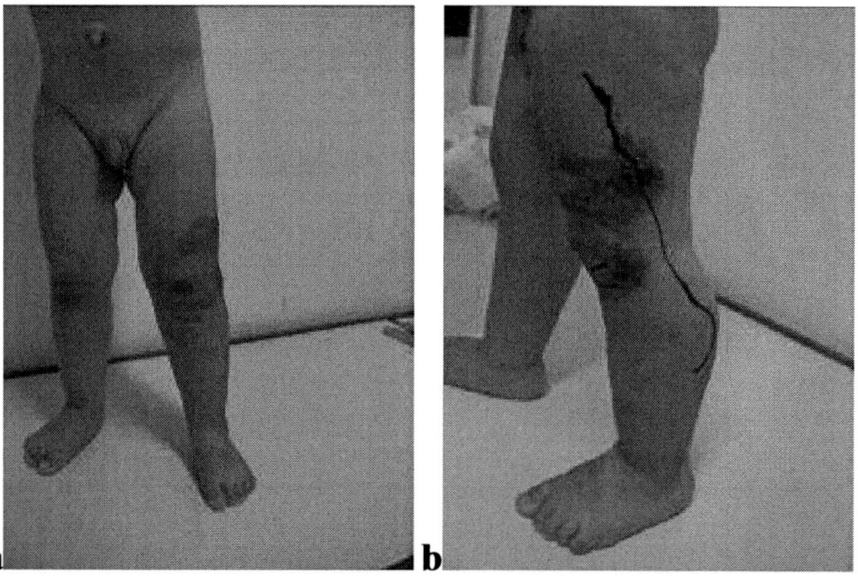

Figure 25. a) Klippel)Trenaunay syndrome of the left lower limb with cutaneous capillary malformations, angiokeratomas, varicose veins and soft tissue and bone hypertrophy b) the course of a persistent lateral embryonic vein.

Significant arteriovenous communications are not found in KTS in many large series [240,241]. Physiologic arteriovenous connections are always trivial and never clinically important. Significant arteriovenous fistulas are the hallmark, distinguishing Parkes Weber syndrome from KTS [242]. Consequently, Parkes Weber syndrome represents a combined high-flow vascular malformation, with important clinical, prognostic and therapeutic implications. However, at first glance both syndromes clinically may appear very similar.

Etiology

Despite the recognition of this condition for more than a century, with hundreds of cases reported, its etiology and pathogenesis are still not well understood. Moreover, there is no consensus on proper investigation or treatment. A better understanding of the underlying pathological processes could help in its management. Servelle [240] proposed that obstruction or atresia of deep veins of the leg produces chronic venous hypertention, which is in turn responsible for the development of port-wine stains, varicose veins, and limb hypertrophy. However, Baskerville et al [243], after performing phlebographic studies, found only 5 limbs out of 36 affected to have atresia of their deep venous system. Following that, they assumed that KTS is a generalized mesodermal abnormalitiy and the anomalies of the deep veins are only a part of the syndrome and not its cause. Others have speculated that KTS may be due to a somatic mutation of a factor critical to vasculogenesis or angiogenesis during embryonic development [262]. A susceptibility gene, AGGF1, was cloned for KTS. AGGF1 encodes a potent angiogenetic factor, and KTS-associated mutations enhance angiogenic activity of AGGF1, defining "increased angiogenesis" as one molecular mechanism for the pathogenesis of KTS.

Incidence

KTS is a congenital angiodysplasia. Males and females are equally affected. The lower limbs are affected in almost 95% of patients, the upper limb accounting for about 5% of patients. Approximately 15% have combined upper and lower limb involvement. Uncommonly, patients may have trunk involvement only [240,241]. The syndrome is rare with estimated worldwide prevalence of over 1500 cases (probably underreported) [242,244]. Most cases are sporadic, and familial trends have not been confirmed, although some cases within the same family have been reported. In a series of 114 patients, two families with familial KTS were documented, as well as the occurance of familial hypertrophy an naevi inflammei in first-degree relatives in other pedigrees [245]. In a report from of 14 patients from Spain, paternal and maternal age and the number of pregnancies were related to the prevalence of KTS, which suggested a variably expressed autosomal dominant inheritance. A report on a child with KTS identified a balanced chromosome translocation and suggests the potential site of localization for KTS to be on chromosome 5q or 11p [246].

Clinical Presentation

In most cases, the patient's family notes the clinical presentation of KTS at birth or in the first few years of life [239]. In a large series of 252 cases with KTS [238], 98% had capillary malformations., 72% had varicosities or VMs, and 67% had limb hypertrophy. Of these 252 patients, 63% had all three features of KTS. Other clinical features such as syndactyly, macrodactyly, polydactyly, and hip dysplasia have been reported in up to 29% of patients with KTS [247]. Clinical symptoms are related to the extent and location of the hypertrophy and VMs, which may vary from mild varicosities to massively enlarged limbs or truncal involvement. KTS may also be associated with lympedema or lymphatic malformations. The lower extremity varicosities tend to be more prominent laterally. Often, in an affected lower extremity, an enlarged, tortuous, superficial venous trunk can be identified laterally, above the knee and the thigh. This represents abnormal persistence of an embryonic lateral vein, which normally regresses at 8 weeks of gestation. Some researchers refer to this lateral trunk as the "Klippel-Trenaunay vein." This vein usually drains into the deep system, often into an Internal iliac tributary of the Profunda femoris vein. Atypical veins, including lateral vein and persistent sciatic vein, were seen in 72% of the patients [244].

Complications associated with this condition are numerous and include thrombosis, pulmonary embolism, coagulopathy, heart failure, hemothorax, central nervous system anomalies [248], gangrene, and bleeding from abnormal vessels of the gastrointestinal tract, kidney, or genitalia. Patients with abnormal lymphatic drainage are particularly at risk for cellulitis and gram-negative bacteremia [249]. Pain is a rather common and debilitating problem in these patients. Common causes of pain in patients with KTS are 1) chronic venous insufficiency 2) cellulitis 3) superficial thrombophlebitis 4) deep vein thrombosis 5) calcification of vascular malformations 6) growing pains 7) intraosseous vascular malformation 8) arthritis 9) neuropathic pain [250].

Affected individuals may also have significant psychological effects because of the disfiguring aspect of their condition [251]. No prospective studies focusing on the relation between severity of the involvement and prognosis have been published, and larger retrospective studies do not emphasize on which factors predict the outcome more accurately.

Few studies have specifically addressed the incidence of lymphatic malformations in KTS. Estimates from published series vary from 15% to 77% [252].

Imaging Studies

The diagnosis of the KTS is rarely made antenatally. It is possible to diagnose KTS during prenatal period with sonography as multiloculated cystic areas and hypertrophy of the involved limb [253].

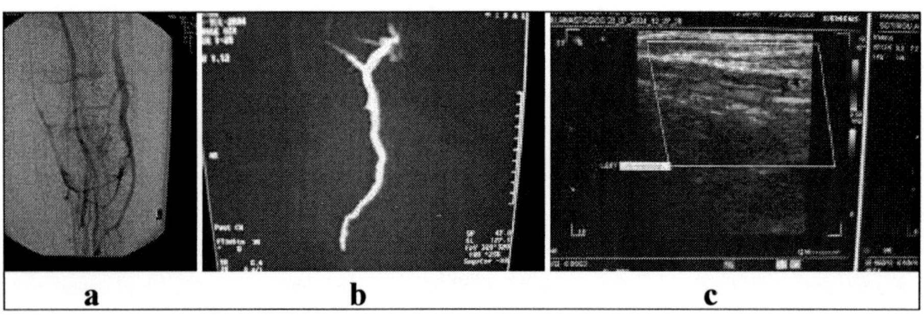

Figure 26. a) MRA of a patient with Klippel)Trenaunay syndrome b) MRP with imaging of the persistent lateral embryonic vein c) Color Ultrasound showin the patency of the lower deep limb vessels

Digital subtraction angiography (DSA) is the gold standart for accurate distinction between of high-flow and low-flow vascular malformations [254]. However less invasive imaging modalities are desisrable, especialy for screening of patients without overt clinical signs of atreriovenous shunting. Before surgical intervention, contrast phlebography, MRI or MR Phlebography (MRP) should document venous anatomy (Fig.26). The primary goal is to confirm patency of the deep venous system before excision of superficial veins. In addition, descending phlebography, with duplex scanning, is used to asses deep venous incompetence in the deep, superficial, and perforator system in the extremity and the pelvis. MRI and MRP provide three dimensional imaging of VMs and are useful in defining the hypertrophy of the bony and soft tissue and the extent and depth of VMs within the subcutaneous or subfascial space.

Grey scale and Doppler US are non-invasive tools to distinguish high-flow from low-flow vascular malformations [255]. Drawbacks of US are the limited ability to display the full extent of large lesions and its operator dependence.

Scanograms (long bone films) are usually performed serially in all patients with KTS to document leg length discrepancy and bony hypertrophy.

Treatment

According to a recent review of the literature, the guidelines in the management of this syndrome suggest nonoperative therapies for most patients.The conservative management includes high compression hose (60-80 mmHg) and pneumatic compression pump (70-100mmHg) to improve the condition of hypoplastic deep venous system. A gradual increment of the pneumatic compression pump pressure from 20 mmHg to 90mmHg with corresponding pressure increment of the compression hose allows the transferring of venous flow from the superficial to the deep venous system. These measures not only progessively enlarge the hypoplastic deep vein, but will also collapse the superficial vein to reduce discoloration and traumatic bleeding from the varices. This helps to diminish the symptoms of venous insufficiency and prevents trauma but has no effect on the size of the limb [244].

The clinical findings observed in adult patients affected by KTS suggest that long-term haemodynamic effects of distal venous hypertention can have serious repercussions, such as disfiguring swollen legs, huge chronic ulcers requiring skin grafts, and rapidly progressive limb overgrowth requiring epiphysiodesis or contralateral limb bone elongation, when leg length discrepancy is more than 2 cm [244,252]. Amputation is used as a last resort. Laser therapy has had limited succes.

According to literature, the removal of superficial varicose vein in order to relieve the distal venous hypertension is controversial in patients with KTS and it is recommended only in selected patients because of the high risk of recurrence of varicosity and the high incidence of associated deep venous system anomalies such as agenesis, atresia, or obstruction of the popliteal, femoral, or iliac vein by external bands. Deep venous system abnormalities are absolute contraindications to surgical excision of superficial atypical varicosities from persistent embryonic veins: their frequency is difficult to assess and differnt authors report percentages of incidence ranging from 0% to 100% [241,244,47].

We and others [244] contest this overconservative attitude, because we consider that only a small percentage of patients with KTS (<10%), have deep venous anomalies. Furthermore, although excision of varicosities is often incomplete, and venous malformation may recur in most patients, an over-all clinical improvement is noted and reexcision may be performed as indicated.

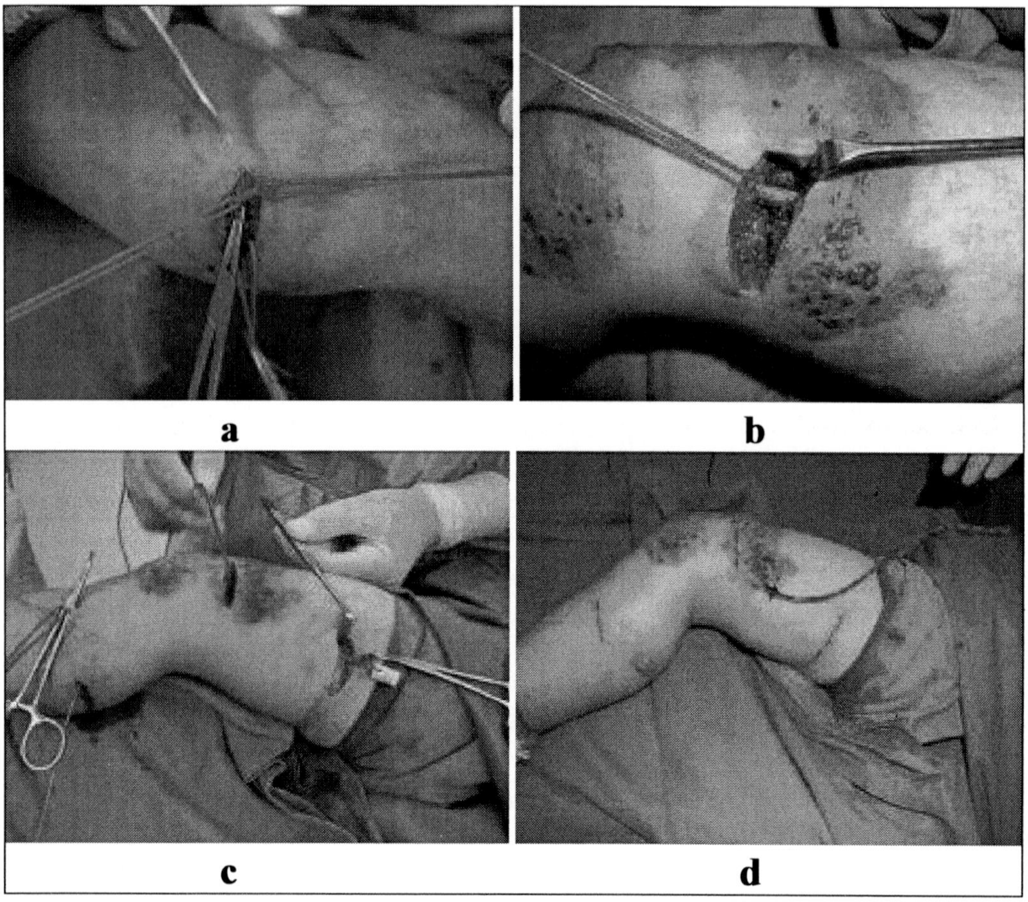

Figure 27. a) Ligation and excision of varicose veins b) Dissection of the lateral embryonic vein c) Excision with the help of a stripper. d) Immediate postoperative view.

The most common venous surgical procedures are stripping of veins, includind lateral embryonic veins, and avulsion and excision of varicosities and VMs (Figure 27, 28). Before surgery, venous anatomy must be confirmed with contrast phlebography, MRI, and MRP. Although 50% [247] of patients with KTS will have recurrent varicosities and it is nearly imposible to remove all varicosities because of the extent of disease, the overall clinical improvement after surgical treatment is good (Figure 29). Although rare, deep venous reconstruction or release of restricting fibrous bands is indicated in a small group of patients [247,256]. In a subset of patients with incompetent perforating veins, open ligation of these veins or obliterationby using endoscopic venous perforator (SEPS) is indicated [257].

Although longer follow-up is needed it seems that early surgical management of venous insufficiency in KTS is safe and effective in preventing or minimizing the long-term hemodynamic effects of distal venous hypertension such as distal chronic dystrophic ulcers and limb over or undergrowth.

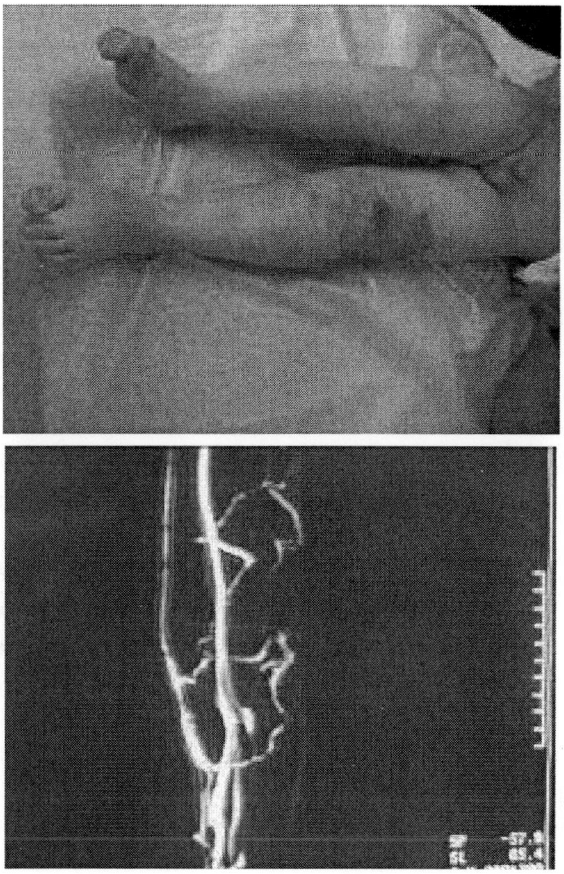

a

b

Figure 28. a) The patient on fig.25, one month after the operation b) postoperative MRA. The venous system is imaged, the lateral embryonic vein has been excised.

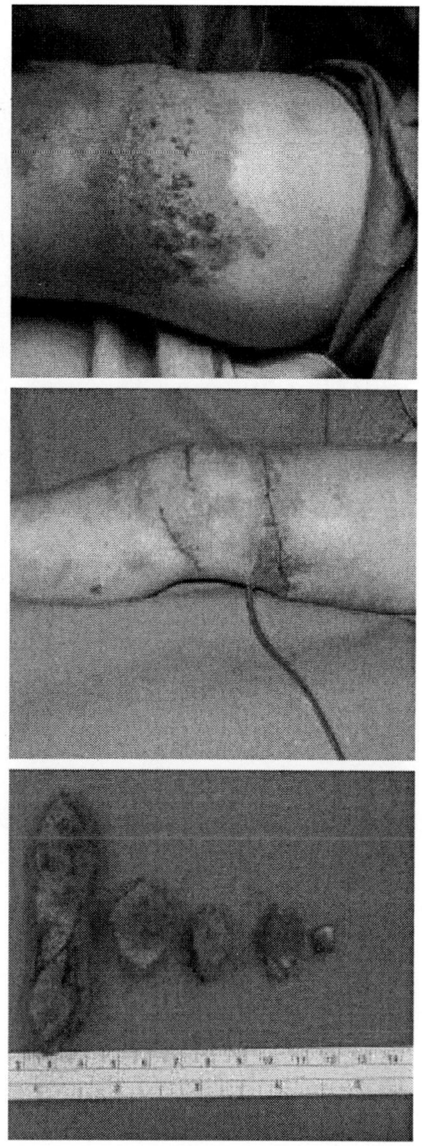

Figure 29. Reoperation on a Klippel-Trenaunay patient for resection of angiokeratomas a) Preoperative view b) Postoperative view c) Resected angiokeratomas.

References

[1] Petropoulos A.S.: *Experimental study on chylothorax in dogs. Modern treatment through the use of the Spitz-Holter valve*. PhD Thesis, Aristotle University of Thessaloniki, Thessaloniki, 1980.

[2] F.H. Garrison. *History of medicine 4th edition* W.B. Saunders eds 1929, Philadelphia and London.

[3] *Surgical Anatomy: The Embryologic And Anatomic Basis Of Modern Surgery* By J. E. Skandalakis (Editor in chief), G. L. Colborn, P. N. Skandalakis, L.J. Skandalakis , R. S. Foster, T. A. Weidman , A. N. Kingsnorth , P. Mirilas (Editors), P.M.P. eds, 2004, Athens.

[4] Eriksson G. [Olaus Rudbeck as scientist and professor of medicine] *Sven Med Tidskr.* 2004;8(1):39-44.

[5] Kaul TK, Bain WH, Turner AM, Taylor MK. Chylothorax: report of a case complication ductus ligation through a median sternotomy and review. *Thorax* 1976;31:610-616.

[6] Marinozzi S. [Rei Medicae Praelectiones Theoricae Proemialium Quastionum. To expert mentor Pauli Manfredi 1695 Paulus Valle SBT: a collection of theoretical medicine of lessons of 1695 to the Rome Studium] *Med Secoli.* 2004;16(2):407-27.

[7] Baum H. Das lymphgefassystem des handes. *Arch Wissprakt Tierheilk*, 1918;44:521-650.

[8] Carvalho R, Rodrigues a, Pereira A. A mise en evidence par la radiographic du systeme lymphatique chez le vivant. *Ann Anat Path* 1931;8:193-197.

[9] Kinmonth JB. Lymphangiography in man. Method of outlining lymphatic trunks at operation. *Clin Sc* 1952;11:13-20.

[10] Davis HK. A statistical study of the thoracic duct in man. *Am J Anat* 1915;17:211-244.

[11] Koehler PR. Complications of lymphography. *Lymphology* 1968; 1:117-120.

[12] Weissleder H, Weissleder R. Lymphedema: evaluation of qualitative and quantitative lymphoscintigraphy in 238 patients. *Radiology* 1988; 167:729-735

[13] Ohhashi T, Mizuno R, Ikomi F, Kawai Y: Current topics of physiology and pharmacology in the lymphatic system. *Pharmacology & Therapeutics* 2005; 105: 165–188

[14] Skandalakis JE, Gray SW, Ricketts RR. *The Lymphatic System. In Embryology for Surgeons*, Skandalakis & Gray editors. 2nd edition, Williams and Wilkins, 1994.

[15] Davis HK. A statistical study of the thoracic duct in man. *Am J Anat* 1915;17:211-244.

[16] Saxer F. Uber die Entwicklung und den Bau der Lymphdrusen und die Enttehung der rotten und weissen Blutkorperchen. *Anat Hefte* 1896;6.

[17] Sabin FR. The development of the lymphatic system. In: Keibel F, Mall FP, eds. *Manual of human embryology, Vol 2.* Philadelphia: JB Lippincott, 1912.

[18] Lewis FT. The development of the lymphatic systen in rabbits. *Am J Anat* 1905;10:95-111.

[19] Huntington GS, McClure CFW. The anatomy and development of the jugular lymph sac in the domestic cat. *Am J Anat* 1910;10:177-311

[20] Kampmeier OF. The development of the jugular lymph sacs in the light of vestigial provisional and definitive phases of morphogenesis. *Am J Anat* 1960; 107:153-176.

[21] Sabin FR. The lymphatic system in human embryos with consideration of the morphology of the system as a whole. *Am J Anat* 1909;9:43.

[22] Wilting J, Papoutsi M, Becker J. The lymphatic vascular system: secondary or primary? *Lymphology.* 2004 Sep;37(3):98-106.

[23] Jeltsch M, Tammela T, Alitalo K, Wilting J. Genesis and pathogenesis of lymphatic vessels. *Cell Tissue Res*. 2003 Oct;314(1):69-84. Epub 2003 Aug 27.

[24] Karkkainen MJ, Haiko P, Sainio K, Partanen J, Taipale J, Petrova TV, Jeltsch M, Jackson DG, Talikka M, Rauvala H, Betsholtz C, Alitalo K. Vascular endothelial growth factor C is required for sprouting of the first lymphatic vessels from embryonic veins. *Nat Immunol* 2004; 5: 74-80.

[25] Wilting J, Tomarev SI, Christ B, Schweigerer L Lymphangioblasts in embryonic lymphangiogenesis. *Lymphat Res Biol*. 2003;1(2):179.

[26] Boardman KC, Swartz MA. Interstitial flow as a guide for lymphangiogenesis. *Circ Res*. 2003 Apr 18;92(7):801-8.

[27] Suami H, Taylor GI, Pan WR. A new radiographic cadaver injection technique for investigating the lymphatic system. *Plast Reconstr Surg*. 2005 Jun;115(7):2007-13.

[28] Podgrabinska S, Braun P, Velasco P, Kloos B, Pepper MS, Skobe M. Molecular characterization of lymphatic endothelial cells. *Proc Natl Acad Sci U S A*. 2002 Dec 10;99(25):16069-74.

[29] Petrenko VM, Kruglov SV. [Thoracic duct valves in man and albino rat] *Morfologiia*. 2004;126(6):40-2.

[30] Zawieja D. Lymphatic biology and the microcirculation: past, present and future. *Microcirculation*. 2005 Jan-Feb;12(1):141-50.

[31] Oliver G. Lymphatic vasculature development. *Nat Rev Immunol* 2004;.4: 35-45.

[32] Schmid-Schonbein GW.The second valve system in lymphatics. *Lymphat Res Biol*. 2003;1(1):25-9; discussion 29-31.

[33] Harland MM, Fedele C, Berens v Rautenfeld D. The presence of myofibroblasts, smooth muscle cells and elastic fibers in the lymphatic collectors of horses. *Lymphology*. 2004 Dec;37(4):190-8.

[34] Speden RN. Adrenergic transmission in small arteries. *Nature*. 1967 Oct 21;216(112):289-90.

[35] Ohhashi T, Azuma T. Effect of potassium on membrane potential and tension development in bovine mesenteric lymphatics. *Microvasc Res*. 1982 Jan;23(1):93-8.

[36] Ohhashi T, Azuma T, Sakaguchi M. Active and passive mechanical characteristics of bovine mesenteric lymphatics. *Am J Physiol*. 1980 Jul;239(1): H 88-95.

[37] Hall JG, Morris B, Woolley G. Intrinsic rhythmic propulsion of lymph in the unanaesthetized sheep. *J Physiol*. 1965 Sep;180(2):336-49.

[38] Benoit JN, Zawieja DC, Goodman AH, Granger HJ. Characterization of intact mesenteric lymphatic pump and its responsiveness to acute edemagenic stress. *Am J Physiol*. 1989 Dec;257(6 Pt 2):H2059-69.

[39] Guyton AC, Taylor AE, Brace RA. A synthesis of interstitial fluid regulation and lymph formation. *Fed Proc*. 1976; Jun;35(8):1881-5.

[40] Young-Kwon Hong, Jay W. Shin, Michael Detmar Development of the lymphatic vascular system: A mystery unravels. *Developmental Dynamics* 2004; 231 (3): 462-473

[41] Strausser JL, Flye MW. Management of nontraumatic chylothorax. *Ann Thorac Surg* 1981; 31:520-526

[42] Young-Kwon Hong, Jay W. Shin, Michael Detmar Development of the lymphatic vascular system: A mystery unravels. *Developmental Dynamics* 2004; 231 (3): 462-473

[43] Tammela T, Enholm B, Alitalo K, Paavonen K. The biology of vascular endothelial growth factors. *Cardiovasc Res.* 2005 Feb 15;65(3):550-63.

[44] Hong YK, Foreman K, Shin JW, Hirakawa S, Curry CL, Sage DR, Libermann T, Dezube BJ, Fingeroth JD, Detmar M. Lymphatic reprogramming of blood vascular endothelium by Kaposi sarcoma-associated herpesvirus. *Nat Genet* 2004; 36: 683-685.

[45] Kunstfeld R, Hirakawa S, Hong YK, Schacht V, Lange-Asschenfeldt B, Velasco P, Lin C, Fiebiger E, Wei X, Wu Y, Hicklin D, Bohlen P, Detmar M. Induction of cutaneous delayed-type hypersensitivity reactions in VEGF-A transgenic mice results in chronic skin inflammation associated with persistent lymphatic hyperplasia. *Blood* 2004; 104: 1048-1057.

[46] Irrthum A., Karkkainen M.J., Devriendt K., Alitalo K., Vikkula M. Congenital hereditary lymphedema caused by a mutation that inactivates VEGFR3 tyrosine kinase, *Am. J. Hum. Genet.* 2000; 67: 295–301.

[47] Oh S.J., Jeltsch M.M., Birkenhager R., McCarthy J.E., Weich H.A. Christ B. et al. VEGF and VEGF-C: specific induction of angiogenesis and lymphangiogenesis in the differentiated avian chorioallantoic membrane, *Dev. Biol* 1997; 188: 96–109.

[48] Karkkainen MJ, Ferrell RE, Lawrence EC, Kimak MA, Levinson KL, McTigue MA, Alitalo K, Finegold DN. Missense mutations interfere with VEGFR-3 signalling in primary lymphoedema. *Nat Genet* 2000; 25: 153-159.

[49] Jackson DG. The lymphatics revisited: new perspectives from the hyaluronan receptor LYVE-1. *Trends Cardiovasc Med* 2003; 13: 1-7.

[50] Schacht V, Ramirez MI, Hong YK, Hirakawa S, Feng D, Harvey N, Williams M, Dvorak AM, Dvorak HF, Oliver G, Detmar M. T1alpha/podoplanin deficiency disrupts normal lymphatic vasculature formation and causes lymphedema. *EMBO J* 2003; 22: 3546-3556

[51] Yuan L, Moyon D, Pardanaud L, Breant C, Karkkainen MJ, Alitalo K, Eichmann A. Abnormal lymphatic vessel development in neuropilin 2 mutant mice. *Development* 2002; 129: 4797-4806.

[52] Northup K.A., Witte M.H. Witte C.L, Syndromic classification of hereditary lymphedema, *Lymphology* 2003; 36; 162–189

[53] Fang J, Dagenais SL, Erickson RP, Arlt MF, Glynn MW, Gorski JL, Seaver LH, Glover TW. Mutations in FOXC2 (MFH-1), a forkhead family transcription factor, are responsible for the hereditary lymphedema-distichiasis syndrome. *Am J Hum Genet* 2000; 67: 1382-1388.

[54] Karkkainen MJ, Saaristo A, Jussila L, Karila KA, Lawrence EC, Pajusola K, Bueler H, Eichmann A, Kauppinen R, Kettunen MI, Yla HS, Finegold DN, Ferrell RE, Alitalo K.. A model for gene therapy of human hereditary lymphedema. *Proc Natl Acad Sci U S A* 2001; 98: 12677-12682.

[55] Ayadi A, Zheng H, Sobieszczuk P, Buchwalter G, Moerman P, Alitalo K, Wasylyk B. Net-targeted mutant mice develop a vascular phenotype and up-regulate egr-1. *EMBO J* 2001;20: 5139-5152.

[56] McColl BK, Stacker SA, Achen MG. Molecular regulation of the VEGF family - inducers of angiogenesis and lymphangiogenesis. *APMIS.* 2004 Jul-Aug;112(7-8):463-80.

[57] Jalili F. Medium chain triglycerides and total parenteral nutrition in the management of infants with congenittal chylothorax. *South Med J* 1987;80:1290-1293.

[58] Van Straaten HL, Gerards LJ, Krediet TG. Chylothorax in the neonatal period. *Eur J Pediatr* 1993;152:2-5.

[59] Azizkhan RG. Chylothorax and other pleural effusions in neonates. In: Puri P, editor. *Newborn surgery. 2nd edition.* London: Arnold, 2003:283-293.

[60] Van Pernis PA. Variations of the thoracici duct. *Surgery* 1949;26:806-809.

[61] Kirkland I. Chylothorax in infancy and childhood. *Arch Dis Child* 1965; 40:186-191.

[62] Fishman SJ, Burrows PE, Upton J, Hendren H. Life-threatening anomalies of the thoracic duct: Anatomic deliniation dictates management. *J Pediatr Surg* 2001; 36:1269-1272.

[63] Randolph JG, Gross RE: Congenital Chylothorax, *Arch Surg* 1957;74:405.

[64] Vain NE, Swarner OW, Cha CC. Neonatal chylothorax: a report and discussion of nine consecutive cases. *J Pediatr Surg.* 1980 Jun;15(3):261-5.

[65] L. S. Wafelman, B. H. Pollock, J. Kreutzera, D. S. Richards, A.A. Hutchison: Nonimmune Hydrops fetalis: Fetal and Neonatal Outcome during 1983-1992 *Biology of the Neonate* 1999;75:73-81

[66] Nakayama H; Kukita J; Hikino S; Nakano H; Hara T Long-term outcome of 51 liveborn neonates with non-immune hydrops fetalis. *Acta Paediatrica, Volume 88*, Number 1, 5 February 1999, pp. 24-28(5)

[67] Ibrahim H, Asamoah A, Krouskop RW, Lewis D, Webster P, Pramanik AK. Congenital chylothorax in neonatal thyrotoxicosis. *J Perinatol.* 1999 Jan;19(1):68-71.

[68] Dunkelman H, Sharief N, Berman L, Ninan T. Generalised lymphangiomatosis with chylothorax. *Arch Dis Child.* 1989 Jul;64(7):1058-60.

[69] JA Noonan, LR Walters and JT Reeves, Congenital pulmonary lymphangiectasia. *Am J Dis Child* 120 (1970), pp. 314–319.

[70] Moerman P, Vandenberghe K, Devlieger H, Van Hole C, Fryns JP, Lauweryns JM Congenital pulmonary lymphangiectasis with chylothorax: a heterogeneous lymphatic vessel abnormality. *Am J Med Genet.* 1993 Aug 1;47(1):54-8.

[71] Bellini C, Mazzella M, Campisi C, Taddei G, Mosca F, Toma P, Villa G, Boccardo F, Sementa AR, Hennekam RC, Serra G. Multimodal imaging in the congenital pulmonary lymphangiectasia-congenital chylothorax-hydrops fetalis continuum. *Lymphology.* 2004 Mar;37(1):22-30.

[72] Lee S, Finn L, Sze RW, Perkins JA, Sie KC. Gorham Stout syndrome (disappearing bone disease): two additional case reports and a review of the literature. *Arch Otolaryngol Head Neck Surg.* 2003 Dec;129(12):1340-3.

[73] Chen E, Larabell SK, Daniels JM, Goldstein S. Distichiasis-lymphedema syndrome: tetralogy of Fallot, chylothorax, and neonatal death. *Am J Med Genet.* 1996 Dec 18;66(3):273-5.

[74] Easa D, Balaraman V, Ash K, Thompson B, Boychuk R. Congenital chylothorax and mediastinal neuroblastoma. *J Pediatr Surg.* 1991 Jan;26(1):96-8.

[75] Schluter G, Steckel M, Schiffmann H, Harms K, Viereck V, Emons G, Burfeind P, Pauer HU. Prenatal DNA diagnosis of Noonan syndrome in a fetus with massive hygroma colli, pleural effusion and ascites. *Prenat Diagn.* 2005 Jul;25(7):574-6.

[76] Fisher E, Weiss EB, Michals K, DuBrow IW, Hastrieter AR, Matalon R. Spontaneous chylothorax in Noonan's syndrome. *Eur J Pediatr.* 1982 May;138(3):282-4.

[77] Yoss BS, Lipsitz PJ.Chylothorax in two mongoloid infants. *Clin Genet.* 1977 Dec;12(6):357-60.

[78] Nanda S, Rajpal M, Reddy BS. Cardio-facio-cutaneous syndrome: report of a case with a review of the literature. *Int J Dermatol.* 2004 Jun;43(6):447-50.

[79] Unusual autosomal recessive lymphatic anomalies in two unrelated Amish families. *Am J Med Genet.* 1997 Dec 19;73(3):286-9.

[80] Ro PS, Hill SL, Cheatham JP. Congenital superior vena cava obstruction causing anasarca and respiratory failure in a newborn: successful transcatheter therapy. *Catheter Cardiovasc Interv.* 2005 May; 65(1):60-5.

[81] Van Veldhuizen PJ, Taylor S. Chylothorax: a complication of a left subclavian vein thrombosis. *Am J Clin Oncol.* 1996 Apr;19(2):99-101.

[82] Villa E, Eynden FV, Le Bret E, Folliguet T, Laborde F. Paediatric video-assisted thoracoscopic clipping of patent ductus arteriosus: experience in more than 700 cases. *Eur J Cardiothorac Surg.* 2004 Mar;25(3):387-93.

[83] Cooper P, Paes ML. Bilateral chylothorax. *Br J Anaesth.* 1991 Mar;66(3):387-90.

[84] Khosa JK, Leong SL, Borzi PA. Congenital cystic adenomatoid malformation of the lung: indications and timing of surgery. *Pediatr Surg Int.* 2004 Jul;20(7):505-8.

[85] Cheah FC, Noraida MH, Boo NY, Amin TY. Chylothorax after repair of congenital diaphragmatic hernia--a case report. *Singapore Med J.* 2000 Nov;41(11):548-9.

[86] Allen EM, van Heeckeren DW, Spector ML, Blumer JL. Management of nutritional and infectious complications of postoperative chylothorax in children. *J Pediatr Surg.* 1991 Oct;26(10):1169-74.

[87] Vera Büttiker, MD; Sergio Fanconi, MD and Réne Burger, MD Chylothorax in Children Guidelines for Diagnosis and Management *Chest.* 1999;116:682-687.

[88] Brissaud O, Desfrere L, Mohsen R, Fayon M, Demarquez J L. Congenital idiopathic chylothorax in neonates: chemical pleurodesis with povidone-iodine (Betadine) Archives of Disease in Childhood Fetal and Neonatal Edition 2003; 88:F531

[89] Coultre C. Chylothorax. In: Ziegler MM, Azizkhan RG, Weber TR editors. *Operative pediatric surgery.* McGraw-Hill, 2003:465-473. Williams MS, Josephson KD.

[90] Eddleman KA, Levine AB, Chitkara U, Berkowitz RL.Reliability of pleural fluid lymphocyte counts in the antenatal diagnosis of congenital chylothorax. *Obstet Gynecol.* 1991 Sep;78(3 Pt 2):530-2.

[91] Kala K. Davis, Gerald J. Berry, Thomas A. Raffin, John L. Faul, M.D. *Lymphatic Research and Biology,* Nov 2004, Vol. 2, No. 3: 131-137

[92] Matsuoka S, Takeuchi K, Yamanaka Y, Kaji Y, Sugimura K, Maruo T. Comparison of magnetic resonance imaging and ultrasonography in the prenatal diagnosis of congenital thoracic abnormalities. *Fetal Diagn Ther.* 2003 Nov-Dec;18(6):447-53.

[93] Liu X, Ashtari M, Leonidas JC, Chan Y. Magnetic resonance imaging of the fetus in congenital intrathoracic disorders: preliminary observations. *Pediatr Radiol.* 2001 Jun;31(6):435-9.

[94] A.S.Petropoulos, X. Sinopidis, G. Karachatzis. The contribution of lymph node lymphangiography to the X-Ray representation of the Thoracic Duct. *Surg Childh Intern* 1998: VI, 4, 241-244

[95] A.S. Petropoulos, I Valioulis, K. Koutsias, H. Papaharalampous, A. Visouli, D. Alupi. *Chylothorax-experimental model in dogs*. Scientific Annals of the Faculty of Medicine, Aristotle University of Thessaloniki, 1993;20:135-148.

[96] A.S. Petropoulos. *Contribution of direct surgical lymph node-lymphangiography on the diagnosis of thoracic duct diseases*. Scientific Annals of the Faculty of Medicine, Aristotle University of Thessaloniki, 1988;17:29-42.

[97] Harisinghani MG, Dixon WT, Saksena MA, Brachtel E, Blezek DJ, Dhawale PJ, Torabi M, Hahn PF. MR lymphangiography: imaging strategies to optimize the imaging of lymph nodes with ferumoxtran-10. *Radiographics*. 2004 May-Jun;24(3):867-78.

[98] Smaropoulos EC, Papazoglou LG, Patsikas MN, Vretou E, Petropoulos AS. Lymphatic regeneration following hind limb replantation:an experimental study in dogs. Lymphatic regeneration following hind limb replantation: an experimental study in the dog. *Eur J Pediatr Surg*. 2005 Oct;15(5):337-42.

[99] Wasmuth-Pietzuch A, Hansmann M, Bartmann P, Heep A.Congenital chylothorax: lymphopenia and high risk of neonatal infections. *Acta Paediatr*. 2004 Feb;93(2):220-4.

[100] Orange JS, Geha RS, Bonilla FA. Acute chylothorax in children: selective retention of memory T cells and natural killer cells. *J Pediatr*. 2003 Aug;143(2):243-9.

[101] Bond SJ, Guzzetta PC, Snyder ML, Randolph JG. Management of pediatric postoperative chylothorax. *Ann Thorac Surg*. 1993 Sep;56(3):469-72; discussion 472-3.

[102] Natrajan S, Hadeli O, Quan SF. Infected spontaneous chylothorax. *Diagn Microbiol Infect Dis*. 1998 Jan;30(1):31-2.

[103] Gonen R, Degani S, Kugelman A, Abend M, Bader D. Intrapartum drainage of fetal pleural effusion. *Prenat Diagn*. 1999 Dec;19(12):1124-6.

[104] Koike T, Minakami H, Kosuge S, Izumi A, Shiraishi H, Sato I. Severe hypoproteinemia in a fetus after pleuro-amniotic shunts with double-basket catheters for treatment of chylothorax. *J Obstet Gynaecol Res*. 2000 Oct; 26(5):373-6

[105] Rejjal AR, Rahbeeni Z, al-Zahrani AF. Prognostic factors and prenatal management in non immune hydrops fetalis are still a dilemma. *J Perinat Med*. 1996;24(5):461-6.

[106] Bartha JL, Comino-Delgado R. Fetal chylothorax response to maternal dietary treatment. *Obstet Gynecol*. 2001 May;97(5 Pt 2):820-3.

[107] Mazzanti L, Prandstraller D, Tassinari D, et al: Heart Disease in Turner's Syndrome. *Helv Paediatr Acta* 1988; 43: 25-31

[108] Marino B, Digilio MC, Toscano A: Congenital heart diseases in children with Noonan syndrome: An expanded cardiac spectrum with high prevalence of atrioventricular canal. *J Pediatr* 1999 Dec; 135(6): 703-6

[109] Laursen HB. Congenital heart disease in Down's syndrome. *Br Heart J*. 1976 Jan;38(1):32-8.

[110] Fernandez Alvarez JR, Kalache KD, Grauel EL. Management of spontaneous congenital chylothorax: oral medium-chain triglycerides versus total parenteral nutrition. *Am J Perinatol.* 1999;16(8):415-20.

[111] Clarke SA, Lakhoo K, Sherwood W: Somatostatin for intractable postoperative chylothorax in a premature infant. *Pediatr Surg Int* 2005 May; 21(5): 390-1

[112] Mohseni-Bod H, Macrae D, Slavik Z: Somatostatin analog (octreotide) in management of neonatal postoperative chylothorax: is it safe? *Pediatr Crit Care Med* 2004 Jul; 5(4): 356-7

[113] Maayan-Metzger A, Sack J, Mazkereth R, Vardi A, Kuint J. Somatostatin treatment of congenital chylothorax may induce transient hypothyroidism in newborns. *Acta Paediatr.* 2005 Jun;94(6):785-9.

[114] Rasiah SV, Oei J, Lui K. Octreotide in the treatment of congenital chylothorax. *J Paediatr Child Health.* 2004 Sep-Oct;40(9-10):585-8.

[115] Mavroudis C. Management of postoperative chylothorax with nitric oxide: a critical review. *Crit Care Med.* 1999 May;27(5):877.

[116] Engum SA, Rescorla FJ, West KW, Scherer LR 3rd, Grosfeld JL. The use of pleuroperitoneal shunts in the management of persistent chylothorax in infants. *J Pediatr Surg.* 1999 Feb;34(2):286-90.

[117] Beghetti M, La Scala G, Belli D, Bugmann P, Kalangos A, Le Coultre C. Etiology and management of pediatric chylothorax. *J Pediatr.* 2000 May;136(5):653-8.

[118] A.S. Petropoulos, N. Vassou. Chylothorax : A new experimental method of surgical treatment. *Acta Paedochirurgica Hellenica* 1995;13:30-35.

[119] A.S. Petropoulos, C. Dimopoulos, A. Avramidou, M. Karageorgaki, K. Tziampiris, K.Kallergis. The surgical treatment of congenital chylothorax and chylous ascites, with internal drainage of chyle using Holter valve. *Pediatr N Gr* 1998;19:53-60.

[120] A.S. Petropoulos. Chylothorax: A new experimental method of surgical treatment. *Galenus* 1996;38:282-291.

[121] Takahashi M, Kurokawa Y, Toyama H, Hasegawa R, Hashimoto Y. The successful management of thoracoscopic thoracic duct ligation in a compromised infant with targeted lobar deflation. *Anesth Analg.* 2001 Jul;93(1):96-7

[122] Browse NL, Allen DR, Wilson NM: Management of chylothorax. *Br J Surg* 1997 Dec; 84(12): 1711-6

[123] Azizkhan RG, Canfield J, Alford BA et al. Pleuroperitoneal shunts in the management of neonatal chylothorax. *J Pediatr Surg* 1983;18:842-8.

[124] Takahashi M, Kurokawa Y, Toyama H, Hasegawa R, Hashimoto Y. The successful management of thoracoscopic thoracic duct ligation in a compromised infant with targeted lobar deflation. *Anesth Analg.* 2001 Jul;93(1):96-7.

[125] Wolff AB, Silen ML, Kokoska ER, Rodgers BM. Treatment of refractory chylothorax with externalized pleuroperitoneal shunts in children. *Ann Thorac Surg.* 1999 Sep;68(3):1053-7.

[126] Rifai N, Sfeir R, Rakza T, Alameh J, Besson R, Lequien P, Storme L. Successful management of severe chylothorax with argon plasma fulguration and fibrin glue in a premature infant. *Eur J Pediatr Surg.* 2003 Oct;13(5):324-6.

[127] Tanemura M, Nishikawa N, Kojima K, Suzuki Y, Suzumori K. A case of successful fetal therapy for congenital chylothorax by intrapleural injection of OK-432. *Ultrasound Obstet Gynecol.* 2001 Oct;18(4):371-5.

[128] Dunkelman H, Sharief N, Berman L, Ninan T. Generalised lymphangiomatosis with chylothorax. *Arch Dis Child.* 1989 Jul;64(7):1058-60.

[129] Kajiyama Y, Iwanuma Y, Tomita N, Amano T, Hattori K, Tsurumaru M. Sealing the thoracic duct with ultrasonic coagulating shears. *Hepatogastroenterology.* 2005 Jul-Aug;52(64):1053-6.

[130] Vasko JS, Tapper RI. The surgical significance of chylous ascites. *Arch Surg* 1967;95:355.

[131] Loiterman DL, Bleicher MA. Chylous ascites: an etiology of peritonitis in infancy. *J Pediatr Surg* 1985;5:538.

[132] Chang JHT et al. Generalized lymphangiomatosis with chylous ascites –Treatment by peritoneo-venous shunting. *J Pediatr Surg* 1980;15:748.

[133] Unger Schandler J. Chylous ascites in infants and children. *Surgery* 1983;93:455-461.

[134] Cohen MM. Klippel-Trenaunay syndrome. *Am J Med Genet* 2000;93:171-175.

[135] Duhra P, Quingley B, Marsh M. Chylous ascites, intestinal lymphangiectasia and the "yellow nail" syndrome. *Gut* 1985;26:1266-1269.

[136] Fox U, Lucani G. Disorders of the intestinal mesenteric lymphatic system. *Lymphology* 1993;26:61-66.

[137] Aalami OO, Allen DB, Organ CH Jr. Chylous ascites: A collective review. *Surgery* 2000;128:761-778.

[138] Varekamp A et al. Chylousd ascites after aortic replacement. *Eur J Surg* 1992;158:623-625.

[139] Jahsman W. Chylothorax: a brief review of the literature, report of 3 non-traumatic cases. *Ann Intern Med* 1944;21:669-678.

[140] Ward P. Interpretation of ascitic fluid data. *Postgrad Med* 1982;71:171-178.

[141] Staats BA, Ellefson RD, Budahn LL, Dines DE, Prakash UB, Offord K. The lipoprotein profile of chylous and nonchylous pleural effusions. *Mayo Clin Proc* 1980;55:700-704.

[142] Pui MH, Yueh TC. Lymphoscintigraphy in chyluria, chyloperitoneum and chylothorax. *J Nucl Med* 1998;39:1292-1296.

[143] Browse N, Wilson N, Russo F at al. Aetiology and treatment of chylous ascites. *Br J Surg* 1992;79:1145-1150.

[144] Mitsunaga T, Yoshida H, Iwai J et al. Successful surgical treatment of two cases of congenital chylous ascites. *J Pediatr Surg* 2001;36:1717-171.

[145] Chye JK, Lim CT, Van der Heuvel. Neonatal ascites-report of three cases and review of the literature. *Pediatr Surg Int* 1997;12:296-298.

[146] Alliet P, Young C, Lebenthal E. Chylous ascites: total parenteral nutrition as a primary therapeutic modality. *Eur J Pediatr* 1992;151:213-214.

[147] Unger SW, Chandler JG. Chylous ascites in infants and children. *Surgery* 1983;93:455-461.

[148] Caty MG, Hilfiker ML, Azizkhan RG, Glick PL. Successful treatment of congenital chylous ascites with a somatostatine analogue. *Pediatr Surg Int* 1996;11:396-397.

[149] Andreou A, Papouli M, Papavasiliou V, Badouraki M. Postoperative chylous ascites in a neonate treated successfully with ocreotide: bile sludge and cholestasis. *Am J Perinatol* 2005;22:401-404.

[150] Mitsunaga T, Yoshida H Iwai J et al. Successful surgical treatment of two cases of congenital chylous ascites. *J Pediatr Surg* 2001;36:1717-1719.

[151] Antao B, Croaker D, Squire R. Successful management of congenital chyloperitoneum with fibrin glue. *J Pediatr Surg* 2003;38:7-8.

[152] Varge J Palmer R, Koff R. chylous ascites in adults. *South Med J* 1985;78:1244-1247.

[153] Weston P et al. Chylous ascites following retroperitoneal lymph node dissection for testis cancer. *Br L Urol* 1992;70;688-689.

[154] Noonan JA, Walters LR, Reeves JT. Congenital pulmonary lymphangiectasis. *Am J Dis Child* 1970;120:314–319.

[155] SJ Wagenaar, J Swierenga and CA Wagenvoort, Late presentation of primary pulmonary lymphangiectasis. *Thorax* 1978; 33: 791–795.

[156] EstherC R.Jr.,Barker MP,Pulmonary Lymphangiectasia: Diagnosis and Clinical Course *Pediatr Pulmonol.* 2004; 38:308–313.

[157] Laurence KM. Congenital pulmonary lymphangiectasis. *J Clin Pathol* 1959;12:12.

[158] France CE, Brown RJ. Congenital pulmonary lymphangiectasis. Report of 11 examples with special reference to cardiovascular findings. *Arch Dis Child* 1971;46:528–532.

[159] P Moerman, K Vandenberghe, H Devlieger et al., Congenital pulmonary lymphangiectasis with chylothorax: A heterogenous lymphatic vessel abnormality. *Am J Med Genet* 1993; 47: 54–58.

[160] Hunter WS, Becroft DM. Congenital pulmonary lymphangiectasis associated with pleural effusions. *Arch Dis Child.* 1984 Mar;59(3):278-9.

[161] Bouchard S, Di Lorenzo M, Youssef S, Simard P, Lapierre JG. Pulmonary lymphangiectasia revisited. *J Pediatr Surg.* 2000 May;35(5):796-800.

[162] Hoeffel JC, Marcon F, Worms AM, Diffuse pulmonary lymphangiectasis with heart defect discovered 4 months post-natally. *Paediatr Paedol* 1992; 27: 25–27.

[163] JES White, D Veale, D Fishwick et al., Generalized lymphangiectasia: Pulmonary presentation in an adult. *Thorax* 1996; 51: 767–768.

[164] RH Cleveland, A radiological update on medical diseases of the newborn chest. *Pediatr Radiol* 1995; 25: 631–637.

[165] Thong MK, Thompson E, Keenan R, et al. A child with hemimegalencephaly, hemihypertrophy, macrocephaly, cutane-ous vascular malformation, psychomotor retardation and intestinal lymphangiectasia—a diagnostic dilemma. *Clin Dysmorphol* 1999; 8: 283–286.

[166] Dumont DJ, Jussila L, et al. Cardiovascular failure in mouse embryos deficient in VAGF receptor-3. *Science* 1998;282:946-949.

[167] Browse NL, Stewart G. Lymphedema: pathophysiology and classification. *J Cariovasc Surg.* 1985;26:91-106.

[168] Olszewski WL. Pathophysiological and clinical observations of obstructive lymphedema in the limbs. In: Clodius L, (ed). *Lymphoedema.* Stuttgart: Georg Thieme;1977:79-102.

[169] Kinmoth JB, Taylor GW, Jantet GH. Chylous complications of primary lymphedema. *J Cardiovasc Surg* 1964;5:327

[170] Crocket DJ. Lymphatic anatomy nad lymphedema. *Br J Plast Surg* 1965;28:12.

[171] Serville M. Surgical treatment of lymphedema: a report of 652 cases. *Surgery* 1987;101:485.

[172] Reed RK, Laurent TC, Taylor AE. Hyaluronian in prenodal lymph from skin: changes with lymph flow. *Am J Physiol* 1990;259:1097-1100.

[173] Piller NB. Macrophage and tissue changes in the developmental phases of secondary lymphoedema and during conservative therapy with benzopyrone. *Arch Histol Cytol* 1990;53:209-218.

[174] Rockson SG. Lymphedema. *Am J Med* 2001;110:288-295.

[175] Ryan T, de Berker D. The interstitium, the connective tissue environment of the lymphatic, and angiogenesis in human skin. *Cli Dermatol.* 1995;13:451-458.

[176] Levinson KL, Feingold E, Ferrel RE et al. Age of onset in hereditary lymphedema. *J Pediatr* 2003;142:704-708.

[177] Fang J, Dagenais SL, Erickson RP et al. Mutations in FOXC2 (MFH-1), a forkhead family transcription factor, are responsible for the hereditary lymphdema-distichiasis syndrome. *Am J Hum Genet* 2000;67:1382-1388.

[178] Szuba A, Rockson S. Lymphedema: anatomy, physiology and pathogenesis. *Vasc Med.* 1997;2:321-326.

[179] Smeltzer DM, Stickler GB, Schirger A. Primary lymphedema in children and adolescents: a follow-up study and review. *Pediatrics.* 1985;76:206-218.

[180] Wolfe JHN, Kinmonth JB. The prognosis of primary lymphedema of the lower limbs. *Arch Surg* 1981;116:1157-1160.

[181] Rockson SG. Precipitating factors in lymphedema: myths and realities. *Cancer* 1998;83(suppl 12):2814-2816.

[182] Mallon E, Powell S, Mortimer P, Ryan Tj. Evidence for altered cell-mediated immunity in postmastectomy lymphoedema. Br J Dermatol 1997;137:928-933.

[183] Lister RK, Black MM, calonje E et al. Squamous cell carcinoma arising in chronic lymphedema. *Br J Dermatol* 1997;136:384-387.

[184] Tiwari A, Cheng KS, Button M, Myint F, Differential diagnosis, investigation, and current treatment of lower limb lymphedema. *Arch Surg* 2003;138:152-161.

[185] Ruffini E, Jorini M, Palumbo B et al. Lymphedema praecox. *Ital J Pediatr* 2004;30:405-408.

[186] Stemmer R. Ein klinisches zeichen zur fruh-und differential-diagnose des lymphodems. *Vasa* 1976;5(3):261-262.

[187] Witte CL, Witte MH, Unger EC et al. Advances in imaging of lymph flow disorders. *Radiographics* 2000;20:1697-1719.

[188] Liu N, Wang C, Sun M. Noncontrast three-dimensional magnetic resonance imaging vs lymphoscintigraphy in the evaluation of lymph circulation disorders: A comparative study. *J Vasc Surg.* 2005 Jan;41(1):69-75

[189] Upperman JS, Barksdale EM Jr. Images in clinical medicine. Congenital lymphedema. *N Engl J Med.* 2004 Feb 5;350(6):e5.

[190] Mikes DM, Cha BA, Dym CL et al. Bioelectrical impedance analysis revisited. *Lympoligy*. 1999;32:157-165.

[191] Kubik S. The role of the lateral upper bundle and the lymphatic watersheds in the formation of collateral pathways in lymphedema. Acta Biologica Academia Scientiarum *Hungaricae*. 1980:31:191-200.

[192] Casley-Smith J, Casley-Smith J. Other physical therapy for lymphedema: pumps, heating, etc. In: Casley-Smith J, Casley-Smith J, eds. *Lymphedema*. Adelaide: Lymphedema Association of Australia; 1991:155-159.

[193] Ogawa Y, Yoshizumi M, Kitagawa T et al. Investigation of the mechanism of lymphcyte therapy in the treatment of lymphedema with special emphasis on cell adhesion molecule (L-selectin). *Lymphology*. 1999;32:151-156.

[194] Casley-Smith JR, Morgan RG, Piller NB. Treatment of lymphedema of the arms and legs with 5,6-benzo-[a]-pyrone. *N Engl J Med*. 1993;329:1158-1163.

[195] Soria P, Cuesta A, Romero H, Martinez FJ, Sastre A. Dietary treatment of lymphedema by restriction of long-chain triglycerides. *Angiology*. 1994;45:703-707.

[196] Gloviczki P. Principles of surgical treatment of chronic lymphedema.*Int Angiol* 1999;18:42-46.

[197] Coffin CM, Dehner LP. Soft tissue tumors in first year of life: a report of 190 cases. *Pediatr Pathol* 1990;19:509-526.

[198] Alqahtani A, Nuyen LT, Flageolo H, Shaw K, Laberge JM. 25 years experience with lymphangiomas in children. *J Pediatr Surg* 1999;34:1164-1168.

[199] King DR, Groner JI, Teich S. Mediastinal cysts and tumors In: Ziegler MM, Azizkhan RG, Weber TR editors. *Operative pediatric surgery*. McGraw-Hill, 2003:407-419.

[200] S. Puig , B. Casati , A. Staudenherz , K. Paya Vascular low-flow malformations in children: current concepts for classification, diagnosis and therapy. *European Journal of Radiology* 2005; 53: 35–45

[201] Mulliken JB, Glowacki J. Hemangiomas and vascular malformations in infants and children: a classification based on endothelial characteristics. *Plast Reconstr Surg* 1982;69:412–22.

[202] Abernethy LJ. Classification and imaging of vascular malformations in children. *Eur Radiol* 2003;13:2483–97.

[203] Burrows PE, Mulliken JB, Fellows KE, Strand RD. Childhood hemangiomas and vascular malformations: angiographic differentiation. *AJR Am J Roentgenol* 1983;141:483–8.

[204] Belov S. Classification of congenital vascular defects. *Int Angiol* 1990;9:141–6.

[205] Puig S, Aref H, Chigot V, Bonin B, Brunelle F. Classification of venous malformations in children and implications for sclerotherapy. *Pediatr Radiol* 2003;33:99–103.

[206] Dubois J, Garel L. Practical aspect of intervention in vascular anomalies in children. *Semin Intervent Radiol* 2002;19:73–87.

[207] Smith RJ, Burke DK, Sato Y et al. OK-432 therapy for lymphangiomas. *Arch Otolaryngol Head Neck Surg* 1996;122:1195-1199.

[208] Enjolras O, Ciabrini D, Mazoyer E, Laurian C, Herbreteau D. Extensive pure venous malformations in the upper or lower limb: a review of 27 cases. *J Am Acad Dermatol* 1997;36:219–25.

[209] Jeltsch M, Tammela T, Alitalo K, Wilting J. Genesis and pathogenesis of lymphatic vessels. *Cell Tissue Res* 2003;314:69–84.

[210] Jussila L, Alitalo K. Vascular growth factors and lymphangiogenesis. *Physiol Rev* 2002;82:673–700.

[211] Breiteneder-Geleff S, Soleiman A, Kowalski H, et al. Angiosarcomas express mixed endothelial phenotypes of blood and lymphatic capillaries: podoplanin as a specific marker for lymphatic endothelium. *Am J Pathol* 1999;154:385–94.

[212] Bloom D, Perkins JA, Manning SC. Management of lymphatic malformations. *Curr Opin Otalaryngol Head Neck Surg* 2004;12:500-504.

[213] Chervenak FA, Isaacson G, Blakemore KJ et al. Fetal cystic hygroma: cause and natural history. *N Engl J Med* 1983;309:109-112.

[214] Levine C. Primary disorders of the lymphatic vessels: a unified concept. *J Pediatr Surg* 1989;24:233-240.

[215] Huang HY, Ho CC, Huang PH et al. Co-expression of VEGF-C and its receptors, VEGFR-2 and VEGFR-3, in endothelial cells of lymphangioma. Implication in autocrine or paracrine regulation of lymphangioma. *Lab Invest* 2001;81:1729-1734.

[216] Galambos C, Nodit L. Identification of lymphatic endothelium in pediatric vascular tumors and malformations. *Pediatr Dev Pathol.* 2005 Mar-Apr;8(2):181-9.

[217] Marler JJ, Fishman SJ, Upton J at al. Prenatal diagnosis of vascular anomalies. *J Pediatr Surg* 2002;37:318-326.

[218] Descamps P, Jourdain O, Paillet C et al. Etiology, prognosis and management of nuchal cystic gygroma: 25 new cases and literature review. *Eur J Obstet Gynecol* 1997;71:3-10.

[219] Pandya P, Brizot ML, Kuhn P et al. First trimester fetal nuchal translucency thickness and risk for trisomies. *Obstet Gynecol* 1994;84:420-423.

[220] Hirakawa S, Hong YK, Harvey N et al. Identification of vascular lineage-specific genes by transcriptional profiling of isolated blood vascular and lymphatic endothelial cells. *Am J Pathol* 2003;162:575-586.

[221] Teksam M, Ozyer U, McKinney A, Kirbas I. MR imaging and ultrasound of fetal cervical cystic lymphangioma: utility in antepartum treatment planning. *Diagn Interv Radiol.* 2005 Jun;11(2):87-9.

[222] Leva E, Pansini L, Fava G, Maestri L, Pansini A, Selvaggio G. The role of the surgeon in the case of a giant neck mass in the EXIT procedure. *J Pediatr Surg.* 2005 Apr;40(4):748-50.

[223] Fung K, Poenaru D, Sobelski DA, Kamal IM. Impact of magnetic resonance imaging on the surgical management of cystic hygromas. *J Pediatr Surg* 1998;33:839-841.

[224] Sandrasegaran K, Lall C, Aisen AA, Rajesh A, Cohen MD. Fast fetal magnetic resonance imaging. *J Comput Assist Tomogr.* 2005 Jul-Aug;29(4):487-98.

[225] Boxen I, Zhang ZM, Filler RM. Lymphoscintigraphy for cystic hygroma. *J Nucl Med.* 1990 Apr;31(4):516-8.

[226] Rothenberg S, Pokorny W. Use of argon beam ablation and sclerotherapy in the treatment of a life-threataning total abdominal lymphangiomatosis. *J Pediatr Surg* 1994;29:322-323.

[227] Puig S, Aref H, Brunelle F. Double-needle sclerotherapy of lymphangiomas and venous angiomas in children: a simple technique to prevent complications. *AJR* 2003;180:1399-1401.

[228] Sanliap I, Karnak I, Tanyel FC at al. Sclerotherapy for lymphangioma in children. *Int J Pediatr Otorynolaryngol* 2003;67:795-800.

[229] Rautio R, Keski-Nisula L, Laranne J et al. Treatment of lymphangioma with OK-432. *Cardiovasc Intervent Radiol* 2003;26:31-36.

[230] Giguere CM, Bauman NM, Sato Y at al. Treatment of lymphangiomas with OK-432 sclerotherapy: a prospecrive multi-institutional trail. *Arch Otolaryngol Head Neck Surg* 2002;128:1137-1144.

[231] Benieghbal B, Davies MR. Guidelines for the successful treatment of lymphangioma with OK-432. *Eur J Pediatr Surg* 2003;13:103-107.

[232] Hall N, Ade-Ajayi N, Brewis C et al. Is intralesional injection of OK-432 effective in the treatment of lymphangioma in children? *Surgery* 2003;133:238-242.

[233] Fujino A, Moriya Y, Morikawa Y et al. A role of cytokines in OK-432 injection therapy for cystic lymphangioma: an approach to the mechanism. *J Pediatr Surg* 2003;38:1806-1809.

[234] Mathur NN, Rana I, Bothra R, Dhawan R, Kathuria G, Pradhan T. Bleomycin sclerotherapy in congenital lymphatic and vascular malformations of head and neck. *Int J Pediatr Otorhinolaryngol*. 2005 Jan;69(1):75-80.

[235] Turner C, Gross S. Treatment of recurrent suprahyoid cervicofacial lymphangioma with intravenous cyclophosphamide. *Am J Pediatr Hematol Oncol*. 1994 Nov;16(4):325-8.

[236] Boulos PR, Harissi-Dagher M, Kavalec C, Hardy I, Codere F. Intralesional injection of Tisseel fibrin glue for resection of lymphangiomas and other thin-walled orbital cysts. *Ophthal Plast Reconstr Surg*. 2005 May;21(3):171-6.

[237] Goetsch E. Hygroma colli cysticum and hygroma axillare. *Arch Surg* 1938;36:394.

[238] Gloviczki P et al. Klippel-Trenaunay syndrome: the risks and benefits of vascular interventions. *Surgery*.1991;110:469.

[239] Jacob AG, Driscoll DJ, Shaughnessy WJ, et al. Klippel-Trenaunay syndrome; spectrum and management. *Mayo Clinic Proc*. 1998;73:28-36.

[240] Servelle M. Klippel-Trenaunay syndrome. 786 operated cases. *Ann Surg*. 1985;201:365-273.

[241] Samuel M, Spitz L. Klippel-Trenaunay syndrome: clinical features, complications and management in children. *Br J Surg*. 1995;82;757-761

[242] Cohen MM Jr. Klippel-Trenaunay syndrome. *Am J Med Genet*. 2000;93;171-175.

[243] Baskerville PA, Ackroyd JS, Browse NL. The etiology of the Klippel-Trenaunay syndrome. *Ann Surg*. 1985;202:624-627.

[244] Nafday SM, Heiden RA, Rai DB. Unusual case of Klippel-Trenaunay syndrome. A case report and review of the literature.*Int J Angiol*. 2000;9:250-253.

[245] Aelvoet GE, Jorens PG, Roelen LM. Genetic aspects of the Klippel-Trenaunay syndrome. *BR J Dermatol*. 1992;126:603-607.

[246] Whelan AJ, Watson MS, Porter FD, Steiner RD. Klippel-Trenaunay-Weber syndrome associated with a 5:11 balanced translocation. *Am J Med Genet*. 1995;59:492-494.

[247] Noel AA, Gloviczki P, Cherry KJ, Rooke TW et al. Surgical treatment of venous malformations in Klippel-Trenaunay syndrome. *J Vasc Surg.* 2000;32:840-847

[248] Torregrosa A, Marti-Bonmati L, Higueras V, Poyatos C, Sanchis A. KTS: frequency of cerebral and cerebellar hemihypertrophy on MRI. *Neuroradiol.* 2000;42:420-423.

[249] Bird LM, Jones MC, Kupperman N, Huskins WC. Gram-negative bacteremia in four patients with Klippel-Trenaunay-Weber syndrome. *Pediatrics* 1996;97:739-741.

[250] Lee A, Driscoll D, Gloviczki P, Clay R, Shaughenessy, Stans A. Evaluation and management of pain in patients with KTS: a review. *Pediatrics* 2005;115:744-749.

[251] Van der Ploeg HM, van der Ploeg MN, van der Ploeg-Stapert JD. Psychological aspects of the KTS. *J Psychosom Res* 1995;39:183-191.

[252] Baraldini V, Coletti M, Cipolat L, Santuary D, Vercellio G. Early surgical management of Klippel-Tranaunay syndrome in childhood can prevent long-term haemodynamic effects of distal venous hypertension. *J Pediatr Surg.* 2002;37:232-236.

[253] Yang JI, Kim HS, Ryu HS. Prenatal sonographic diagnosis of Klippel-Trenaunay-Weber syndrome: a case report. *J Reprod Med.* 2005;50:291-294.

[254] Ziyeh S, Spreer J, Rossler J et al. Parkes Weber or KTS? Non-invasive diagnosis with MR projection angiography. *Eur Radiol* 2004;14:2025-2029.

[255] Paltiel HJ, Burrows PE, Kozakewich HP, Zurakowski D, Mulliken JB. Soft-tissue vascular anomalies: utility of US for diagnosis. *Radiology* 2000;214;747-754.

[256] Taheri Sa, williams J, Boman L, Pisano S. Superficial femoral vein transposition in KTS. *J Pediatr Surg* 1989;24:494-496.

[257] Gloviczki P, Bergan JJ, Rhodes JM, Canton LG, Harmsen S et al. Mid-term results of endoscopic perforator vein interruption for chronic venous insufficiency: lessons learned from the North America Subfascia Endoscopic Perforator Surgery (NASEPS) Registry. *J Vasc Surg* 1999;29:485-502.

In: New Developments in Birth Defects Research
Editor: Nelson A. Gaslem, pp. 69-86
ISBN 1-60021-400-2

Chapter 2

DIAGNOSIS, TREATMENT AND PROGNOSIS OF NEURAL TUBE DEFECTS IN CONTEMPORARY VIEW

***Krzysztof Preis*[1,*], *Malgorzata Swiatkowska-Freund*[1] and *Iwona Janczewska*[2]**

[1]Department of Obstetrics, [2]Department of Neonatology, Medical University of Gdansk

ABSTRACT

Aim of the Study

Follow-up of the development of children born with neural tube defect.

Material and Method

We performed a follow-up study of 54 infants born with myelomeningocoele between 1991 and 2001 in the Department of Obstetrics of the Medical University of Gdansk.The selected group consisted of children that lived until the end of the observation period – till 28.02.2003. We analyzed: fetal age at diagnosis, the time of delivery, mode of delivery, the newborn`s Apgar score after birth, birth weight, the location of defect, mortality, the further development – sphincters function, motoric abilities.

* Correspondence concerning this article should be addressed to Krzysztof Preis, Kliniczna 1a, 80-402 Gdansk, Poland

Results

In the period between 1991 – 2001 22 534 births took place in the Department of Obstetrics of the Medical University of Gdansk. Most of the analyzed defects were diagnosed between 31st and 35th week pf pregnancy. Almost 54% of children were still born (13%) or died till the end of observation (40,1%). There was significant correlation between high level of spina bifida, presence of other malformations or late diagnosis and mortality. Most of the children had no ability of locomotion, some of them used wheelchairs or braces and only 3 of them needed no help in walking. Bladder and bowel problems were most common when spinal defect was localized in lumbo-sacral region.

Keywords: Neural Tube Defects, Birth defects, Spina bifida, Myelomeningocoele, Hydrocephaly, Fetal malformations, Treatment, Outcome

Neural tube closing disturbances are the cause of malformations of the spine, spinal cord and meninges. They result in different types of the spina bifida. There are many types of that malformation and many different classifications of it regarding its localization, damaged parts involved, direction and extent of dysrrhaphia as well as the content of a coele [19,26,29,34,47].

In the following study the MacMahon classification was used [22]:

1. Closed spina bifida (oculta).
2. Cystic spina bifida (coele):
   a. myelomeningocoele,
   b. meningocoele.

1. Spina bifida oculta (closed) develops as a result of the defect in closing of the vertebral canal posterior elements. Spinal cord remains normal. It is localized in lumbo-sacral, lumbal or sacral region in 80% of cases. Increased amount of hair, vascular naevi or dermatoid cysts can frequently be seen on the skin above the lesion. Sometimes cystis pilloidalis or skin-neural fistula is present. This kind of lesions is seldom accompanied by any symptoms. Only some malformations of foot or worse sphincters' control in the late childhood may be observed [9,19].
2. Dislocation of structures normally closed in the vertebral canal is called a coele [19].
   a. Myelomeningocoele is diagnosed in 95 % of neural tube defects. The most common localization is the lumbo-sacral region, but it can also be found in the cervical region (4 – 8%) and the rarest is the thoracic one. If the defect is closed, it is covered by meninges and skin. There is a cerebro-spinal fluid with neural elements inside the coele – destroyed spinal cord and spinal nerves. The skin and the neural tissue in the coele are dysplastic [6,19,26]. Myelomeningocoele causes neurological impairment in all cases [26]. Its seriousness depends on localization of a lesion, its size and exposition of the neural tissue on the amniotic fluid destructive influence [13,44]. Morphological appearance of the coele influences the clinical image of the malformation. It consists of the motor and sensor deficiency, bladder and anus

insufficiency. Deformations of lower limbs are results of muscle dysfunction. Neurological deficiency is usually responsible for serious mobile impairment – the most of children are unable to walk, but some of them have the femoral muscles strong enough [6,19,47,49]. Bones lesion leads to deformations, adhesions and absence of the vertebrae. In most of the cases, the myelomeningocoele coexists with Chiari II syndrome and hydrocephaly [32,41]. In the 1/3 of patients, the posterior cerebral dysfunction can be diagnosed and it presents as headache, strabismus, upper limbs weakness, swallowing problems, stridor or breathlessness. The last symptom is responsible for the 1/3 of neonatal deaths in these patients [32].

Myelomeningocoele is a cause of the neurogenic urinary bladder in many of these patients. It presents as the dysfunction of the urinary bladder filling and emptying or urinary incontinence. In consequence, we can observe recurrent urinary tract infections, refluxes and hydronephrosis [19]. We can also observe neurogenic colono-anal canal presenting as fecal incontinence, lesion and collapsing of anus or even colon [19].

b. Some authors distinguish also a myelocoele. It is the result of lack in closure of the neural tube, usually involving more than 2-3 vertebrae. Deformed spinal cord and cerebro-spinal fluid are in a direct contact with the amniotic fluid. Neural tissue becomes destroyed and inactive [19].

Meningocoele is diagnosed in 4 – 5% of all neural tube defects. Coele contains meninges and cerebro-spinal fluid only covered by skin or epidermis. Defect involves usually only one vertebra and spinal cord remains untouched. Sometimes happens, that spinal nerves or "horse tail" are partially or completely moved into the coele. The dislocated neural structures are normal and usually no neurological impairment is observed. Only in cases of a large meningocoele, changes in cerebro-spinal fluid pressure may lead to neurological disorders and secondary hydrocephaly may develop [9,29].

Tethered cord syndrome usually coexists with dysrrhaphic malformations. It appears as the effect of the end of spinal cord immobilization by a coele, cystis pilloidalis, or adhesions after surgical correction procedure. A spinal cord becomes stretched and therefore ischemic as a result of changes in the spine during the child's growing. The additional neurological deficit appears as a consequence of this mechanism. In a patient able to walk the difficulties with walking and muscle weakness usually can be observed first. Next symptoms are the backache, scoliosis and sometimes the sensor deficits. Urine and fecal incontinence can increase [37].

Early prenatal diagnosis is essential in managing pregnancies with neural tube defects [45]. Diagnostic methods applied to that type of malformations are biochemical screening using the alpha-fetoprotein assessment and the ultrasound imaging [15,16]. Invasive test – alpha-fetoprotein and acetylocholinestherase evaluation in the amniotic fluid – is also possible. Ultrasound screening performed in the 12–14th week of pregnancy is a mean to detect neural tube defects, especially when they are big. The smaller malformation can be missed at this time. The second ultrasound, performed at about the 20th week of pregnancy is the one dedicated to smaller malformations, and all of them should be detected at that time

[12,46]. It is essential to visualize both, the longitudinal and the transverse scans of the whole spine. The proper plan of ossification points of each vertebra should be visualized. Except the obvious appearance of the spine defect, some cerebral markers of this kind of malformation can be found: lemon sign (adapted frontal bones), banana sign (cerebellum moved to the back and elongated) and ventriculomegaly or hydrocephaly [24,35]. Depending on the author, the ultrasound examination allows to diagnose about 40–90% of neural tube defects. Biochemical screening – alpha-fetoprotein (AFP) elevated above 2.5 multiples of median (MoM) – allows to rise the detection rate to as high as 96% [15]. Due to wide introduction of biochemical tests – so called "triple test" (using AFP assessment as a component) for assessing the risk of the Down syndrome, more present neural tube defects are suspected by this way and then patients are forwarded to detailed ultrasound examination. If there are any indications for a fetal karyotyping, the amniocentesis should be carried out. Then the alpha-fetoprotein and the acetylocholinesterase levels are assessed in the amniotic fluid. Elevated alpha-fetoprotein and acetylocholinesterase levels or the presence of its neural isoenzyme is strongly associated with the neural tube defects [15].

Early diagnosis is very important for the appropriate management of pregnancy and delivery. There are some options for parents to choose [46]. When parents decide to continue the pregnancy, observation of the cerebral ventricles is essential. Sometimes, it is indicated to deliver the baby some time earlier due to increasing hydrocephaly. The way of delivery is chosen according to the fetal position, size of the head and of the coele. There are some data confirming the better neurological status of babies born by the cesarean section (breech presentation, coele bigger than 4 cm), but there are also some papers showing the opposite results [33,49]. Very convincing is the paper of Ralis, showing additional lesions of nerves and muscles in the autopsy of the fetuses born vaginally when comparing to the group born by caesarean section [33].

In addition, no difference between groups of children born vaginally or by cesarean section was found shortly after delivery but it was found at the age of 24 months – children born by elective cesarean section did better than those born vaginally [49]. Because of a potential destroying influence of the amniotic fluid on a neural tissue, the time of delivery should be set at no later than in the 37th week of pregnancy.

A few years ago, first experiences with intrauterine fetoscopic or open surgery of coele began (Figure 1.). In this kind of treatment the early diagnosis is crucial due to the shorter exposure of the neural tissue to the amniotic fluid influence, lower uterine contractility during and after surgery. It is still experimental method but seems very promising. First results suggested the lower incidence of hydrocephaly as the only benefit of the surgery. Last data from Philadelphia proved, that the neurological impairment in babies after early intrauterine surgical procedure corresponds to approximately two spinal levels lower damage in comparison to the children that underwent surgery in the neonatal period [50]. We still have to wait for the greater number of operated individuals and, perhaps, for the multicenter studies assessing not only the shorter outcome but also the long-term results for which few years must pass [6,31,41].

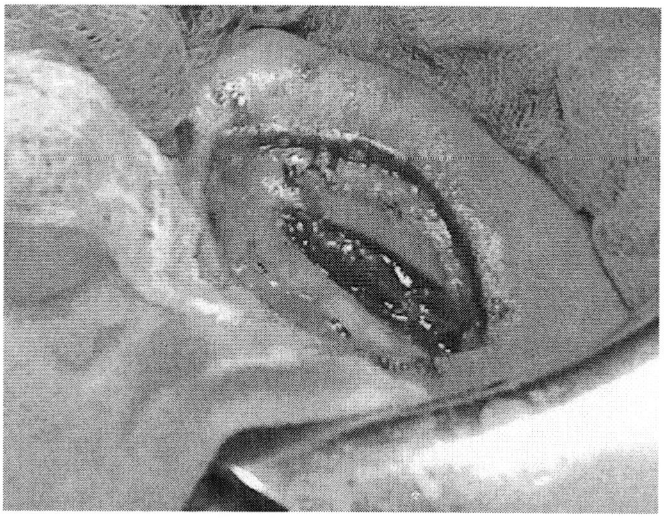

Figure 1. Myelocoele just before in utero closure.

There are experiments carried out on the use of biodegradable matrices for the coverage of the neural tube defect [10]. The other proposed method is to perform the amniotic fluid exchange to replace it by saline fluids to avoid the damaging influence of the amniotic fluid on the neural tissue [28]. Also, the methods of enhancement for re-closure capacity by the intraamniotic administration of the human embryonic stem cells are studied [17].

Events of first hours after the delivery are very important for neonates with the open neural tube defects. The lesion should be closed as early as it is possible [19,20]. Prevention of rupture of coele sac and infection is of a great importance for the future neurological development of a child. Reconstructing the proper surrounding of the spinal cord – cerebro-spinal fluid, muscle and skin protection – is the clue to sustain its motor and sensor function. Additionally, the surgery corrects the shape of the back, what helps in rehabilitation and care [20].

The hydrocephaly surgical treatment introduction in the proper time is very important, to avoid further destruction of the brain [29].

In 2–3 weeks time after the delivery, the size of the neurological impairment in child is assessed. The baby is then qualified to orthopedic and urologic treatment and rehabilitation [2]. Ability to walk depends on the level of the coele and of the coexisting defects. The most of children with spina bifida located below the L-2 level are able to walk [19]. Urine incontinence and recurrent urinary tract infections may lead to renal impairment and death. Early survey of the urinary tract state and its proper management according to the function improves the children's outcome. In 90% of newborns, the urinary tract has no structural defect and there is a chance to avoid its further destruction [49].

Material and Method

In the Department of Obstetrics of the Medical University of Gdansk, 22.534 deliveries took place between 1991 and 2001. Neural Tube Defects were found in 54 neonates. A retrospective analysis of medical records of each pregnancy course and delivery was performed. Questionnaires were sent to families of these children. Questions about the actual condition, the motor and physiologic functions, the intellectual development and the school ability were asked. We gathered also information from pediatricians taking care for these children.

The pregnancy course, the time of defect diagnosis, the prenatal diagnostic tests, the time and the mode of delivery were analyzed. Data about neonate – the Apgar score at delivery, his weight and head circumference, the type of Neural Tube Defect, his status while discharge home were assessed. From Pediatric Surgery records, the time and the type of surgical procedure performed as well as the status of his urinary bladder and the anus function were analyzed. Information about present (February 2003) status of these children was collected from the questionnaires.

Coele was qualified according to the localization (cervical, thoracic, thoraco-lumbal, thoraco-lumbo-sacral, lumbal, lumbo-sacral, sacral, total) and its coverage by the skin/epithelium (open or closed). Motor function was qualified as: 1. walking ability, 2. walking with orthopedic means aid, 3. wheelchair mobility, 4. no motor ability at all. Intellectual development was qualified as: normal, slightly impaired or heavily impaired. Sphincters' function was normal or impaired. In children with the urinary bladder dysfunction two subgroups were created – catheterized every few hours (Clean Intermittent Catheterization - CIC) or/and diaper users. Those using diapers and CIC were qualified as CIC. School ability was assessed by parents as: regular school ability, special school demand, home teaching demand, no teaching ability at all.

Statistic Chi^2 test, logistic regression, T-Student test, Cox' proportional hazard test were used to analyze the collected data.

RESULTS

From 1991 to 2001, in the Department of Obstetrics 22.534 deliveries took place. Central nervous system malformations were found in 112 neonates. In this group, 54 children were diagnosed as having the neural tube defects.

The lumbo-sacral region was the most frequent localization of dysrrhaphia – in 18 cases. The next – lumbal and thoraco-sacral localization appeared in 16 children (8 children in each group), thoraco-lumbal in 7 patients, total dysrrhaphia in 6 cases, sacral - in 4 cases, cervical in 2 cases and on the last position the thoracic one in 1 case (Figure 2.).

Children born with spina bifida are in a high risk of death. In our material, we had 7 stillbirths (13%). In the group of 47 born alive, 12 children died before the end of the observation period but later than in the first day after delivery (22.2%), 10 died in the first day of life (18.6%), 22 were alive at the end of the observation period (40.7%) and 3 (5.5%) were lost to the follow-up. In the last group, the latest observation was done in the ages of 1 month, 13 months and 3 years and 3 months.

Most often, the death occurred in the first month of life – in 16 cases (73% of all deaths), 4 children died till the end of the first year of life (18%), and only two of them (9%) died after one year of life.

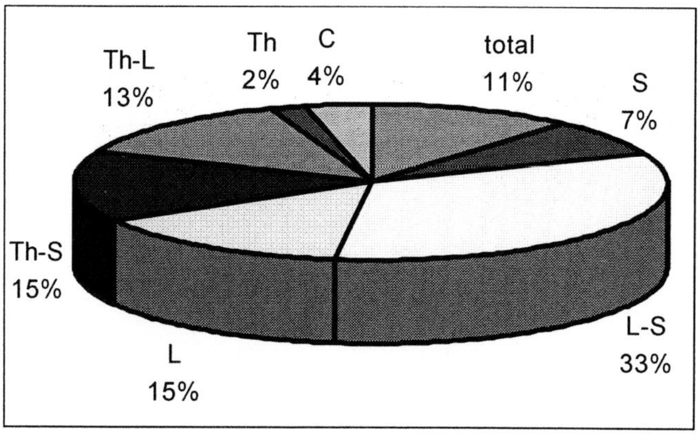

Figure 2. Freuquency of localization of spina bifida in newborns.

In the analyzed group 30 neonates (55.6%) were delivered at term and 24 (44.4%) – prematurely.

In the premature group we had 6 (25%) stillbirths, 10 (41%) neonates died in the first day of life, 4 (16.7%) children survived until the end of the follow-up period. In the group of term deliveries only one child died in the first day of life, 18 of them (60%) survived until the end of the follow-up period.

In the analyzed group, there were 9 neonates (16.7%) with delivery weight below 1500g, 10 (18.5%) - of weight 1500-2499g and 35 (64.8%) - of 2500g and above. The lowest birth weight was 990g and the highest 3900g with the mean of 2762g. In the group of very low birth weight (<1500g) there were 4 stillbirths (44.5%). Four of them (44.5%) died in the first day of life and only one child survived till the end of the observation period. The higher birth weight we observed the lower rate of stillbirths and early deaths occurred. In the group of 1500-2499g only one fetus died "in utero", 5 neonates (50%) died in the first day of life, one child died after the first day of life and 3 of them (30%) survived. In the group of birth weight 2500g and above, we observed 2 cases (5.7%) of stillbirths, 2 cases (5.7%) of deaths in the first day of life, but 10 children (28.6%) died later. Until the end of the follow-up period, 18 children (51.4%) survived.

Low birth weight and prematurity increased the risk of death, but the correlation was not statistically significant.

Time of the Diagnosis

In most of the cases, the spinal defect was diagnosed prenatally (44 cases – 81.5%). The most frequent time of diagnosis ranged from the 30th until the 35th week of pregnancy and the mean was 32nd week. The malformation was diagnosed after the delivery in 10 neonates (18.5%) (Figure 3.).

There was statistically significant correlation between the time of diagnosis and the risk of death: the later diagnosis, the higher mortality rate of children. The correlation between the level of defect in a vertebral column and the mortality rate was also confirmed.

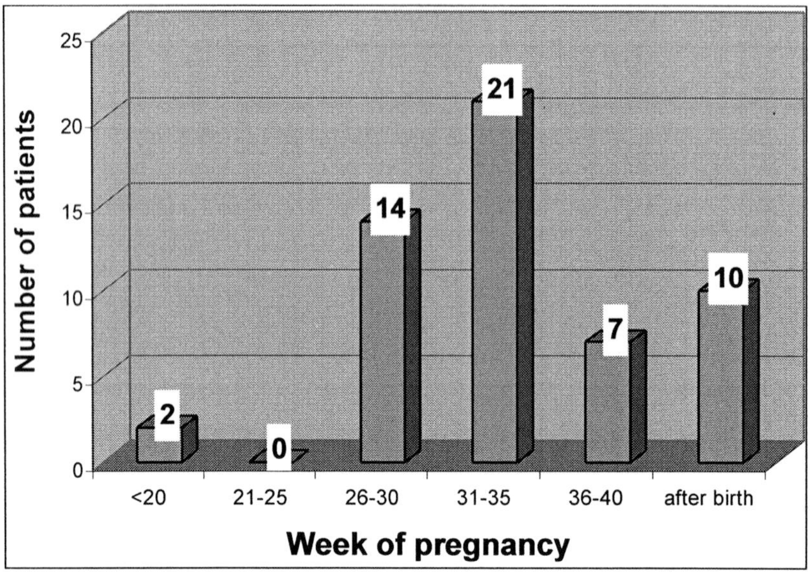

Figure 3. Week of pregnancy at the time of spina bifida diagnosis.

Coexisting Malformations

Other central nervous system defects were found in 9 (16.6%) of neonates with spina bifida. We found statistically significant rise of mortality rate in this group (81% vs. 18% in children with isolated spina bifida). In 14 cases (25.9%), other coexisting malformations were diagnosed. Defects of other systems caused higher mortality rate in children (53% vs. 18% respectively).

Hydrocephaly

To analyze the clinical appearance of hydrocephaly in children with spina bifida, six neonates with anencephaly were excluded. In the remaining group of 48 children, hydrocephaly was present at birth in 33 cases (69%). The head circumference at birth was measured in 44 neonates. In 6 cases (13.6%), it measured below the 10th percentile, in 13 cases (29.6%) it was between the 10th and 90th percentile and in 25 neonates (56.8%) – more than the 90th percentile.

In the group of small head circumference, 3 children (50%) developed hydrocephaly and needed drainage, one child had no symptoms of ventriculomegaly and two children (32.3%) died in the first day of their life.

In the group of children with normal head circumference, 10 neonates (77%) needed implantation of drainage system and only one of them had no symptoms of hydrocephaly.

In the group of higher head circumference, 15 children (60%) needed surgical treatment due to hydrocephaly and only one remained without drainage. Nine children (36%) died before the introduction of treatment.

To assess, if a hydrocephaly increased after the surgical treatment of a myelomeningocoele, all stillbirths and children with many other accompanying defects who died in the first day of life were excluded. Thus, a group of 36 neonates was analyzed. In 25 cases (70%), hydrocephaly was present at birth. After surgery 4 children died (11%), hydrocephaly was observed in 30 cases (83%). Only 2 of them (5.5%) had no evidence of hydrocephaly.

Presence of hydrocephaly according to the level of spina bifida was assessed. We found no correlation between the level of the defect and the ventriculomegaly.

Time of the Surgery

Surgery of the myelomeningocoele was performed in the first day of life in 26 cases (70.3%), in 3 cases (8.1%) in the second day, in 2 cases (5.4%) in the 3rd day of life, in 2 cases (5.4%) in the 4th day of life. No surgery was done in 3 cases because of the poor condition of children – one of them died in the first day of life and two of them – in the second day. One child with closed spina bifida and cystis pilloidalis needed no surgery.

Presentation of a Fetus and the Mode of Delivery

32 neonates were born from cephalic presentation (59.6%), and 22 from breech presentation (40.8%). 29 (53%) vaginal deliveries took place in the analyzed group and 25 (46.3%) cesarean sections were done. Neonates born by cesarean section had a little better Apgar score after delivery comparing to these born vaginally. The difference was not statistically significant. There was correlation between the route of delivery and the mortality rate: risk of death was 50% lower for children born by cesarean section, but the difference was not statistically significant. 13 children (52%) survived until the end of the follow-up period in the group born by a cesarean section and 12 (41.4%) in the group born vaginally. No statistically significant difference was found.

Follow-up of Children with Spina Bifida

In the group of children born with spina bifida and alive until the end of the follow-up period, 15 (68.4%) of them showed normal mental development. In two cases only (9%), deep mental retardation was observed.

Gestational age at delivery and Apgar score after birth correlated with the mental development of these children. These born after the 37th week of pregnancy and achieving higher Apgar score were more likely to have normal mental development. Results are on the border of statistical significance. There was no correlation between the delivery route and mental development.

In the analyzed group, 3 children (13.7%) were able to walk, 5 of them (22.7%) used orthopedic aids (braces) to walk, 5 (22.7%) - used wheelchair and 9 children (40.9%) were not able to move at all. We found out that children with lower vertebral level of the spinal defect were more likely to walk, but the difference was no statistically significant. The ability to walk was observed in children with defect in the lumbo-sacral region.

No influence of the time and the mode of delivery as well as Apgar score on the ability to walk were found.

In the survivals group there were children from 2 to 12 years of age. 15 of them aged from 4 to 12 years. Only 15% of them were able to walk, 26.7% used braces, 33% - wheelchairs, 26.7% had no locomotion ability at all. In the group of 7 younger children (below 4 years of age), 28.6% had some ability to move: one of them was moving at home in vertical position, one of them used braces. Children experienced intensive rehabilitation including walking exercises. Five of children in this group (71.4%) had no ability to move.

In the group of 22 survivals, fecal control was full in 9 patients (40.9%) and no control was observed in 12 children (54.5%). There was statistically significant correlation between level of the spinal defect and anal sphincter function – the lower defect, the more frequent fecal incontinence (Figure 4).

Neurogenic urinary bladder was diagnosed in 21 children (95.5%) in the group of survivals. Only one child was able to control urine. There was statistically significant correlation between level of the spina bifida and the urinary bladder sphincters control – the lower defect, the more urinary bladder dysfunctions. In the group of the neurogenic urinary bladder in 12 children (54.5%) intermittent catheterization was advised (CIC) and in 7 of them (31.9%) diapers were necessary.

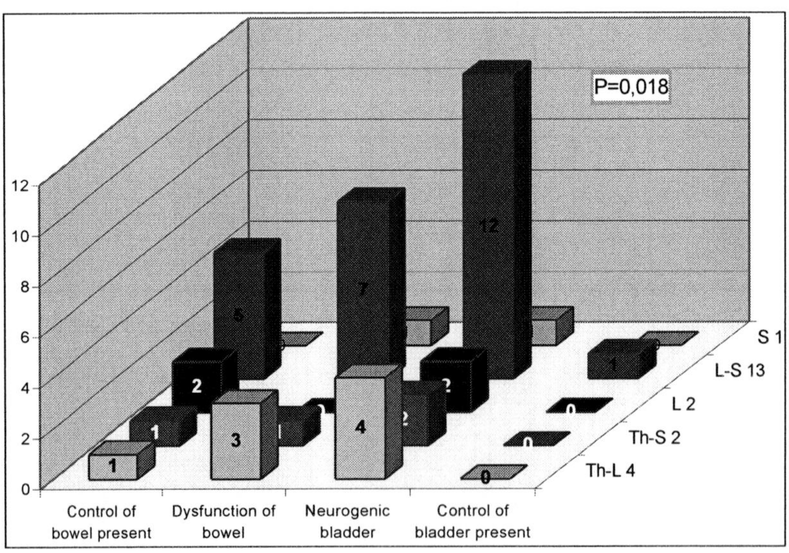

Figure 4. Bowel and bladder function in the children with myelomeningocoele in relation to the defect level.

Complications and Death Causes

In the group of 37 children, who underwent surgical treatment, 6 patients (16.2%) needed drainage revision, in 4 patients drainages were exchanged, one of them died of respiratory distress in the 6th month of life. One of these children had new drainage inserted for 3 times (in the 3rd, 4th and 7th year of life – the last one led to the gall bladder due to the peritoneal adhesions). One of the patients had the drainage changed for 8 times, and died in the 5th year of life due to neuroinfection.

12 children died (32.4%) in this group. The most often cause of death was a respiratory distress – 8 cases (21.6%). That was the reason for 67% of cases of the children's mortality. It was diagnosed in the neonatal or infant period only. It was the cause of 5 deaths in the first month of life and of 3 deaths from the 3rd to 8th month of life. Remaining 4 patients (10.8%) died due to infectious complications – all of them were neuroinfection and one additionally of peritonitis.

In the total population of children with spina bifida, we found 22 survivals (40.7%). In 12 (22.2%) the dysfunction of both sphincters was observed and in 21 children (38.8%) – the neurogenic urinary bladder. Only 8 children reached "social" level of motor function, 5 (9.2%) use wheelchair and 9 children (16.6%) have no motor ability.

There were 8 children in the school age (7 to 12 years), 4 of them were at the regular schools, three in the special schools, one studied at home. There were 4 children 6 years old, one was in the regular preschool, one studied at home, two remained at home without teaching. In the younger group, there was one child 5 years old and one 4 years old (on the wheelchair) attending regular daycare.

DISCUSSION

The Central Nervous System defects are very important in overall morbidity and mortality of the fetuses and newborns. Their clinical consequences are always very serious. They are very often the cause of death, physical impairment and mental retardation. The most frequent malformations in this group are neural tube defects. In our material, the incidence (2.4/1000) was much higher than in the literature, because we analyzed the children born in the referral center [43].

According to the literature polihydramnios associates 50% of neural tube defects, however it more likely coexists with cases of acrania than with the isolated open spina bifida [34]. In our material, the polihydramnios was found in 8 children (21,6%) of all 37 cases of isolated myelomeningocoele and in 15 children (27,8%) of all open spina bifida cases including these coexisting with acrania (54 children).

Spina bifida is a frequent cause of stillbirths and deaths after delivery. Presence of other malformations increases the mortality [39,48].

In the analyzed group there was slightly higher number of girls (59.3%), the same percentage is reported in the literature [39,48]. The most frequent localization of the spinal defect was the same in our material and in the literature – lumbo-sacral, the next was lumbal, thoraco-lumbal and thoraco-sacral [8,19,39]. We found quite high incidence of thoraco-lumbal and thoraco-sacral spina bifida (13 and 15%). Cochrane and Mizai found even higher incidence of 18.9% and 20% respectively [8,27].

The mortality rate in the group of children born with spina bifida in the literature is cited from 14% to 18% [25,36,39]. In our material, we found 53% mortality rate. In the group of neonates with spina bifida, the most of deaths occur in the first month of life. In some papers, the mortality in the first month of life is as high as 77% of all deaths [27]. In our material, it was 73%.

Lee-Yang analyzing survival rate in the group of 235 neonates born with spina bifida found, that low birth weight increases the mortality rate [48]. In our group, we found slight correlation between the low birth weight and the mortality.

The role of early prenatal diagnosis is more often accentuated in the literature. For the last few years, thanks to the modern diagnostic methods, mainly ultrasound examination, many malformations are diagnosed prenatally, what makes possible the "in utero" treatment. It is a chance for early defect correction and prevention of its further consequences [24]. Since late 90th, the "in utero" surgical treatment of spina bifida has been tried. The purpose of the treatment is shortening of the period of neural tissue exposure to the amniotic fluid destructive influence [31,43]. Bruner and Tulipan proved, that surgery performed "in utero" decreases the hydrocephaly frequency and dysfunction of the posterior fossa [6,41]. Decreasing the extent of neurological impairment is also a possible benefit of the prenatal treatment according to Walsh [50].

The frequency of prenatal diagnosis of spina bifida ranges from 40% to 80% [24]. Myelomeningocoele is relatively easy to diagnose prenatally, if the skilled sonographer follows the continuity of the vertebral column, vertebral ossification centers and skin shape. In the analyzed group, spina bifida was diagnosed before birth in the 81.5% of cases, similarly to the literature data. However, the problem was, that it was diagnosed between the 30th and 35th week of pregnancy, what influenced the rise in the mortality rate of children.

Termination of pregnancy (TOP) in most countries is usually allowed in cases of fetal severe malformations that could significantly affect the babies' future life. The gestational age limit to which this procedure can be performed depends on a country. In some countries this limit is described as "before the ability of baby for the extrauterine life", in others the "late TOP" is allowed. The decision made up by the future parents should be based on the multidisciplinar counseling including opinions of pediatric surgeon, geneticist and psychologist. Due to the correlation between the high spina bifida localization and its poor outcome, in these cases TOP is strongly recommended [11,30].

In the analyzed group, we found correlation between the spine defect level and the mortality rate – the lower defect, the lower mortality rate – similar to that presented by Lee-Yang [48]. Presence of other malformations increased mortality rate in children, other authors described the same pattern [19,48].

In some papers it was written, that only 25% of neonates with spina bifida had hydrocephaly at birth [1]. Other authors found hydrocephaly in the 62 – 80% of neonates [19,23,39]. In our material 69% of them presented hydrocephaly at birth. To assess how many of children required surgical treatment, children stillborn and died in the first day of life were excluded. In this extracted group, 70% of them presented hydrocephaly at birth, and 4 of them died after spine defect surgery. All the remaining children required surgical drainage of hydrocephaly (84%) or neurosurgery (1 case). In the group without hydrocephaly at birth, 82% developed hydrocephaly later and needed further treatment. The results are consistent with other authors. In a group described by Bell hydrocephaly developed in the 82% of the children born without symptoms, in the group of McLoan - in 86% [4,25]. The studies indicate the high risk of the hydrocephaly development in children born with small head circumference. Very promising are the results of prenatal surgery of myelomeningocoele significantly decreasing risk of hydrocephaly [6,41].

As only some children present hydrocephaly at birth, the routine management is the spine defect surgery after birth and the ventricles drainage only if the hydrocephaly develops [42]. Some authors suggest performing the both surgeries at the same time [49]; some even suggested that spine surgery results in hydrocephaly development [3]. Not all the authors present the same opinion [21]. In our group, the 83% of children after a spine surgery required hydrocephaly treatment. It was performed in the 13th to 71st day after the spine surgery.

Many authors indicate the correlation between the localization of the spinal defect and the hydrocephaly – it appears the most often in the children with thoracic spinal defect [4]. Lorber wrote that it happens more often in the lumbal defects [21]. Other authors did not find any correlation, just as we found in our group [27].

The most of children born with myelomeningocoele (94.6%) were transferred to the Pediatric Surgery Department in the first day of life, as it is recommended by most of the authors [20,25]. Lorber divided children with myelomeningocoele into groups with good and poor prognosis. It resulted in surgical treatment in the first group and conservative treatment in the second group. Mortality rate in the group with good prognosis was 14%, in the other group – 100% [21]. The modern management of myelomeningocoele consists of early (up to 48 hours) spinal defect closure and hydrocephaly treatment with ventricles shunting when needed [25,43]. In the first 48 hours of life, 78.5% of our patients underwent spinal defect surgery; the latest surgery was performed in the 4th day of life in 5.4% of the children.

Despite of wide diagnostic possibilities, there are many controversies in the delivery management of patients with the diagnosed spina bifida in fetus. The mode of delivery depends on the size of the defect and the risk of the coele injury at the vaginal delivery [24]. Spinal cord injury during a delivery in many papers is presented as a risk factor for the poor neurological condition [38]. Some authors underline the benefits of the cesarean section route: aseptic environment and lower risk of spinal cord and coele injury, when others describe no difference between the groups born vaginally and abdominally [7,16]. Liu et al. at the University of Washington observed the influence of the mode of delivery on the motor function of children with myelomeningocoele for 19 years. He found, that when the coele is flat (<1cm) the elective cesarean section gives no benefit to a child. The elective cesarean section is beneficial only in patients with myelomeningocoele rising more than 1cm above the spine level and allows the better motor functions development [18]. In the retrospective analysis of 200 children with myelomeningocoele, no difference was found between the group exposed to the labor and those born by elective cesarean section. However, at the age of 24 months of life 2.2 higher cerebral palsy rate was found in the group of vaginal labor trial if compared to the elective cesarean section group [8].

In analyzed group, 60% were born vaginally. Children born by cesarean section had slightly higher Apgar score in the first minute after delivery. Cesarean section decreased the mortality rate for 50%, but the difference was not statistically significant. We also found no difference in motor functions and mental development between children born vaginally and abdominally. Delivery after the 37th week and the higher Apgar score decreased frequency of mental retardation and motor dysfunction, although the difference was not statistically significant.

There is no way of the urinary bladder dysfunction treatment giving satisfying voiding. Regular catheterization of a urinary bladder is the most effective in preventing renal dysplasia. Regular catheterization leads to acceptable level of urinary continence. In our material in almost all children, the neurogenic urinary bladder was diagnosed. In 54.5%, Clean Intermittent Catheterization (CIC) was applied, the latest at 2 years of age. No child catheterized urinary bladder himself/herself. In the McLon group 85% of children achieved "social" urine continence using CIC [25]. In 28 years of Hunt observation 75% of patients achieved satisfying urine and fecal continence. The 40.9% of children with myelomeningocoele achieved fecal control [14]. Treatment of urination and defecation dysfunctions is difficult, requires a lot of patience from patients and from physicians. Permanent rehabilitation gives results sometimes after many years. Worse results in children in our material may be due to low availability of rehabilitation and consultation in Poland.

The main death reason in the group of children with spina bifida is the respiratory distress, especially in the neonatal and infant period [25,45]. In the analyzed group, it was the cause of 66.6% of deaths. Although in no patient the Chiari II syndrome was diagnosed, apnea, swallowing problems and respiratory insufficiency suggested presence of the syndrome in some children. In our material most of the deaths caused by respiratory distress occurred in the early period.

Infection of the draining system is still a big problem. Its incidence is approximately 5 to 15%, and mortality rate ranges 30 – 40% [5,40]. In the analyzed group, 4 children died due to infections (10.8%). In one child, drainage to the gall bladder was performed due to peritonitis and adhesions.

The poor overall results in managing the neural tube defects in children cause that this malformation entitles to terminate the pregnancy (TOP) in its early point. In countries where the early prenatal screening is widely applied and the diagnosis can be set by the end of the first trimester or in the beginning of the second one such solution can be considered. The background for such conduct are the results of long term outcome confirmed in this paper allowing to treat this malformation as sublethal and leading to various range of disability which is usually severe. Thus, the strict diagnosis at the earliest possible pregnancy period should be set to assess the prognosis and to present future parents what kind and what extent of disability they should expect. Then, the prenatal counseling should be carried out with the support of psychologist and perhaps the contact with the society of disabled children should be enabled. The approach of parents to the problem and good understanding of it can allow them the proper decision making fitting to their psychological, ethical and religious profile. There are countries like Netherlands, where late termination of pregnancy in the cases of myelomeningocoele is accepted and most of the neonates with poor prognosis are not qualified to the surgery [11,30].

Depending on accessibility to early prenatal diagnosis and prenatal policy, the results will differ due to preselection of the analyzed group. If more severe cases are terminated in the early pregnancy, then the postnatal outcome would be better. Thus paradoxically, in countries where the prenatal diagnosis is not effective or TOP is generally not accepted the results are worse but seem to describe the problem more accurately.

CONCLUSION

1. Spina bifida is associated with high mortality rate, most of the deaths occurred in the first year of life.
2. Low birth weight, prematurity, coexistence of other malformations and early prenatal diagnosis increase the risk of death.
3. The level of the spine defect correlates with the mortality rate and the sphincters function.
4. Mental development depends on the neonate condition after delivery.
5. Mode of delivery has no influence on the further child's development.
6. The high incidence of spine surgery in the early postnatal period (94% referred to Pediatric Surgery Department in their first day of life) is a result of good cooperation of interdisciplinary specialists and underlines the necessity of such cooperation.

REFERENCES

[1] Barszcz S: Hydrocephaly in children. In: Roszkowski M*: Hydrocephaly in children.* EMU Warsaw 2000; 108-123.

[2] Bartecki B. Rehabilitation in children with myelomeningocoele. XVI Symposium of Polish Society of Pediatric Surgery Gorzow (1991) 41.

[3] Bell WO, E Arbit, RAR Fraser. On-stage meningomyelocoele closure and ventriculoperitoneal shunt placement. *Surg Neurol 27* (1987) 233.

[4] Bell WO, TE Summer, FM Volberg: The significance of ventriculomegaly in the newborn with myelodysplasia. *Child's Nerv Syst 3* (1987) 239.

[5] Bidzinski J. Infection prophylaxis in neurosurgery. *Neur Neurochir Pol 27*, 1 (1993) 85.

[6] Bruner JP, N Tulipan, RL Paschal: Fetal Surgery for Myelomeningocoele and the Incidence of Shunt-Dependent Hydrocephalus. *JAMA 282* (1999) 1819.

[7] Chervenak FA, L Duncan, IR Ment: Perinatal management of myelomeningocoele. *Obstet Gynecol 63* (1984) 376.

[8] Cochrane D, B Irwin, K Chambers: Clinical Outcomes that Fetal Surgery for Myelomeningocoele Needs to Achieve. *Eur J Pediatr Surg 11 Suppl I* (2001) 18.

[9] Dambska M, H Traczynska-Kubin: *Pediatric neurology.* Czochanska J. PZWL Warsaw 1990, 301-25.

[10] Eggink AJ, LA Roelofs, WF Feitz, RM Wijnen, RA Mullaart, JA Grotenhuis, TH van Kuppevelt, MM Lammens, AJ Crevels, A Hanssen, PP van den Berg. *Fetal Diagn Ther. 20* (2005) 335-40.

[11] EUROCAT Working Group. Prevalence of neural tube defects in 20 regiond of Europe and the impact of prenatal diagnosis, 1980-1986. *J Epidemiol Community Health 45* (1991) 52-8.

[12] Hackeloer BJ. Ultrasonography in pregnancy. *Ginekologia Praktyczna 3* (1998) 5.

[13] Heffez DS, J Aryanpur, GM Hutchins, JM Freeman: The paralysis associated with myelomeningocoele: clinical and experimental data implicating a preventable spinal cord injury. *Neurosurgery 26* (1990) 987.

[14] Hunt G. Open spina bifida: The Cambridge cohort in their twenties. *Eur J Pediatr Surg 2 Suppl I* (1992) 39.

[15] Jezuita J, J Siemaszko: Ultrasonographic assessment of central nervous system in I trimester with vaginal probe. *Pol Tyg Lek XLIX; 809* (1994) 186.

[16] Kolble N, TAG Huisman, M Stallmach M Meuli, FZR Imahorn, R Zimmermann: Prenatal diagnosis of the fetus with lumbal myelocystocoele. *Ultrasound Obstet Gynecol 18* (2001) 536.

[17] Lee DH, S Park, EY Kim, SK Kim, YN Chung, BK Cho, YJ Lee, J Lim, KC Wang. Enhancement of re-closure capacity by the intra-amniotic injection of human embryonic stem cells in surgically induced spinal open neural tube defects in chick embryos. *Neurosci Lett 364* (2004) 98-100.

[18] Liu SL, DB Shurtleff, RG EllenbogenJD Loser, R Kropp: 19-year Follow-Up of Fetal Myelomeningocoele Brought to Term. *Eur J Pediatr Surg 9 Suppl I* (1999) 12.

[19] Lodzinski K: Dysrrhaphia. In: Poradowska W: *Pediatric surgery*. PZWL, Warsaw 1992.

[20] Lodzinski K, Z Dudkiewicz, S Jaworski: Evolution of myelomeningocoele treatment. XVI Symposium of Polish Society of Pediatric Surgery Gorzow (1991) 17.

[21] Lorber J. Results of Treatment if Myelomeningocele. *Develop Med Child Neurol 13* (1971) 279.

[22] Mac Mahon RA: *Pediatric Surgery*. PZWL Warsaw 1990.

[23] Mandat K. Simultaneous and Sequential Treatment of Newborns with Open Myelomeningocoele and Concomitant Hydrocephalus. *Surg Childh Intre II, 3* (1994) 174.

[24] Marianowski L, R Debski: Prenatal diagnosis of congenital malformations. *Ultrasonografia pediatryczna* (1999) 364.

[25] McLone DG, TP Naidich: *Myelomeingocoele: outcome and late complications. Ped Neurosurg: Surgery of the Developing Nervous System*; Saunders Philadephia 1989; 53-70.

[26] Mikiel-Kostyra K: Classification and definitions of neural tube defects. In: Brzezinski ZJ: *Prevention of congenital neural tube defects*. Institute of Mother and Child, Warsaw 1998.

[27] Mirzai H, Y Ersahin, S Mutluer, A Kayahan: Outcome of patients with myelomeningocoele. *Child's Nerv Syst 3* (1987) 239.

[28] Olguner M, FM Akgur, T Ozdemir, T Aktug, E Ozer. Amniotic fluid exchange for the prevention of neural tissue damage in meylomeningocoele: an alternative minimally invasive metod to open in utero surgery. *Pediatr Neurosurg 33* (2000) 252-56.

[29] Osemlak J: Morphology and classification of dysrrhaphic malformations of central nervous system. *Ped Pol 9-10* (1992); Suppl 466.

[30] Paintin D. Abortion after 24 weeks. *Br J Obstet Gynaecol 104* (1997) 398-400.

[31] Polis L. K Szaflik: In utero treatment of hydrocephaly. *Neurologia Dziecieca 8*; 16 (1999) 23.

[32] Pollack IF, D Pang, AL Albright D Krieger: Outcome following hindbrain decompression of symptomatic Chiari malformations in children previously treated with myelomeningocoele closure and shunts. *J Neurosurg 77* (1992) 881.

[33] Ralis ZA. Traumatizing effect of breech delivery on infants with spina bifida. *J Pediatr 87* (1975) 613.

[34] Romero R, G Pilu, P Jeanty, A Ghidini, JC Hobbins: *The Central Nervous System in Prenatal Diagnosis of Congenital Anomalies. Appleton and Lange*, Connecticut 1988, 1-80.

[35] Roszkowski T. Diagnosis of fetal malformations. *Klinika 5*; 1 (1998) 33.

[36] Roszkowski T, S Barszcz, Z Turkowski. Operative cerebral endoscopy in hydrocephaly treatment. *Neur Neurochir Pol 31* (1997) 805.

[37] Roszkowski M, L Skobejko, S Barszcz: Diagnosis and surgical treatment of Tethered spine syndrome. *Postepy pediatrii LXXI; 2* (1996) 135.

[38] Stark G, M Drummond: Spina bifida as an obstetric problem. *Develop Med Child Neurol Suppl 22* (1970) 157.

[39] Steinbok P, B Irvine, D Cohrane, BJ Irvin: Long-term outcome and complications of children born with myelomeningocoele. *Child's Nerv Syst 8* (1992) 92.

[40] Stoba Cz. M Krolak. Drainage of ventricles to the gall bladder as an alternative management in complications during hydrocephaly treatment. XVI Symposium of Polish Society of Pediatric Surgery Gorzow (1991) 83.

[41] Sutton LN, NS Adzick, LT Bilaniuk: Improvement in Hindbrain Herniation Demonstrated by Serial Fetal Magnetic Resonance Imaging Following Fetal Surgery for Myelomeningocoele. *JAMA 282* (1999) 1826.

[42] Swank M. L Dias: Myelomeningocele: a review of the orthopedic aspects of 206 patients treated from birth no selection criteria. *Developmental Medicine and Child Neurology 34* (1992) 1047.

[43] Szaflik K: Intensive fetal therapy. In: Breborowicz GH: *High Risk Pregnancy*. PAN Poznan 2000; 439.

[44] Tulipan NB, JP Bruner: Myelomeningocoele repair in utero. *Pediatr Neurosurgery 28* (1998) 177.

[45] Wilczynski J, K Szaflik, M Respondek-Liberska, T Stetkierwicz: Malformations of the fetus – management. In: Breborowicz GH: *High Risk Pregnancy*. PAN Poznan 2000.

[46] Vial Y, Ch Tran, MC Addor, P Hohlfeld:. Screening for fetal malformations: performance of routine ultrasonography in the population of the Swiss Canton of Vaud. *Swiss Med Wkly 131* (2001) 490.

[47] Wocjan J: Congenital nervous system malformations and genetic disorders. In: Bidzinski J: *Neurosurgery*. PZWL, Warsaw 1998.

[48] Wong LY, LJ Paulozzi: Survival of infants with spina bifida: a population study 1979-94. *Paediatric and Perinatal Epidemiology 4* (2001) 374.

[49] Wosko IP: *Orthopedic and rehabilitation problems in children with myelomeningocoele*. Folium Lublin 1995.

[50] Walsh DS, Adzick NS. Foetal surgery for spina bifida. *Semin Neonatol 8* (2003) 197-205.

In: New Developments in Birth Defects Research
Editor: Nelson A. Gaslem, pp. 87-109

ISBN 1-60021-400-2

Chapter 3

NEW INSIGHTS IN TREATMENT OF OSTIUM SECUNDUM ATRIAL SEPTAL DEFECT: FROM GENETIC BACKGROUND TO MYOCARDIAL FUNCTION

Marco Pascotto, Giuseppe Santoro*, Giovanbattista Capozzi, Giovanni Di Salvo, Giuseppe Pacileo, Carlo Pisacane, Maria Giovanna Russo and Raffaele Calabrò

Division of Cardiology, 2nd University of Naples, "Monaldi" Hospital, Naples, Italy.

ABSTRACT

Ostium Secundum Atrial Septal Defect (osASD) is a common, sometimes familial, form of congenital heart disease, accounting for approximately 10% of all congenital cardiac defects. Atrial septal defect is very well tolerated in most cases, and its diagnosis is often made during routine clinical evaluation in asymptomatic patients. In the last decade, percutaneous closure by device implantation has been proposed as the one-stop choice for ASD treatment. When compared to surgery, percutaneous approach is less invasive, does not require cardiopulmonary by-pass, preserves pericardial and atrial integrity, allows shorter admission time and faster reintegration to daily life and is less psychologically stressing for patients (especially in pediatric age). Mid-term follow-up studies underscore that percutaneous treatment is as effective as surgery in terms of ASD closure but is associated with less early and late complications (e.g. arrhythmias, unresolved right side dilation). Since percutaneous ASD closure has been routinely available for about 10 years, long term follow up studies are still warranted.

However, transcatheter option might be considered as an "unbiased" tool to study the impact of ASD closure on cardiac electro-geometric remodeling, allowing to differentiate

* Correspondence concerning this article should be addressed to Dr. Giuseppe Santoro, MD. E-mail: santoropino@tin.it; Phone/Fax +39-081-7064275; Via Vito Lembo, 14, 84131 – Salerno, Italy.

the hemodynamic consequences of shunt disappearance from the artificial changes resulting from surgery. Indeed, improvements in cardiac electrical analysis (QT and PR dispersion, signal-averaged EKG, Monophasic Action Potential invasive recording) and imaging technologies (e.g. Doppler Tissue Imaging, Strain/Strain Rate, Integrated Backscatter, 3-D Echo, MRI) brought new insights both in patho-physiology of right ventricular volume overload and time-course of its normalization after percutaneous ASD closure. These data might help the clinical decision-making on timing for percutaneous ASD treatment in the era of device closure, In fact, while all symptomatic patients and asymptomatic adults should be treated as soon as ASD is diagnosed, the indication in asymptomatic children is usually given by subjective ultrasound or EKG signs of right heart suffering. In fact, it is unclear if all children significantly benefit from early treatment when benefits have to be weighed over risks related to dealing with growing hearts. Recent data show that in asymptomatic children, despite the general idea, ASD closure might be safely deferred to early adulthood with no difference in terms of cardiac remodeling and mid-term clinical endpoints. Indeed, it appears that traditional parameters do not select children who might most benefit from early treatment. In general, volume overload associated with ASD appears to be responsible for very mild, if any, impairment of cardiac function in childhood to early adulthood. In this age range, it appears that percutaneous ASD closure completely reverses to normal any adaptive cardiac remodeling. In conclusion, new advances in diagnostic technologies might help to better understand the patho-physiologic consequences of atrial shunt disappearance as well as to clarify the most appropriate timing for ASD closure in childhood.

Keywords: Atrial Septal Defect, device closure, RV function

Introduction

In the past decade ostium secundum Atrial Septal Defect (osASD) has been a field of growing interest by the research community. A medline research on PubMed (National Institute of Health) using "Atrial septal defect" as key word shows over 3200 published papers in the last 10 years as compared to 2100 articles in the previous decade. Several important features might be responsible for this undoubted rise of interest for this cardiac malformation:

1) osASD is a relatively common malformation, accounting for almost 1/4 of all congenital heart diseases (CHD) with high prevalence both in children and adults.
2) osASD is a relatively well tolerated defect associated with long term morbidity in untreated adults.
3) osASD is potentially responsible for paradoxical right-to-left shunt which can determine a life threatening condition in selected patients.
4) osASD closure is considered as a "single step treatment" with positive impact on patient prognosis.

Moreover, both imaging modalities and endovascular approaches have recently experienced a very steep technical improvement which, in turn, has provided cardiologists with a very powerful tool of investigation and treatment.

In this paper, some interesting data providing new insights in osASD will be discussed. Ostium secundum ASD is the most common form of atrial septal defect, making up approximately 69% of all ASDs. This type of defect results from either developmental failure of the septum primum or secondary fenestration in the septum primum. Despite its epidemiological weight, patent foramen ovale cannot be considered as a form of osASD, thus it will not be discussed in the present chapter.

EPIDEMIOLOGY

It is well known that osASD is a relatively frequent congenital heart disease, accounting for 6-10% of all cardiac anomalies and twice as common in females as in males (Campbell *Br Heart J* 1970, Dickinson *Br Heart J* 1981, Feldt *Mayo Clin Proc* 1971). The occurrence of congenital heart disease in a total of 43 studies was reviewed recently, and the overall incidence of osASD was found to be ~2-3/10000 live births (Hoffman *J Am Coll Cardiol* 2002). According to these data osASD would be second only to ventricular septal defect (VSD) as the leading congenital cardiac malformation. It is somehow difficult to carry out a survey on osASD epidemiology. Diagnosis in newborns is fairly easy when a murmur is present, but often osASD is silent at cardiac auscultation, thus potentially causing its underestimation. On the other hand, small osASD often undergo spontaneous closure early in life, thus it is advisable to defer its epidemiological evaluation after the first year of life. Recently, a regional Italian study conducted after the first year of life reported interesting data, highlighting isolated osASD as the most frequent congenital heart disease (about 23% of all) with an incidence of about 0.3% (Capozzi *It Heart J* 2002). Thus, despite regional differences it is conceivable that osASD is the first congenital heart malformation in several countries. In fact, unlike VSD which is usually associated with a loud murmur, osASD diagnosis is often missed at auscultation due to faint murmurs.

GENETICS

Ostium secundum ASD is usually a sporadic and not genetically transmitted malformation. However, familial distribution of osASD is suggested by several small studies (Bizarro *Circulation* 1970, Li *Ann Genet* 1991, Ferencz *J Am Coll Cardiol* 1989, Ferreira *Arq Bras Cardiol* 1999, Benson *Circulation* 1998, Megarbane *Am J Med Genet* 1999). Moreover, the association between osASD and anomalies of the upper extremities is a well-known feature of the Holt-Oram syndrome (Holt *Br Heart J* 1960). However there are few data from large cohorts underscoring the familial distribution of congenital heart disease in patients with osASD. Boughman et al (*Am J Med Genet* 1987) previously showed a 4.9% recurrence rate of CHD in the nuclear family (parents and sibs) of 61 patients with osASD. More recently, Caputo et al (*Eur Heart J* 2005) extended the investigation up to third-degree relatives in a large cohort of 583 patients with osASD. Their main finding is a higher recurrence rate of CHD (18.7%) in patients with osASD than in controls for each degree of relatedness. Moreover, their data underscore a trend towards a higher familial recurrence of isolated osASD in patients with isolated osASD than in patients with non-isolated osASD, thus suggesting a different genetic background for isolated and non-isolated osASD.

Recently, several studies on family with high prevalence of osASD were able to identify different genes potentially causing osASD. In particular, mutations in the cardiac homeobox gene NKX2-5 and gene GATA4 were characterized by different groups (Schott *Science* 1998, Elliott *J Am Coll Cardiol* 2003, Hirayama-Yamada *Am J Med Genet* 2005). Moreover, a mutation in alpha-myosin heavy chain 6 (MYH6) was identified in a large family with dominantly inherited ASD (Ching *Nature Genetics* 2005). Interestingly, the wild type cardiac transcription factor TBX5 strongly modulates MYH6 expression whereas mutated TBX5 (causing Holt-Oram syndrome) does not, which provides evidence linking a transcription factor, a structural protein a congenital heart disease.

Pathophysiology

Ostium secundum ASD is a relatively simple malformation responsible for pathophysiological adaptation and maladaptation of both cardiac muscle and pulmonary circulation.

Dimension of osASD in Childhood

It is well known that osASD is often present in newborns. However, as derived from natural history and echocardiographic studies, significant changes in osASD size could be found over a long-term follow-up. Since the heart does not complete its macroscopic development until about 16 years of age, it is conceivable that also osASD size may change during cardiac remodeling. In most cases, small osASDs undergo spontaneous closure during the first year of life. However, in up to 65% of patients, this septal defect may enlarge during childhood, with a >50% increase in about 30% of patients and an osASD enlargement up to > 20 mm in 13% of patients (McMahon Heart 2002). This concept has to be considered if follow-up evaluation or when defect closure is planned.

Atrial Shunt Direction

The shunt across osASD is mostly responsible for the related structural and functional changes involving both the heart and lungs. Indeed, blood mostly flows from left to right across the septal defect during the cardiac cycle with maximal velocity in late systole. Nevertheless, Doppler investigation underscores the existence of right-to-left shunt in early systole. This pattern of directional flow corresponds to the pressure pattern existing between the atria throughout the cardiac cycle (Levin *Circulation* 1968). These data strongly underline that right-to-left shunt is present despite ultrasound might fail to demonstrate it. This concept should not be underestimated, due to the unquestionable risk of paradoxical embolism associated with osASD. The shunt direction is very sensitive to the pressure gradient between the atrial chambers, thus a bidirectional or right-to-left shunt will be present if severe pulmonary hypertension develops. This is a remarkable finding in the natural history of patients with untreated osASD since pulmonary overflow causes increased pre-capillary resistances and pulmonary hypertension.

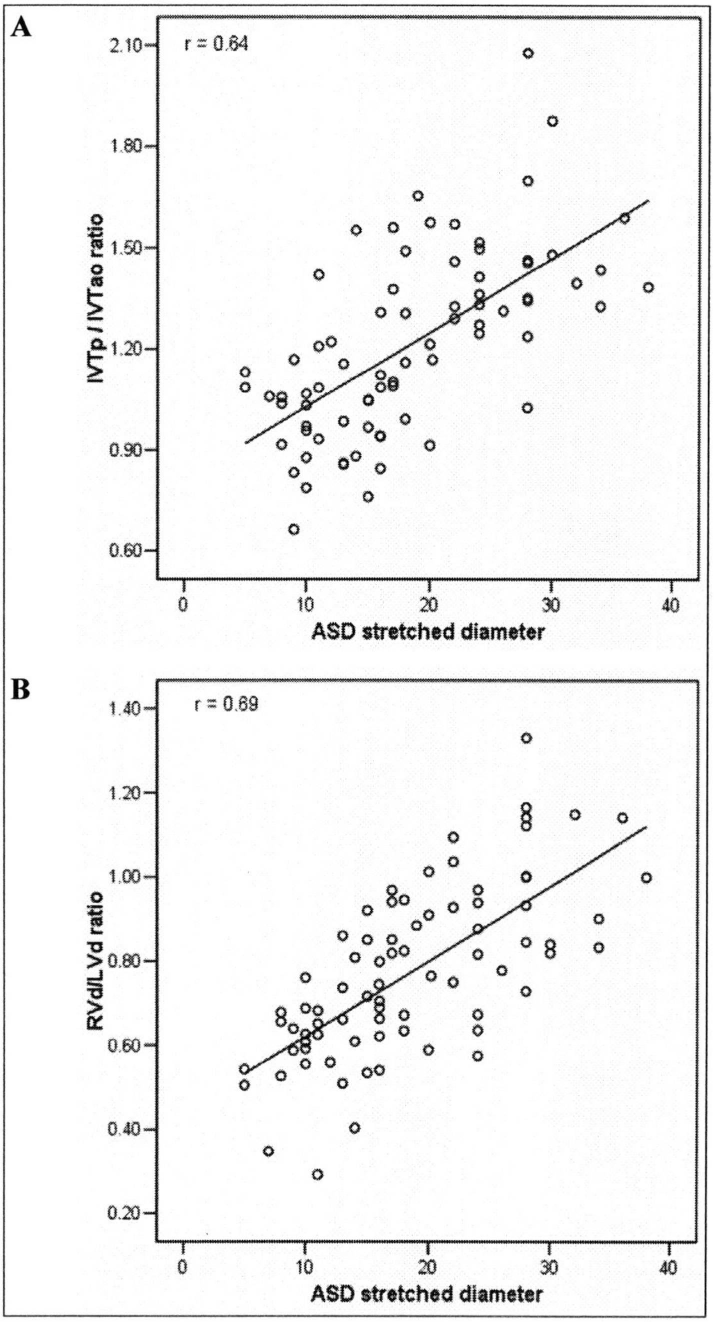

Figure 1. (A) Scatter-plot depicting the relation between osASD stretched diameter and the non-invasive surrogate of pulmonary-to-systemic flow ratio (Qp/Qs). In the absence of pulmonary hypertension, atrial septal defect size is mainly responsible for the increased pulmonary-to-systemic

overflow. (B) Scatter-plot depicting the relation between osASD stretched diameter and right (RV) to left (LV) ventricular diameter ratio, used as an index of overload related cardiac remodeling. In the absence of pulmonary hypertension, defect size is mainly responsible for cardiac remodeling associated with volume overload. Abbreviations: osASD: ostium secundum atrial septal defect; VTIp: pulmonary Velocity-Time-Integral; VTIao: aortic Velocity-Time-Integral; RVd/LVd: right-to-left ventricular diameter ratio as evaluated by parasternal M-Mode analysis.

Atrial Shunt Magnitude

As already pointed out, flow usually shunts from left to right across the defect and this is likely due to the ASD size (Fuse *Am J Cardiol* 2001) as well as a small but constant left-to-right pressure gradient between the atria and the different compliance between the right and left heart. The higher right ventricular compliance is always considered as the major actor in directing atrial flow shunt. This is certainly true in diastole when the atrio-ventricular valves are opened and all 4 cardiac chambers behave as a single chamber, but the higher right ventricular compliance cannot be responsible for the magnitude of systolic left-to-right shunt. In fact, compliance is by definition a diastolic property. Thus, it is likely that left-to-right atrial shunt in systole is mainly due to the higher pull-down effect exerted on the atrio-ventricular plane by the right ventricle compared to the left ventricle. This can be easily showed by ultrasound M-Mode analysis of tricuspid versus mitral annulus plane systolic excursion (TAPSE vs MAPSE). Indeed, we have analyzed (Pascotto *Am J Cardiol 2004*, Pascotto *Am J Cardiol 2005*) TAPSE and MAPSE in 41 patients with osASD and we have consistently found that TAPSE is higher than MAPSE (21.6±5.0 mm vs 13.9±3.2 mm, $p < 0.001$, respectively). Thus, higher right ventricular compliance in diastole and wider tricuspid excursion in systole are usually responsible for directing the shunt from left to right. Since most patients with osASD show preserved right ventricular diastolic and systolic function, it is conceivable that the actual size of osASD is the major predictor of the amount of blood shunting from left to right. As a matter of fact, by keeping a pressure gradient constant between two chambers the flow across the connecting port will be directly related to the actual size of the port. Indeed, we have found in our population at multivariate regression analysis that osASD diameter is the only predictor of both the shunt entity and the heart remodeling (Figure 1).

As already stated, pulmonary pressure and right ventricular compliance strongly affect the magnitude of interatrial shunt, so that both worsening pulmonary hypertension and ventricular compliance cause concomitant and progressive reduction in left-to-right shunt until bidirectional and right-to-left shunt happens.

Volume Overload and Cardiac Remodeling

In the presence of osASD, both the right atrium and ventricle are forced to handle a blood surplus compared to the left cardiac chambers. Indeed, despite the fact that the left atrium is directly involved in the short-circuit, it experiences a mild, if any, volume overload and dilation. This is mostly due to the small but continuous pressure gradient forcing the flow from left to right.

The presence of congenital osASD exposes the right heart to a long lasting volume overload so that a very important issue to address is how the right ventricle adapts structurally and functionally over time. Despite the fact that time can be partially responsible for progressive dilation of both right atrium and ventricle, it appears that cardiac dimensions are weakly related to patient age ($R^2=0.38$ $p<0.001$, personal data) with no relation at all after age of 30. Unlike age, we have found that osASD size shows a good linear positive relation with ventricular dimension ($R^2=0.66$ $p<0.001$, personal data). This finding suggests that cardiac remodeling mostly happens "early" in life, probably before age of 30.

Despite the striking macroscopic remodeling involving the right heart, it is unclear what happens at the histological and cellular level. Unfortunately, to the best of our knowledge, no data are available from animal models of osASD and it would be unethical to take in vivo human samples of the right ventricular free wall. Thus, it is unclear what kind of ultrastructural remodeling the right ventricle experiences dealing only with volume overload. It is well known that fibrosis, hypertrophy and apoptosis happens in mixed models of right ventricular volume and pressure overload, but pulmonary hypertension is usually a late sequel in the natural history of osASD. Moreover, ultrasound characterization of the right ventricle by integrated backscatter failed to show increased fibrosis in patients with moderate osASD (Pacileo *Am J Cardiol* 2004). So, even if it is reasonable that some ultrastructural adaptation is present, we lack data on its extent and reversibility.

Right Ventricular Function

Children and young adults seem to tolerate well the volume overload in terms of both diastolic and systolic right ventricular function. Despite the presence of chamber dilation as a compensatory reaction to volume overload, the right ventricle apparently does not show any sign of dysfunction. This is not surprising if one thinks of the Frank-Starling relation. In fact, analysis of ventricular performance by Doppler Myocardial Imaging underscores the tendency of the right ventricle to react by increasing its myocardial velocities with volume overload (Pascotto *Am J Cardiol* 2004). However, right ventricular function is strongly affected by pulmonary vascular resistance._Thus, development of pulmonary hypertension over time results in progressive worsening of right ventricular performance.

Left Ventricular Function

It is well established that chronic right ventricular volume overload is associated with impairment of left ventricular performance (Flamm *Am J Med* 1970, Popio *Am J Cardiol* 1975). This is mainly due to the mechanical disadvantage of a non-circular short axis configuration over radial function (Walker *Am J Cardiol* 2004). Unlike radial function, regional longitudinal left ventricular function in children and young adults seems to be slightly affected by right ventricular overload associated with osASD, as suggested by preserved Doppler Myocardial velocities of the left ventricular inferior and lateral wall (Pascotto *Am J Cardiol* 2005) and mild reduction of the septal velocities (Giardini *Am J Cardiol* 2005). Overall, resting global left ventricular function is usually normal or slightly impaired in children and young adults suffering of osASD.

Despite reassuring data on resting function, the cardiac performance under stress is affected in adult patients. Cardio-pulmonary exercise stress showed depressed functional capacity in asymptomatic or mildly symptomatic adults with osASD (Brochu *Circulation* 2002, Giardini *J Am Coll Cardiol* 2004). On the other hand, a small study on younger patients failed to show any impairment of functional capacity in osASD patients (Rhodes *Am J Cardiol* 2002).

Pulmonary Vascular Adaptation-Maladaptation

It is well established that chronic volume overload results in dilation of the entire pulmonary vascular bed. At the histological level, medial hypertrophy is present in the muscular pulmonary arteries and veins (Ishii *J Am Coll Cardiol* 1995). Luckily, osASD causes irreversible hypertensive pulmonary vascular disease in fewer than 10% of patients, with a striking preponderance in female sex (Yamaki *Chest* 1986). Nevertheless, mild-to-moderate increase in pulmonary arterial pressure is not an uncommon finding at Doppler evaluation, but this is not necessarily consistent with irreversible pulmonary hypertension. In fact, when pulmonary vascular resistance is evaluated one will underscore the frequent reversibility of that finding.

Diagnosis

Clinical signs and symptoms rely on the main patho-physiological aspect related to osASD, namely the left-to-right flow shunt across the atrial defect and its consequences (Porter *Heart Disease in Infants, Children and Adolescents, Including the Fetus and Young Adults* 1995). Depending on the magnitude and duration of right heart volume overload, there is a progressive right chamber enlargement along with pulmonary microvascular adaptation, which in turn may cause over time pulmonary hypertension, congestive heart failure and arrhythmias.

Clinical signs and symptoms associated with osASD are often subtle and once ASD is suspected imaging modalities are warranted in order to confirm the diagnosis. Indeed, in most cases the presenting finding is a murmur while others are quite rare. Physical examination is often unremarkable, thus underdiagnosis would be frequent by looking at physical findings (hyperactive right ventricular impulse, split fixed second heart sound, systolic and diastolic flow murmurs) or EKG abnormalities (right axis deviation, right atrial enlargement, and evidence of right ventricular volume overload). Indeed, it appears that, in all, 30% of patients have either one or no typical physical findings, 18% have normal EKG findings, and 7% have no physical or EKG findings (Christensen *Ped Cardiol* 2005). Thus, although it is well known that variations can occur in the clinical signs and symptoms typical of osASD, dependence on classical physical and or EKG findings may result in under-diagnosis of a significant number of patients. These data underline how imaging modalities are irreplaceable in diagnostic decision making.

From a therapeutic perspective, not only osASD presence but also its size, defect rims and relation to surrounding structures, as well as flow shunt quantification, right chamber overload and pulmonary arterial pressure have to be characterized. Traditionally, osASD diagnosis is made by trans-thoracic 2-dimensional ultrasound investigation which is usually able to detect most osASD characteristics when handled by expert sonographers. Several direct and indirect ultrasound findings are associated with osASD. The investigation of the atrial septum is possible from multiple views but those providing a perpendicular alignment to the septum, such as parasternal and subcostal views, are more likely to detect and characterize the defect. First, a bidimensional morphological study is advisable, followed by color-Doppler investigation to uncover the shunt across the septal defect. It is important to differentiate osASD from patent foramen ovale in which the edges still overlap without lacking of septal tissue. Often the suspicion is driven by indirect signs of right chambers volume overload characterized by atrial and ventricular dilation along with flattening of the ventricular septum. Moreover, pulmonary artery dilation is often visualized as well as increased Doppler-derived flow across the tricuspid and pulmonary valve. Variable degrees of tricuspid regurgitation are often discovered from which right ventricular systolic pressure can be determined, the latter usually being in the normal range in children and increased in patients with long-lasting large osASD. Indeed, further investigation is often necessary by transoesophageal echocardiography to obtain more detailed morpho-functional insights and a comprehensive overlook of the diverse aspects of osASD. Thus, transoesophageal echocardiography is considered unanimously the most useful and widely available tool for osASD diagnosis and characterization. Recently, new imaging modalities, such as magnetic resonance imaging (MRI) and 3D-echocardiography have been introduced in the clinical arena, providing very accurate tool for morphological evaluation of atrial septum.

MRI is very accurate in detecting osASD (Piaw *Cardiovasc Intervent Radiol* 2005). Sensitivity and specificity of MRI are extremely high due to the very good spatial resolution of this technique (~0.1 mm), thus MRI might become the gold standard non-invasive technique for osASD diagnosis. Unfortunately, MRI is not widely available, it is time consuming, it is very expensive and it needs multiple expertises from radiologists, cardiologists and technicians. Thus, echocardiography is still unanimously considered the first imaging modality for osASD diagnosis.

The recent development of 3-dimensional echocardiography has guaranteed new insights in the study of osASD (Pepi *Am J Cardiol* 2004). Three-dimensional off-line reconstruction from transesophageal acquisition offers a detailed "surgical-like" view of the atrial septum. This approach potentially provides detailed information regarding the number of defects, defect size, shape and position, relation to surrounding structures (namely AV valves, systemic and pulmonary veins, coronary sinus, ascending aorta), as well as shunt quantification that, in turn, are very helpful for guiding the choice between percutaneous and surgical treatment. In addition, dynamic display of the three-dimensional image is able to demonstrate movement of the atrial septum, and changes in the defect size and shape during the cardiac cycle, information that cannot be directly obtained with conventional 2-

dimensional echocardiography (Maeno *Heart* 2000) (Figure 2). These changes vary sensibly among patients and appear unpredictable with no correlation with patient's age, defect size, heart rate and shunt ratio (Maeno *Heart* 2000). Despite promising data from small clinical studies (Hofmann *J Am Soc Echocard* 2004, Marx *Echocardiography* 2001, Tamborini *Am J Cardiol* 2002), 3-dimensional echocardiography suffers from tedious and time consuming computer work. Recently, real-time transthoracic 3-dimensional echocardiography has been implemented on several ultrasound systems, providing a more rapid evaluation of the 3D characteristics of osASD (Cheng *Am Heart J* 2004, Mehmood *Echocardiography* 2004, Acar *Cardiol Young* 2003) and potentially guiding percutaneous interventions (Roman *Circulation* 2004). It is likely that those promising preliminary data will encourage large clinical studies to better define the potential role of three-dimension echocardiography in the clinical arena.

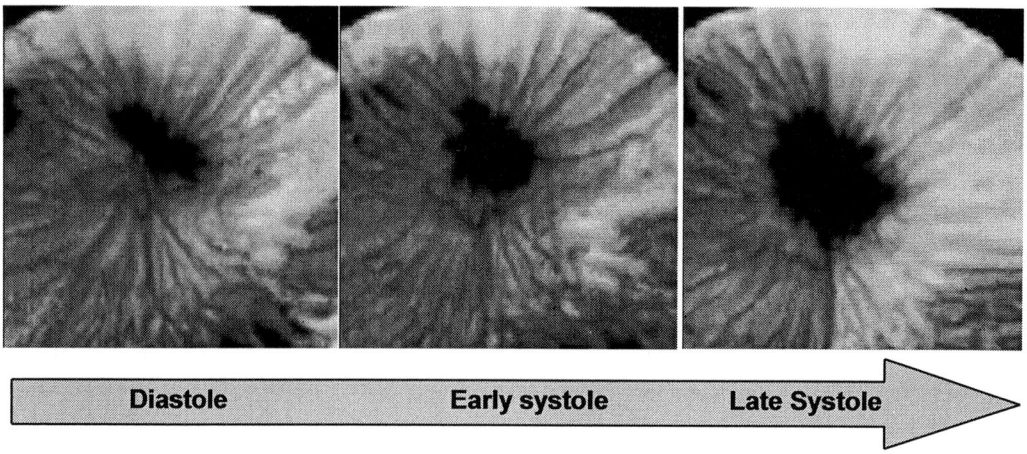

Figure 2. Right atrial en-face 3-dimensional view of an osASD (transoesophageal acquisition). The defect shape and dimensions as well as its surrounding rims are very well detailed. Moreover, 3-dimensional analysis nicely shows diastolic-to-systolic variation of both defect shape and size. Maximal osASD area is seen in systole, minimal in diastole. Abbreviations: osASD: ostium secundum atrial septal defect.

Treatment

Surgical Closure

Treatment of osASD relied on surgical closure for several decades, thus efficacy of any new approach has to be compared to long term follow-up coming from several surgical series (McNamara *Am J Cardiol* 1982, Meyer *Am J Cardiol* 1982, Meijboom *Am J Cardiol* 1993, Murphy *N Eng J Med* 1990, Roos-Hesselink *Eur Heart J* 2003). Surgical osASD closure is very efficacious with a success rate close to 100% and an excellent survival rate at long term follow-up. It appears unlike to experience major cardiac events late after surgical osASD closure since reports of heart failure, pulmonary hypertension, symptomatic ventricular arrhythmias and stroke are merely anecdotic. Nevertheless, surgery carries out some risks and complications related to the invasiveness of the approach. Indeed, not only does surgery requires off-pump circulation and chest opening, but pericardiotomy and atriotomy is warranted to approach the interatrial orifice.

New surgical techniques have been recently introduced in order to obtain a less invasive approach to osASD closure. Indeed, osASD can be treated by a right thoracotomy with a mini-invasive approach (Rosengart *Ann Thorac Surg* 1993, Black *Ann Thorac Surg* 1998, Formigari *J Am Coll Cardiol* 2001). This technique is doable in a consistent number of patients, might be better tolerated due to shorter in-hospital time and less psychological trauma associated with a smaller surgical scar. The efficacy seems to be similar to conventional medial sternotomy, but long term follow-up results are not available yet. More recently, thoracoscopic osASD closure has been attempted with good result and high aesthetical compliance in a limited number of patients (Casselman *Heart* 2005). However, both mini-invasive and thoracoscopic surgery rely on pericardial and atrial opening, as well as cardiopulmonary bypass. Again, large scale studies and long term follow up are warranted before definitive conclusions might be drawn.

It is suggested that age at operation is a major risk factor predicting future complications (Murphy *N Eng J Med* 1990), and recent data confirmed that patients undergoing osASD closure at young age do better in terms of late complications (Roos-Hesselink *Eur Heart J* 2003). Despite the evidence that ASD surgery results in a significant improvement of symptoms (Ghosh *Heart* 2002, Doty *Am J Cardiol* 1984), it often fails to completely revert the electrical and geometric cardiac abnormalities due to the long-standing volume overload. Despite significant changes in electrocardiographic signs of volume overload (Karpawich *Am J Cardiol* 1985, Terada *Jpn J Thorac Cardiovasc Surg* 2000), most postsurgical patients continue to experience arrhythmias (Gatzoulis *N Engl J Med* 1999, Brandenburg *Am J Cardiol* 1993). In addition, persistence of RV enlargement has been reported in >80% of pediatric and up to 77% of adult patients over a midterm follow-up (Pearlman *Am J Cardiol* 1978, Meyer *Am J Cardiol* 1982, Ning *Can J Surg* 1984). Each time, these findings have been ascribed to chronic myopathic changes from long-lasting volume overload, functional postsurgical anomalies, or geometric modifications due to pericardial opening (Dhillon *Heart* 2002, Pearlman *Am J Cardiol* 1978, Satoh *J Cardiovasc Electrophysiol* 1996, Gatzoulis *Circulation* 1995).

Indeed, arrhythmias and incomplete right heart remodeling appear to be the more frequently reported complications, even in patients treated at young age. Roos-Hesselink et al reported symptomatic supraventricular tachyarrhythmias in 8% and pacemaker implantation in 5% of their patients at a mean follow up of 26 years after osASD closure at young age. Moreover, 24-hours Holter monitoring showed signs of sinus node dysfunction in 27-39% and ventricular arrhythmias in 25-43% of asymptomatic in those patients. As far as right heart remodeling concerns, Roos-Hesselink et al reported right atrial and right ventricular dilation in as many as 19% and 24% of their patients, respectively. It is possible but not unquestionably proven that pericardiotomy and atriotomy might play a role in this lack of remodeling. Thus, despite very good outcome in children, surgery is still associated with long term sequels in a consistent number of patients.

Percutaneous Closure

In the last decade percutaneous osASD closure has gained rising consideration in the clinical arena and it is now a widely accepted option for osASD treatment. This technique relies on catheter-based release of a complex-shaped device within the interatrial orifice to correct the defect. There are several device approved for clinical use, with published data on a consistent number of patients. The most used ones are the Amplatzer Septal Occluder (AGA Medical, Golden Valley, Minnesota, USA), the CardioSeal (Nitinol Medical Technologies Inc., Boston, Massachusetts, USA), the Sideris ASD buttoned device (Custom Medical Devices, Amarillo TX, USA), the Angel Wings DAS device (Microvena Corporation, White Bear Lake, MN, USA), the ASDOS device (Osypka Corp., Grenzack-Wyhlen, Germany) and the Helex device (W.L. Gore, Flagstaff, AZ, USA), with different structure, implantation techniques, closure philosophy and indications. From the interventionalist standpoint, the osASD may be classified as "simple", if small-sized and central with adequate rims, and "complex", if large, with deficient rims, multiple or located inside a floppy aneurysmatic septum (Figure 3). However, by tailoring the occluding device to septal anatomy, all these types of osASD may be percutaneously approached with a high rate of success (Figure 4) (Rao *Can J Cardiol* 1995, Suarez de Lezo *Cathet Cardiovasc Interv* 2000, Kauliz *Cardiol Young* 2001, Du *J Interv Cardiol* 2002, Santoro *J Cardiovasc Med* 2006, in press).

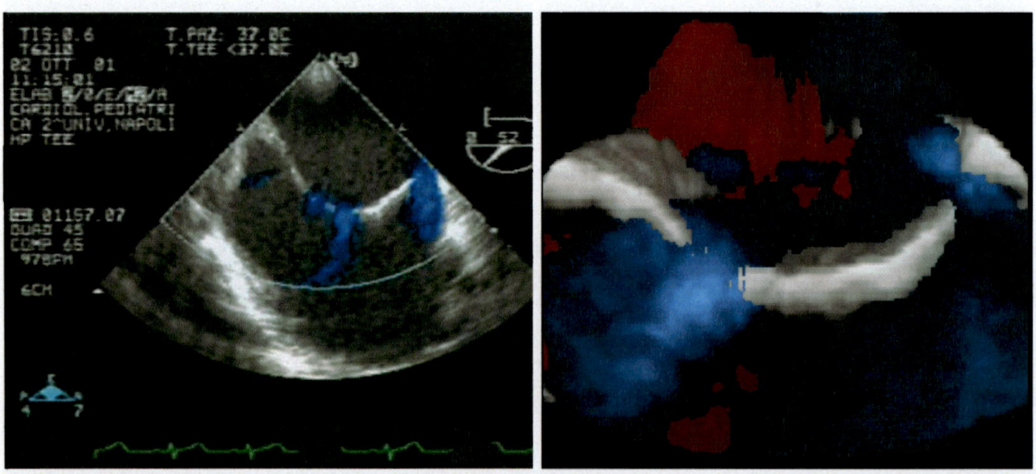

Figure 3. Color-Doppler transoesophageal (TEE) 2-dimensional (A) and 3-dimensional (B) reconstruction of multi-perforated atrial septal aneurysm with 4 different defects responsible for left-to-right shunt. Despite the ability of 2-dimensional TEE to study the interatrial septum, 3-dimensional reconstruction with Color-Doppler might be helpful for a better characterization of complex anatomical pattern.

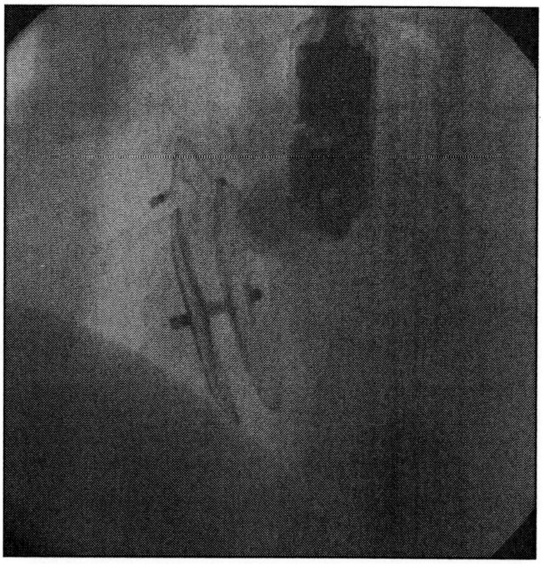

Figure 4. Percutaneous treatment of a "complex" atrial septal defect. This patient showed a multifenestrated atrial septum that was treated with two Amplatzer Septal Occluder devices.

Device Implantation Procedure

All procedures are usually performed under general anesthesia with endotracheal intubation and continuous transoesophageal echocardiographic (TEE) monitoring. Recent advance in the implantation technique is the use of intracardiac echocardiography to guide device positioning and deployment (see below). Techniques of transcatheter ASD closure has been extensively detailed in literature (Butera *J Am Coll Cardiol* 2003; Du *J Am Coll Cardiol* 2002; Fischer *Heart* 2003; Kaulitz *Cardiol Young* 2001; Omeish *J Interv Cardiol* 2001; Pedra *J Invasive Cardiol* 2004; Rao *Can J Cardiol* 2001; Rao *J Invasive Cardiol* 2001; Santoro *J Cardiovasc Med* 2006; Suarez De Lezo *Catheter Cardiovasc Interv* 2000; Zhong-Dong, *J Am Coll Cardiol* 2002). Briefly, after percutaneous femoral vein entry and full eparinization (100 UI/Kg or 5000 UI in adult patients), a complete hemodynamic evaluation is performed, followed by left atrial angiography in hepato-clavicular projection to delineate the atrial septum. Then, a sizing balloon is introduced over an extra-stiff guide positioned in the left upper pulmonary vein to measure the balloon-stretched diameter with either the pulling or static technique. The occluding device is usually chosen according to the atrial septum morphology and ASD size, screwed on the dedicated cable and delivered trough the appropriate-size sheath, previously positioned inside the left upper pulmonary vein. Under fluoroscopic and TEE guidance, both discs of the device are deployed across the septal defect and, after the device release, a repeat TEE evaluation assess any residual post-procedural shunt. Residual shunt is generally classified as intra-prosthetic, trivial (<1mm), mild (1-2mm), moderate (2-4mm) and severe (>4mm). Antibiotic prophylaxis is given for 48 h and patients are usually discharged home 36-48 h after the procedure. Aspirin (3-5 mg/Kg/die) is started 24 h before the ASD closure and continued for 6 months.

Recently, intracardiac echocardiographic guidance has been proposed as a valid alternative to the transoesophageal guidance since it does not need general anesthesia and it allows shorter fluoroscopy time (Bartel *Circulation* 2003). Unfortunately, the latter approach necessitates an adjunctive large venous catheter which makes the procedure more invasive and less feasible, especially in small children.

Since the first international experience reported more than 10 years ago (Rao *Am Heart J* 1994), many studies have showed the efficacy of the transcatheter approach on large cohorts of patients worldwide (Berger *Cardiol Young* 1999, Du *J Am Coll Cardiol* 2002, Chessa *J Am Coll Cardiol* 2002, Butera *J Am Coll Cardiol* 2003, Fisher *Heart* 2003, Masura *J Am Coll Cardiol* 2005). Despite the initial concern regarding the efficacy of percutaneous closure versus surgery, overwhelming data have showed that the percutaneous approach has very high success rate which is similar to surgery. The Amplatzer Investigators (Du *J Am Coll Cardiol* 2002) showed in a non-randomized multicenter study that the early, primary and secondary efficacy success rates for surgical versus device closure of osASD were not statistically different; however, the complication rate was lower (7.2% vs 24.0%) and the length of hospital stay was shorter (1.0±0.3 vs 3.4±1.2 days) for device closure than for surgical repair. Despite the impressive results of percutaneous intervention, concern has been raised on very large osASD where technical problems might be present. A recent paper (Lopez *Catheter Cardiovasc Interv* 2005) showed that percutaneous approach was efficacious in most patients treated, but a not negligible unsuccessful rate (15%) was encountered when a 40 mm device had to be implanted.

Still device closure of osASD carries out a low but quantifiable risk of short- and long-term complications we have to be aware of. In large studies, the most frequent complications described were the embolization/malposition of the device (up to 3.5%) and cardiac arrhythmias requiring minor treatment (up to 3.4%). Then, several other uncommon complications have been described, namely pericardial effusion, thrombus formation with systemic emboli, erosion of the non-coronary sinus of Valsalva, erosion of atrioventricular leaflets, etc (Harper *Catheter Cardiovasc Interv* 2002; Chun *Catheter Cardiovasc Interv* 2003; Divekar *J Am Coll Cardiol* 2005). No device-related deaths have been described so far. Most of the abovementioned complications are short-term complications, and there are anecdotic reports of device embolization or thrombus formation on the device after 1 year follow-up (Ruge *Circulation* 2005).

Effect of Percutaneous Closure on Geometric and Electrical Cardiac Remodeling

We do know that the right ventricle undergoes a progressive macroscopic dilation and that osASD closure usually determines an almost complete normalization (Figure 5). Several groups have showed a positive cardiac remodeling after percutaneous closure of osASD with kinetics of reduction, starting early after device implantation and continuing up to 6 months (Veldtman *J Am Coll Cardiol* 2001, Du *Am J Cardiol* 2001, Kort *J Am Coll Cardiol* 2001, Santoro *Am J Cardiol* 2004). Moreover, a different trend of remodeling was described depending on the RV region explored. Indeed, the outlet portion showed a steep remodeling early after device implantation followed by little but still significant reduction as compared to the muscular inlet portion which showed a progressive and steady remodeling in the first 6 months after osASD closure (Pascotto *Int J Cardiol* 2005). Initial data on a small number of patients suggested a negative correlation between patient's age and right ventricular remodeling following percutaneous osASD closure (Du *Am J Cardiol* 2001). This issue is still a field of discussion as subsequent studies failed to show any correlation (Kort *J Am Coll Cardiol* 2001) or underscored similar remodeling in asymptomatic children or young adults (Santoro 2006 *Heart*, in press). This is further supported by the lack of clear data showing irreversible osASD-related changes in right cardiac ultrastructure. Thus it is unclear if closure at very young age (early childhood) carries out any substantial benefit in terms of cardiac remodeling as compared to adolescent age. Consequently, the opportunity of postponing osASD closure without risks might be important in selected small size children.

As already stated, right ventricular function appears to be preserved in most patients suffering of osASD. Indeed, right ventricle positively reacts to volume overload in terms of performance by increasing both systolic and diastolic Doppler Tissue Imaging velocities. Conversely, transcatheter osASD closure causes a sudden drop in preload which induces right ventricular adaptation and normalization of myocardial function as assessed by Doppler Tissue Imaging (Pascotto *Am J Cardiol* 2004). This is especially true in case of percutaneous closure compared to surgical treatment. Indeed, Strain analysis showed better preservation of right ventricular function in patients undergoing device implantation as compared to surgical treatment with the former group having values substantially similar to the control group (Di Salvo *Am J Cardiol* 2005).

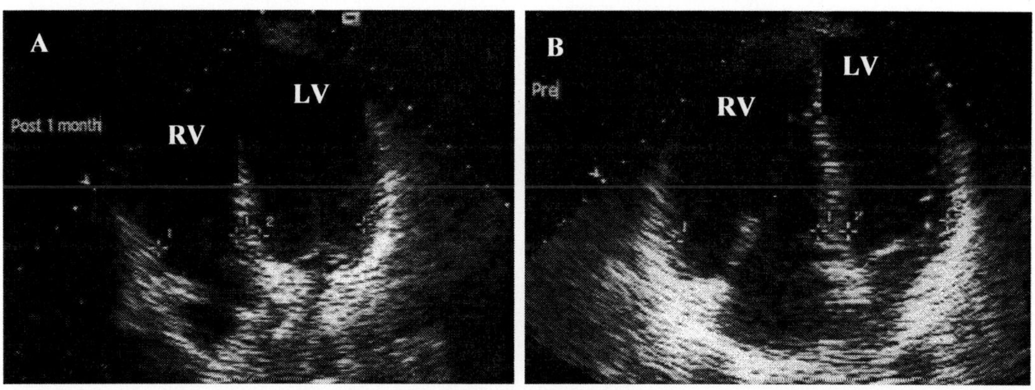

Figure 5. Four-chamber view showing right (RV) and left (LV) ventricular remodeling associated with percutaneous osASD closure. (A) Marked dilation of right ventricle in a young woman with a large osASD (22 mm). The RV and LV diameters in 4-chamber view were 4.73 cm a 3.63 cm, respectively. (B) Cardiac remodeling 1 month after percutaneous osASD closure in the same patient. After device implantation the RV and LV diameters reduced to 3.30 cm and 4,22 cm, respectively. Abbreviations: LV, left ventricle; RV, right ventricle.

Despite long-term volume overload of the right heart might affect left ventricular function over time, it appears that left ventricular performance is usually preserved, as suggested by normal regional Doppler Tissue Imaging velocities. Thus, resting left ventricular function should not change significantly after device implantation. This is confirmed by the unchanged or increased left ventricular myocardial velocities early after transcatheter closure, suggesting preservation or improvement of regional function after the procedure (Pascotto *Am J Cardiol* 2005, Giardini *Am J Cardiol* 2005). Moreover, radial and longitudinal Strain analysis underscored normal regional left ventricular function in patients treated percutaneously but not in those treated surgically. In the former group of patients a slight reduction of systolic regional function might be present only at the septal level (Di Salvo *Am J Cardiol* 2005). Overall, resting global left ventricular function is usually normal or slightly impaired in children and young adults suffering of osASD, with normal function after osASD closure (Giardini *J Am Coll Cardiol* 2004, Walker *Am J Cardiol* 2004, Pascotto *Am J Cardiol* 2005).

The chronic, long-lasting volume overload or the presence of a relatively stiff prosthesis could potentially affect right and left atrial functions. To focus on this issue, analysis by Strain Rate imaging in a small cohort of patients was recently performed at least 6 months after either percutaneous or surgical closure of osASD. Unlike surgical patients who showed biatrial mechanical impairment, both left and right atrial function appeared to be preserved in the percutaneous group (Di Salvo *J Am Soc Echocardiogr* 2005).

Overall, resting cardiac function does not usually show remarkable signs of impairment in patients with osASD. Conversely, cardio-pulmonary exercise stress showed depressed functional capacity in asymptomatic or mildly symptomatic adults with osASD (Brochu *Circulation* 2002, Giardini *J Am Coll Cardiol* 2004). The impairment of functional capacity appears to be reversible since device closure of osASD resulted in normalization of the cardio-pulmonary exercise parameters. The same results could not be duplicated in children, in whom functional capacity was preserved before and remained unchanged after transcathater osASD closure (Rhodes *Am J Cardiol* 2002).

A consistent number of patients with right cardiac volume overload due to osASD experience episodes of supraventricular arrhythmias which persists in some patients after device implantation. EKG studies showed that osASD device closure resulted in significant electrical changes, both at atrial or ventricular level. Analysis of EKGs recording before and after osASD closure underscored that osASD is associated with changes in both electrical conduction, expressed as PQ dispersion (Guray *Ann Noninvasive Electrocardiol* 2004), and repolarization period, expressed as QT dispersion (Santoro *Am J Cardiol* 2004). The underlying mechanisms leading to electrical abnormalities rely on chronic right atrial and ventricular stretch which triggers electrical remodeling. Electrophysiologic analysis showed modest increase in atrial effective refractory period, conduction delay at the crista terminalis, and sinus node dysfunction. When the same analysis was done after osASD closure, a trend towards shortening of effective refractory period was recorded while conduction delay at the crista terminalis was still present beyond intervention, the latter potentially contributing to the long term atrial arrhythmic substrate (Morton *Circulation* 2003). Again, surface EKG analysis showed pre-closure increased dispersion of atrial activation (P dispersion) followed by a significant decrease after percutaneous osASD closure (Santoro *Proceedings of the IV World Congress of Pediatric Cardiology and Cardiac Surgery* 2005). Not only is the right atrium involved in electrical remodeling, but also the right ventricle experiences an electrical response to overload. Diastolic stretch associated with overload results in a shortening of the right ventricular Monophasic Action Potentials, the latter increasing in duration immediately after osASD closure (Santoro *Am J Cardiol* 2004). Moreover, surface EKG analysis performed before and after transcatheter osASD closure showed significant reduction of late potentials, evaluated by signal-averaged EKG, and dispersion of ventricular repolarization (QT dispersion) (Cerrato *Annual Meeting of the Italian Society of Cardiology* 2003, Santoro *Am J Cardiol* 2004). Thus, the volume overload relief is also associated with changes in ventricular electrophysiology as a result of a "mechano-electrical feedback" (Santoro *Am J Cardiol* 2004).

Conclusion

Ostium secundum atrial septal defect is a common congenital heart disease frequently diagnosed in adulthood. It is generally very well tolerated in childhood and early adulthood but implies a significant risk of late complications. Despite the general idea that osASD related volume overload impairs cardiac performance, it appears that in most cases the cardiac function is preserved until early adulthood and that the defect closure reestablish a "normal" anatomy and function. Nevertheless, osASD closure is necessary to avoid long term complications. The introduction in the clinical arena of percutaneous osASD closure by device implantation represents a major step towards patient's safety and compliance. Thus, percutaneous intervention must be nowadays considered as the first therapeutic option in each patient carrying a suitable atrial defect anatomy. Surgery should be considered only when anatomy is unfavorable or when the percutaneous attempt fails. Despite the general agreement on percutaneous osASD treatment, timing might be still field of discussion in early childhood. Despite the fact that device implantation can be performed in small children we still miss evidence of benefits from early treatment in children. Indeed, cardiac anatomy and function revert to normal even when percutaneous intervention is delayed to early adulthood. Moreover we do not know if devices affect cardiac development in young children and eventually new devices with better profile might be approved in this era of rapid technological improvements. Thus it could be wise to delay the intervention to adolescent or early adulthood, at least in asymptomatic children. More data are warranted to clarify this issue.

References

Acar P, Roux D, Dulac Y, Rouge P, Aggoun Y. Transthoracic three-dimensional echocardiography prior to closure of atrial septal defects in children. *Cardiol Young* 2003; 13: 58-63.

Bartel T, Konorza T, Arjumand J, Ebradlidze T, Eggebrecth H, Caspari G, Neudorf U, Erbel R. Intracardiac echocardiography is superior to conventional monitoring for guiding device closure of interatrial communications. *Circulation* 2003: 107: 795-797.

Benson DW, Sharkey A, Fatkin D, Lang P, Basson CT, McDonough B, Strauss AW, Seidman JG, Seidman CE. Reduced penetrance, variable expressivity, and genetic heterogeneity of familial atrial septal defects. *Circulation* 1998; 97: 2043–2048.

Berger F, Ewert P, Bjornstad PG, et al. Transcatheter closure as standard treatment for most interatrial defects: experience in 200 patients treated with Amplatzer septal occluder. *Cardiol Young* 1999; 9 :468 –73.

Bizarro RO, Callahan JA, Feldt RH, Kurland LT, Gordon H, Brandenburg RO. Familial atrial septal defect with prolonged atrioventricular conduction:a syndrome showing the autosomal dominant pattern of inheritance. *Circulation* 1970; 41: 677-83.

Black MD, Freedom RM. Minimally invasive repair of atrial septal defects. *Ann Thorac Surg* 1998; 65: 765-7.

Boughman JA, Berg KA, Astemberski JA, Clark EB, McCarter RJ, Rubin JD, Ferencz C. Familial risks of congenital heart defect assessed in a population based epidemiologic study. *Am J Med Genet* 1987; 26: 839–849.

Brandenburg RO Jr., Holmes DR Jr., Brandemburg RO, McGoon DC. Clinical follow-up study of paroxysmal supraventricular tachyarrhythmias after operative repair of secundum type atrial septal defect in adults. *Am J Cardiol* 1983; 51: 273–276.

Brochu MC, Baril JF, Dore A, Juneau M, De Guise P, Mercier LA. Improvement in exercise capacity in asymptomatic and mildly symptomatic adults after atrial septal defect percutaneous closure. *Circulation* 2002; 106: 1821-6.

Butera G, De Rosa G, Chessa M, Rosti L, Negura DG, Luciane P, Giamberti A, Bossone E, Carminati M. Transcatheter closure of atrial septal defect in young children. *J Am Coll Cardiol* 2003; 42: 241-5.

Campbell M. Natural history of atrial septald effect. *Br Heart J* 1970; 32: 820-6.

Capozzi G, Del Vasto R, Grieco M, Iacono C, Pisacane C, Caputo S, Pascotto M, Russo MG, Calabrò R. Evaluation of incidence of congenital heart defect: is it useful a regional registry? *Ital Heart J* 2002; 3: S34.

Caputo S, Capozzi G, Russo MG, Esposito T, Martina L, Cardaropoli D, Ricci C, Argiento P, Pacileo G, Calabrò R. Familial recurrence of congenital heart disease in patients with ostium secundum atrial septal defect. *Eur Heart J* 2005

Casselman FP, Dom H, De Bruyne B, Vermeulen Y, Vanermen H. Thoracoscopic ASD closure is a reliable supplement for percutaneous treatment. *Heart* 2005: 91: 791-794.

Cerrato F, Santoro G, Pascotto M, Cappelli Bigazzi M, Palladino MT, sarubbi B, Caso I, Russo MG, Calabrò R. Early disappearance of late-onset potentials after transcatheter atrial septal defect closure. *It Heart J* 4(6): C365; 2003

Cheng TO, Xie MX, Wang XF, Wang Y, Lu Q. Real-time 3-dimensional echocardiography in assessing atrial and ventricular septal defects: an echocardiographic-surgical correlative study. *Am Heart J* 2004; 148: 1091-5.

Chessa M, Carminati M, Butera G, et al. Early and late complications associated with transcatheter occlusion of secundum atrial septal defect. *J Am Coll Cardiol* 2002; 39: 1061–5.

Ching YH, Ghosh TK, Cross SJ, Packham EA, Honeyman L, Loughna S, Robinson TE, Dearlove AM, Ribas G, Bonser AJ, Thomas NR, Scotter AJ, Caves LS, Tyrrell GP, Newbury-Ecob RA, Munnich A, Bonnet D, Brook JD. Mutation in myosin heavy chain 6 causes atrial septal defect. *Nature Genetics* 2005; 37: 423-8..

Christensen DD, Vincent RN, Campbell RM. Presentation of atrial septal defect in pediatric population. *Ped Cardiol* 2005 [Epub ahead of print].

Chun DS, Turrentine MW, Moustapha A, Hoyer MH. Development of aorta-to-right atrial fistula following closure of secundum atrial septal defect using the Amplatzer septal occluder. *Cath Cardiovasc Interv* 2003; 58: 246-51.

Dhillon R, Josen M, Henein M, Redington AN. Transcatheter closure of atrial septal defect preserves right ventricular function. *Heart* 2002; 87: 461–465.

Dickinson DF, Arnold R, Wilkinson JL. Congenital heart disease among 160 480 liveborn children in Liverpool 1960 to 1969. Implications for surgical treatment. *Br Heart J* 1981; 46: 55-62

Di Salvo G, Drago M, Pacileo G, Carrozza M, Santoro G, Cappelli Bigazzi M, Caso P, Russo MG, Carminati M, Calabro R. Comparison of Strain Rate imaging for quantitative evaluation of regional left and right ventricular function after surgical versus percutaneous closure of atrial septal defect. *Am J Cardiol* 2005; 96: 299-302.

Di Salvo G, Drago M, Pacileo G, Rea A, Carrozza M, Santoro G, Cappelli Bigazzi M, Caso P, Russo MG, Carminati M, Calabro R. Atrial function after surgical and percutaneous closure of atrial septal defect: a strain rate imaging study. *J Am Soc Echocardiogr* 2005; 18: 930-3.

Divekar A, Gaamangwe T, Shaikh N, Raabe M, Ducas J. Cardiac perforation after device closure of atrial septal defects with the Amplatzer septal occluder. *J Am Coll Cardiol* 2005; 45: 1213-8.

Doty DB, Wright CB, Hiratzaka LF, Eastham CL, Marcus ML. Coronary reserve in volume-induced right ventricular hypertrophy from atrial septal defect. *Am J Cardiol* 1984; 54: 1059–1063.

Du ZD, Cao QL, Koenig P, Heitschmidt M, Hijazi ZM. Speed of normalization of right ventricular volume overload after transcatheter closure of atrial septal defect in children and adults. *Am J Cardiol* 2001; 88: 1450-3.

Du ZD, Cao QL, Rhodes J, Heitschmidt M, Hijazi ZM. Choice of device size and results of transcatheter closure of atrial septal defect using the Amplatzer septal occluder. *J Interv Cardiol* 2002; 15: 287-292

Du ZD, Hijazi ZM, Kleinman CS, Silverman NH, Larntz K, the Amplatzer investigators. Comparison between Transcatheter and surgical closure of secundum atrial septal defect in children and adults. *J Am Coll Cardiol* 2002; 39: 1836-1844

Elliott DA, Kirk EP, Yeoh T, Chandar S, McKenzie F, Taylor P, Grossfeld P, Fatkin D, Jones O, Hayes P, Feneley M, Harvey RP. Cardiac homeobox gene NKX2-5 mutations and congenital heart disease: associations with atrial septal defect and hypoplastic left heart syndrome. *J Am Coll Cardiol* 2003; 41: 2072–2076.

Feldt RH, Avasthey P, Yoshimatsu F, Kurlandt LT, Titus JL. Incidence of congenital heart disease in children born to residents of Olmsted Country. *Mayo Clin Proc* 1971; 46: 794-9.

Ferencz C, Boughman JA, Neill CA, Brenner JI, Perry LW. Congenital cardiovascular malformations: questions on inheritance. *J Am Coll Cardiol* 1989; 14: 756–763.

Ferreira C, Farah LM, Povoa RM, Luna Filho B, Costa A, Ferreira Filho C. Recurrence of atrial septal defect in three generations. *Arq Bras Cardiol* 1999; 73: 211–218.

Fischer G, Stieh J, Uebing A, Hoffmann U, Morf G, Kramer HH. Experience with transcatheter closure of secundum atrial septal defects using the Amplatzer septal occluder: a single center study in 236 consecutive patients. *Heart* 2003; 89: 199 –204.

Flamm MD, Cohn KE, Hancock EW. Ventricular function in atrial septal defect. *Am J Med* 1970; 48: 286–294.

Formigari R, Di Donato RM, Mazzera E, Carotti A, Rinelli G, Parisi F, Pasquini L, Ballerini L. Minimally invasive or interventional repair of atrial septal defects in children: experience in 171 cases and comparison with conventional strategies. *J Am Coll Cardiol* 2001; 37: 1707-12.

Fuse S, Tomita H, Hatakeyama K, Kubo N, Abe N. Effect of size of a secondum atrial septal defect on shunt volume. *Am J Cardiol* 2001; 88: 1447-50.

Gatzoulis MA, Freeman MA, Siu SC, Webb GD, Harris L. Atrial arrhythmia after surgical closure of atrial septal defects in adults. *N Engl J Med* 1999; 340: 839–846.

Gatzoulis MA, Till JA, Somerville J, Redington AN. Mechano-electrical interaction in tetralogy of Fallot. QRS prolongation relates to right ventricular size and predicts malignant ventricular arrhythmias and sudden death. *Circulation* 1995; 92: 231–237.

Ghosh S, Chatterjee S, Black E, Firmin RK. Surgical closure of atrial septal defects in adults: effect of age at operation on outcome. *Heart* 2002; 88: 485–487.

Giardini A, Donti A, Formigari R, Specchia S, Prandstraller D, Bronzetti G, Bonvicini M, Picchio FM. Determinants of cardiopulmonary functional improvement after transcatheter atrial septal defect closure in asymptomatic adults. *J Am Coll Cardiol* 2004; 43: 1886-91.

Giardini A, Moore P, Brook M, Stratton V, Tacy T. Effect of transcatheter atrial septal defect closure in children on left ventricular diastolic function. *Am J Cardiol* 2005: 95: 1255-7.

Guray U, Guray Y, Mecit B, Yilmaz MB, Sasmaz H, Korkmaz S. Maximum p wave duration and p wave dispersion in adult patients with secundum atrial septal defect: the impact of surgical repair. *Ann Noninvasive Electrocardiol* 2004; 9(2): 136-41.

Harper RW, Mottram PM, McGaw DJ. Closure of secundum atrial septal defects with the Amplatzer septal occluder device: techniques and problems. *Catheter Cardiovasc Interv* 2002; 57: 108-24.

Hitayama-Yamada K, Kamisago M, Akimoto K, Aotsuka H, Nakamura Y, Tomita H, Furutani M, Imamura S, Takao A, Nakazawa M, Matsuoka R. Phenotypes with GATA4 or NKX2.5 mutations in familial atrial septal defect. *Am J Med Genet A* 2005; 135: 47-52.

Hoffman JIE, Kaplan S. The incidence of congenital heart disease. *J Am Coll Cardiol* 2002;39:890-1900

Hoffmann T, Franzen O, Koschyk DH, Von Kodolitsch Y, Goldmann B, Meinertz T. Three-dimensional color Doppler echocardiography for assessing shunt volume in atrial septal defects. *J Am Soc Echocardiogr* 2004; 17: 1173-8.

Holt M, Oram S. Familial heart disease with skeletal malformation. *Br Heart J* 1960; 22: 236-42.

Ishii M, Kato H, kawano T, et al. Evaluation of pulmonary arterial histopathologic findings in congenital heart disease: an in vitro study using intravascular ultrasound imaging. *J Am Coll Cardiol* 1995; 26: 272-6.

Kannan BRJ, Francis E, Sivakumar K, Anil SR, Kumar RK. Transcatheter closure of very large (> or = 25 mm) atrial septal defects using the Amplatzer septal occluder. *Catheter Cardiovasc Interv* 2003; 59: 522-527

Karpawich PP, Antillon JR, Cappola PR, Agarwal KC. Pre- and postoperative electrophysiologic assessment of children with secundum atrial septal defect. *Am J Cardiol* 1985; 55: 519–521.

Kaulitz R, Peuster M, Jux C, Paul T, Hausdorf G. Transcatheter closure of various types of defects within the oval fossa using the double umbrella device (CardioSEAL) – feasibility and echocardiographic follow-up. *Cardiol Young* 2001; 11: 214-222

Kort HW, Balzer DT, Johnson MC. Resolution of right heart enlargement after closure of secundum atrial septal defect with transcatheter technique. *J Am Coll Cardiol* 2001; 38: 1528-32.

Levin RA, Spach MS, Boineau JP, Canent RV Jr, Capp MP, Jewett PH. Atrial pressure-flow dynamics in atrial septal defects (secundum type). *Circulation* 1968; 37: 476-88.

Li VS, Distefano G, Garozzo R, Romeo MG, Sciacca P, Mollica F. Autosomal dominant atrial septal defect of ostium secundum type. *Ann Genet* 1991; 34: 14–18.

Lopez K, Dalvi BV, Balzer D, Bass JL, Momenah T, Cao QL, Hijazi ZM. Transcatheter closure of large secundum atrial septal defects using the 40 mm Amplatzer septal occluder: Results of an international registry. *Catheter Cardiovasc Interv* 2005 [Epub ahead of print].

Maeno YV, Benson LN, McLaughlin PR, Boutin C. Dynamic morphology of the secundum atrial septal defect evaluated by three dimensional transoesophageal echocardiography. *Heart* 200; 83: 673-7

Marx GR, Sherwood MC, Fleishman C, Van Praagh R. Three-dimensional echocardiography of the atrial septum. *Echocardiography* 2001 Jul; 18(5): 433-43.

Masura J, Gavora P, Podnar T. Long term outcome of transcatheter secundum-type atrial septal defect closure using Amplatzer Septal Occluders. *J Am Coll Cardiol* 2005; 45: 505-7.

McMahon CJ, Feltes TF, Fraley JK, Bricker JT, Grifka RG, Tortoriello TA, Blake R, Bezold LI. Natural history of growth of secundum atrial septal defects and implications for transcatheter closure. *Heart* 2002 Mar; 87(3): 256-9.

McNamara DG, Latson LA. Long-term follow-up of patients with malformations for which definitive surgical repair has been available for 25 years or more. *Am J Cardiol* 1982; 50: 560–8.

Megarbane A, Stephan E, Kassab R, Ashoush R, Salem N, Bouvagnet P, Loiselet J. Autosomal dominant secundum atrial septal defect with various cardiac and noncardiac defects: a new midline disorder. *Am J Med Genet* 1999; 83: 193–200.

Mehmood F, Vengala S, Nanda NC, Dod HS, Sinha A, Miller AP, Khanna D, Misra VK, Lloyd SG, Upendram S, Bodiwala K, McMahon WS, Kasliwal RR, Chouhan N, Govinder M, Pacifico AD, Kirklin JK, McGiffin DC. Usefulness of live three-dimensional transthoracic echocardiography in the characterization of atrial septal defects in adults. *Echocardiography* 2004; 21: 707-13.

Meijboom F, Hess J, Szatmari A et al. Long term follow-up (9–20 years) after surgical closure of atrial septal defect at young age. *Am J Cardiol* 1993; 72: 1431–3.

Meyer RA, Korfhagen JC, Covitz W et al. Long-term follow-up study after closure of secundum atrial septal defect in children: an echocardiographic study. *Am J Cardiol* 1982; 50: 143–8.

Morton JB, Sanders P, Vohra JK, Sparks PB, Morgan JG, Spence SJ, Grigg LE, Kalman JM. Effect of chronic right atrial stretch on atrial electrical remodeling in patients with an atrial septal defect. *Circulation* 2003; 107: 1775-82.

Murphy JG, Gersh BJ, McGoon MD et al. Long-term outcome after surgical repair of isolated atrial septal defect. *N Engl JMed* 1990; 323: 1645–50.

Ning SB, Fazal H, Cook D, Wood MM, Wood MM, Duncan WJ, Rowe RD. Right ventricular size and ventricular septal motion after repair of atrial septal defect in children. *Can J Surg* 1984; 27: 395–398.

Omeish A, Hijazi ZM. Transcatheter closure of atrial septal defect in children & adults using the Amplatzer Septal Occluder. *J Interv Cardiol* 2001; 14: 37-44

Pacileo G, Limongelli G, Verrengia M, Gimeno J, Di Salvo G, Calabro R. Backscatter evaluation of myocardial functional and textural findings in children with right ventricular pressure and/or volume overload. *Am J Cardiol* 2004; 93: 594-7.

Pascotto M and Santoro G, Cerrato F, Caputo S, Cappelli Bigazzi M, Iacono C, Carrozza M, Russo MG, Caianiello G, Calabro R. Time-course of cardiac remodeling following transcatheter closure of atrial septal defect. *Int J Cardiol* 2006 in press [Nov. 2005 Epub ahead of print].

Pascotto M, Caso P, Santoro G, Caso I, Cerrato F, Pisacane C, D'Andrea A, Severino S, Russo MG, Calabro R. Analysis of right ventricular Doppler Tissue Imaging and load dependence in patients undergoing percutaneous closure of atrial septal defect. *Am J Cardiol* 2004; 94: 1202-5.

Pascotto M, Santoro G, Caso P, Cerrato F, Caso I, Caputo S, Cappelli Bigazzi M, D'Andrea A, Russo MG, Calabro R. Global and regional left ventricula function in patients undergoing transcatheter closure of secundum atrial septal defect. *Am J Cardiol* 2005; 96: 439-42.

Pearlman AS, Borer JS, Clark CE, Henry WL, Redwood DR, Morrow AG, Epstein SE. Abnormal right ventricular size and ventricular septal motion afteratrial septal defect closure: etiology and functional significance. *Am J Cardiol* 1978; 41: 295–301.

Pedra CA, Pedra SR, Esteves CA, Cassar R, Pontes SC Jr, Braga SL, Fontes VF. Transcatheter closure of secundum atrial septal defects with complex anatomy. *J Invasive Cardiol* 2004; 16: 117-122.

Pepi M, Tamborini G, Bartorelli AL, Trabattoni D, Maltagliati A, De Vita S, Andreini D, Pontone G. *Am J Cardiol* 2004; 94: 1343-7.

Piaw CS, Kiam OT, Rapaee A, Khoon LC, Bang LH, Ling CW, Camion H, Hian SK. Use of non-invasive contrast magnetic resonance imaging for estimation of atrial septal defect size and morphology. A comparison with transesophageal echo. Cardiovasc Intervent Radiol 2005 (Epub ahead of print)

Popio KA, Gorlin R, Teichholz LE, Cohn PF, Bechtel D, Herman MV. Abnormalities of left ventricular and geometry in adults with an atrial septal defect. Ventriculographic, hemodynamic and echocardiographic studies. *Am J Cardiol* 1975; 36: 302–308.

Porter CJ, Feldt RH, Edward WD. Atrial septal defects. Emmanoulides GC, Riemenschneider TA, Allen HD, Gutgessel HP. 5th ed. *Heart Disease in Infants, Children and Adolescents, Including the Fetus and Young Adults.*Baltimore, MD: Williams & Wilkins 1995: 687-703.

Rao PS, Ende DJ, Wilson AD, Smith PA, Chopra PS. Follow-up results of transcatheter occlusion of atrial septal defects with buttoned device. *Can J Cardiol* 1995; 11: 695–701

Rao PS, Sideris EB, Hausdorf G, et al. International experience with secundum atrial septal defect occlusion by the buttoned device. *Am Heart J* 1994; 128: 1022–35.

Rao PS. Catheter closure of atrial septal defects. *J Invasive Cardiol* 2003; 15: 398-400

Rhodes J, Patel H, Hijazi Z. Effect of transcatheter closure of atrial septal defect on the cardiopulmonary response to exercise. *Am J Cardiol* 2002; 90: 803–6.

Roman KS, Nii M, Golding F, Benson LN, Smallhorn JF. Images in cardiovascular medicine. Real-time subcostal 3-dimensional echocardiography for guided percutaneous atrial septal defect closure. *Circulation* 2004; 109: e320-1.

Roos-Hesselinka JW, Meijbooma FJ, Spitaelsa SEC, van Domburgan R, van Rijenc EHM, Utensc EMJW, Bogersb AJJC, Simoons ML. Excellent survival and low incidence of arrhythmias, stroke and heart failure long-term after surgical ASD closure at young age. A prospective follow-up study of 21–33 years. *Eur Heart J* 2003 24: 190-197.

Rosengart TK, Stark JF. Repair of atrial septal defect through a right thoracotomy. *Ann Thorac Surg* 1993; 55: 1138-1140.

Ruge H, Wildhirt SM, Libera P, Vogt M, Holper H, Lange R. Left atrial thrombus on atrial septal defect closure device as a source of cerebral emboli 3 years after implantation. *Circulation* 2005; 112: e130-1.

Santoro G and Pascotto M, Caputo S, Cerrato F, Cappelli Bigazzi M, Palladino MT, Iacono C, Carrozza M, Russo MG, Calabro R. Similar cardiac remodelling after transcatheter closure of atrial septal defect in children and adults. *Heart* 2006 in press.

Santoro G, Cappelli Bigazzi M, Iacono C, Gaio G, Caputo S, Pisacane C, Caianiello G, Russo MG, Calabrò R. Transcatheter Closure of "Complex" Atrial Septal Defects: Feasibility and Mid-term Results. *J Cardiovasc Med* 2006 (In press)

Santoro G, Caso I, Caputo S, Gaio G, Cappelli Bigazzi M, Carrozza M, Palladino MT, Caianiello G, Russo MG, Calabrò R. Divergent electro-geometric atrial remodelling early after percutaneous atrial septal defect closure. *IV World Congress of Pediatric Cardiology and Cardiac Surgery Proceedings* 2005; C57

Santoro G, Pascotto M, Sarubbi B, Cappelli Bigazzi M, Calvanese R, Iacono C, Pisacane C, Palladino MT, Pacileo G, Russo MG, Calabro R. Early electrical and geometric changes after percutaneous closure of large atrial septal defect. *Am J Cardiol* 2004; 93: 876-80.

Satoh T, Zipes DP. Unequal atrial stretch in dogs increases dispersion of refractoriness conducive to developing atrial fibrillation. *J Cardiovasc Electrophysiol* 1996; 7: 833–842.

Schott JJ, Benson DW, Basson CT, Pease W, Silberbach GM, Moak JP, Maron BJ, Seidman CE, Seidman JG. Congenital heart disease caused by mutations in the transcription factor NKX2-5. *Science* 1998; 281: 108–111.

Suarez De Lezo J, Medina A, Pan M, Romero M, Segura J, Pavlovic D, Hernandez E, Delgado A, Caballero E, Siles JR, Franco M, Mesa D, Lafuente M. Transcatheter occlusion of complex atrial septal defects. *Catheter Cardiovasc Interv* 2000; 51: 33-41

Tamborini G, Pepi M, Susini F, Trabattoni D, Maltagliati A, Berna G, Onorato E, Bartorelli AL. Comparison of two- and three-dimensional transesophageal echocardiography in patients undergoing atrial septal closure with the amplatzer septal occluder. *Am J Cardiol* 2002; 90: 1025-8.

Terada Y, Mitsui T, Sato M, Horigome H, Tsukada K. Right ventricular volume unloading evaluated by tangential magnetocardiography. *Jpn J Thorac Cardiovasc Surg* 2000; 48: 16–23.

Veldtman GR, Razack V, Siu S, El-Hajj H, Walker F, Webb GD, Benson LN, McLaughlin PR. Right ventricular form and function after percutaneous atrial septal defect device closure. *J Am Coll Cardiol* 2001; 37: 2108-13

Walker RE, Moran AM, Gauvreau K, Colan SD. Evidence of adverse ventricular interdependence in patients with atrial septal defect. *Am J Cardiol* 2004; 93: 1374–377.

Yamaki S, Horiuchi T, Miura R, Suzuki Y, Ishizawa E, Takahashi T. Pulmonary vascular disease in secundum atrial septal defect with pulmonary hypertension. *Chest* 1986; 89: 694-8.

Zhong-Dong Du, Hijazi ZM, Kleinman CS, et al., for the Amplatzer Investigators. Comparison between transcatheter and surgical closure of secundum atrial septal defect in children and adults. *J Am Coll Cardiol* 2002; 39: 1836–44.

In: New Developments in Birth Defects Research
Editor: Nelson A. Gaslem, pp. 111-136
ISBN 1-60021-400-2

Chapter 4

DUPLICATION OF THE ALIMENTARY TRACT

Anil. T. George*

Department of General Surgery
Torbay General Hospital
Torquay, United Kingdom TQ2 7AA

ABSTRACT

Duplications of the alimentary tract make up a group of rare and interesting malformations that vary in size, location and presenting symptoms. Since 1733, when *Calder* published the first reported case of intestinal duplication, more than 500 cases have been published, to date. *Ladd,* in 1937, introduced the term "duplication" and described three features to define the same. Most duplications are possibly "enterogenous cysts" as the actual doubling of the alimentary tract is seen in only a few cases. The aetiology of duplications is still evolving with different theories suggesting different causes for this unusual condition.

Duplications are classified as either tubular or cystic and can occur anywhere along the alimentary tract with colonic mucosa being reported in cysts located in the tongue to gastric mucosa being identified in the rectum. Communication of these duplications with the normal intestinal tract may vary but are more frequently seen with the tubular type.

Clinical presentations of these uncommon anomalies depend upon the location and size of the duplication and some duplications can remain quiscent and persist into adulthood. Though excision remains the preferred treatment, it may not be always a possible option due to co-existing malformations in other organ systems. Further details are given in the discussion of the various types of duplications.

Keywords: Duplications; foregut; midgut; hindgut; enterogenous cysts

* Correspondence concerning this article should be addressed toanilthomasgeorge@hotmail.com

Introduction

Duplication of the alimentary tract makes up a group of rare and interesting malformations that vary greatly in size, location and presenting symptoms. In 1733, *Calder* [1] reported the first such abnormality which was presented as an "intestinal duplication cyst". Later, reports over the next two centuries [2] gave descriptions of enterogenous cysts, giant diverticulae, ileum duplex, inclusion cyst and giant thoracic cyst to a similar spectrum of abnormalities. In 1937, *Ladd* [3] coined the term "duplications" of the alimentary tract to encompass the spectrum of these abnormalities and suggested applying this to congenital anomalies which demonstrated a well developed smooth muscle coat, shared a common blood supply with the native bowel and involved the mesenteric side of the alimentary tract with at least one point of intimate attachment to the bowel [3]. However, the majority of duplications might best be described as 'enterogenous cysts' since only in a small proportion of these cases is there actually doubling of the alimentary tract.

Pathology

Duplications are hollow structures involving the mesenteric side of the associated gastrointestinal (GI) tract [4] and lie between the two leaves of the mesentery. This differentiates them from a *Meckel's* diverticulum which represents the persistent intestinal end of an omphalo-mesenteric duct found attached in close proximity to the terminal ileum and which is usually completely or partially lined by gastric mucosa.

Current nomenclature for duplications relies on the anatomic location of the duplication in relation to the normal intestinal tract and not on the histological features of the mucosal lining [5]. Duplications may be cystic or tubular, non-communicating or more rarely communicating [6]. Communication with the native bowel varies and may be present proximally, distally or at multiple sites. Cystic duplications are usually non-communicating while the tubular types usually communicate to the adjacent bowel. Though the epithelium lining these duplications often mimics that of the adjacent bowel, presence of heterotrophic epithelium can be observed occasionally. Islands of colonic mucosa have been described at the base of the tongue and rests of gastric mucosa near the anus [7].The presence of well formed gastric mucosa in these duplications increases the risk for erosion, peptic ulceration, haemorrhage and perforation [8-11]. Ectopic gastric mucosa is more commonly associated with the tubular type of duplication compared to the cystic type [12]. Other types of heterotrophic mucosa include pancreatic tissue rests which have been identified in duplications of the stomach, ileum and the colon [13].

The contents of the duplication can vary according to the type of epithelium lining the duplication and also with the presence or absence of communicating tracts to the adjacent bowel. If a communicating tract is present, seepage of the intestinal contents from the normal bowel to the duplicated segment occurs. In the absence of any significant connection to the native bowel, the duplication usually fills up with a clear alkaline fluid [14] or may contain mucus, chyle or cellular debris. Inactivated pancreatic enzymes can be found in duplications lined by ectopic pancreatic tissue [13].

Synchronous duplications at different sites along the GI tract have been reported to occur with 5% to 10% prevalence in most series [7,15-17]. Patients with duplications of the bowel have increased co-existant anomalies of other organ systems especially vertebral anomalies like bifid or fused spines and myelo-meningocele [18,19]. Associations with abdominal abnormalities like polysplenic syndrome, pancreatic divisum, imperforate anus and genital abnormalities have also been reported [20-24]. Enteric cystic duplications have been associated with a higher incidence of duodenal and ileal atresias [6,13,17,25,26] and intestinal malrotations [27].

Duplications are seen in 1 of every 4500 autopsies [28]. Most series report the small intestine as the most common site for duplication. Though duplications have been associated with multiple co-existent organ abnormalities, no genetic tendency has been demonstrated, so far.

Embryology

Explanations for this interesting and rare multitude of abnormalities have moved far from the suggestion of a previous era that these cysts and malformations originated from a primary *Meckel's* diverticulum. Many theories have been proposed to account for these uncommon malformations; however, no single theory adequately explains all the known duplications.

Keibe [29] in 1905 followed by *Lewis* and *Thyng* [30] in their 1907 paper, pointed to the presence of tiny buds of intestinal epithelium protruding into the sub-epithelial connective tissue in 4 to 23mm human embryos and foetal alimentary tracts of sheep and other animals though a clinical suggestion was made only in relation to intestinal diverticulae. These nodes or diverticulae, as described by *Lewis* and *Thyng* were found in various positions around the bowel circumference and were not reported to occur on the colon. However, in contrast intestinal duplications almost always occur on the mesenteric side of the bowel and do occur on the colon, though with less incidence than on the small bowel. Neither the presence of heterotrophic mucosa in the duplications nor the existence of long tubular duplications could be satisfactorily explained by this postulation.

Bremer [31] in 1944 suggested that duplications might be the result of abnormal re-canalisation of the intestinal lumen following the "solid stage" of development of the primitive gut that occurs in the sixth or seventh week of gestation where the vacuoles fuse to form two lumina instead of one. However, this too failed to explain the specificity of the location of duplications on the mesenteric side of the bowel compounded by the fact that the 'solid–cord' state of bowel development was largely confined to the duodenum [32].

Other theories postulated included the 1961 environmental theory of *Mellish* and *Koop* [33] suggesting that duplications and twinning in lower orders could be triggered by trauma or hypoxia as the initial event. Based on the work of Louw [34], they concluded that vascular insufficiency could lead to recognised GI duplications in humans.

Paddock and *Arensman* [20] in 1982 suggested an association between the occurrence of bowel duplication and atresias in children with polysplenia, which led to thoughts that duplications could represent an abortive reparative effort by the body.

Split Notochord Theory

A close association observed by *Saunders* [35] between thoracic duplications and vertebral malformations led to the "split notochord" theory which is by far the most satisfactory among the many theories which tried to explain the origin of GI duplications. This theory was first proposed by *Fallon* and modified by *Bentley* and *Smith* [36] and suggested the splitting of the notochord to be the initial step in a series of events that would ultimately lead to duplication of the intestine.

The notochord theory is based on events that have begun by about the third week of embryonic life when the notochord begins to develop. The primitive notochord develops as a proliferation of cells from the ectodermal primitive streak. The narrow column of cells develops into a midline structure that serves to separate the developing yolk sac and the amniotic cavity. By the fourth week of gestation the notochordal plate of the developing embryo migrates dorsally and cleaves off from the endoderm due to the in-growth of the developing mesodermal cells from either side.

Failure of separation of the endoderm can cause the advancing notochord to split. This may cause the developing spinal column to be deficient ventrally and lead onto the vertebral anomalies seen. In association, a rudimentary tract resembling a diverticulum can develop along with the primitive gut. As the embryo continues to grow this tract can remain patent or as in most cases, may close and heal in varying degrees. Rarely, it may persist as a remnant fibrous tract, which could cause mal-rotation in the developing foetus.

Though the dorsal location of the duplications is explained by this theory, the absence of synchronous spinal defects in many of the GI duplications makes this theory less tenable [37] and may suggest a yet undiscovered mechanism as a model for the origin of these duplications.

Emura et al [38] showed that the 'split notochord' theory could explain gastrointestinal duplications, by simulating the partial separation of the developing notochord in *Cynopus pyrrhogaster* embryos which induced these animals to develop gastrointestinal duplications and enteric cysts along with vertebral anomalies, spina bifida, split cord malformations and subcutaneous manifestations.

Twinning

The association of tubular duplications especially that of the terminal ileum and colon with doubling of other body parts has been referred to as *partial* or *abortive twinning* [39,40].The wide spectrum of these complex abnormalities vary from a complete twinning of the lower trunk *(Figure 1a&b)* and limbs [41] to a simple doubling of the hindgut structures. 'Partial twinning' anomalies usually involve anomalies of the urogenital system [42,43] along with the GI tract duplications though associated duplications of the liver and the biliary tract [44-46] have been seen *(Figure 2a&b)*. Though a complete duplication of the colon can open as a fistula into the perineum or into the genitourinary (GU) tract, they can remain quiescent in the abdomen and may be discovered much later [44] or not at all.

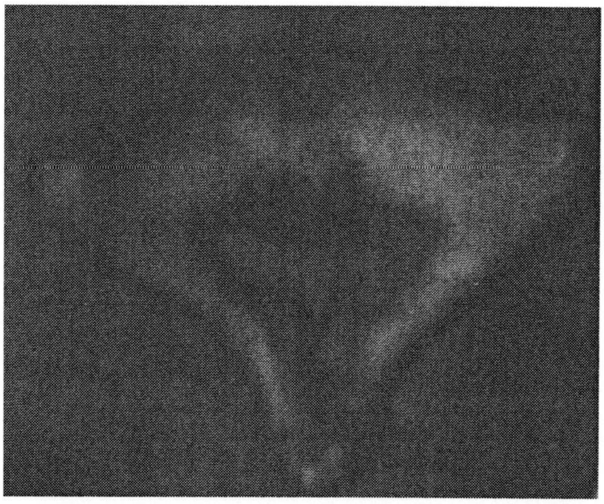

Figure 1 (a): Complete duplication of the lower limbs and genitalia from the first reported case of epigastric heterophagus twinning.

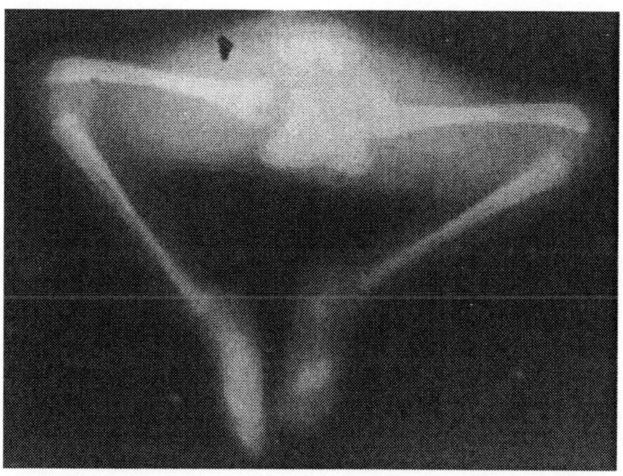

Figure 1 (b). Well formed pelvic and lower limb bones in the detached twin.

Gastric Duplications

Gastric duplications are rare and account for only about 4 to 5 % of all abdominal duplications [47]. These duplications are usually located in close relation to the greater curvature of the stomach but they usually do not communicate with the cavity of the stomach [48]. The incidence of gastric duplications is twice as common in females as in males [49]. Multiple duplications may be present in 15 to 20% of patients [50].

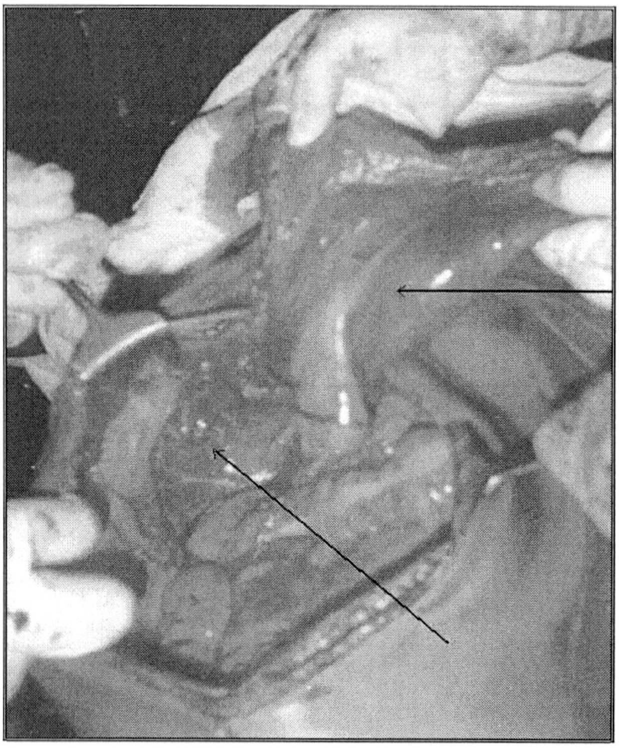

Figure 2 (a). Accessory lobe of the liver in the falciform ligament Arrows point to the accessory lobe and the normal liver.

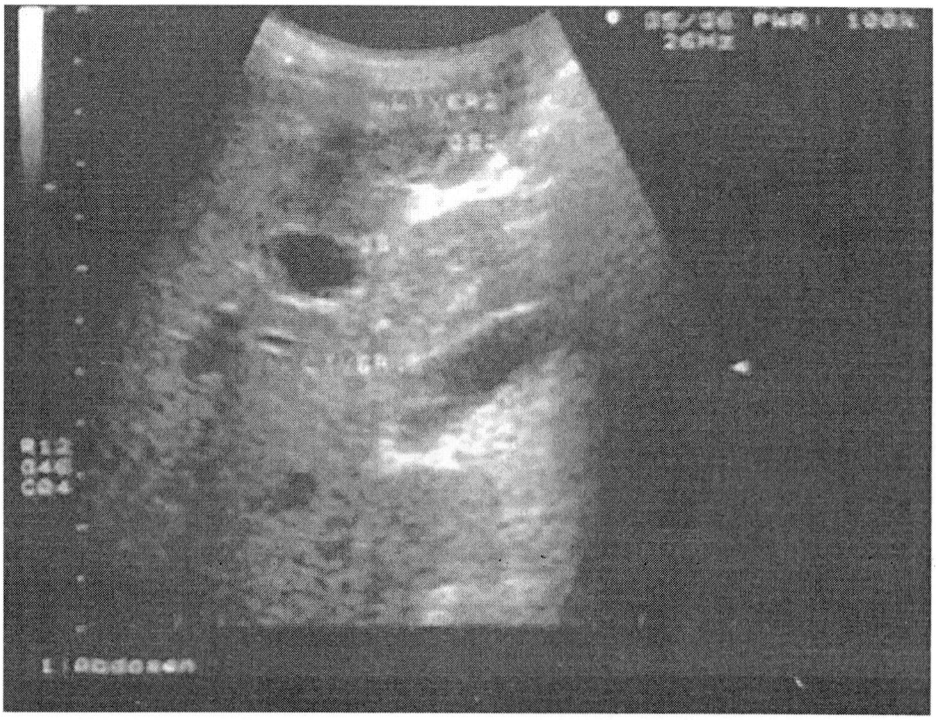

Figure 2 (b). Ultrasonography showing a duplication of the liver and the gall bladder

Although presentation can occur during the neonatal period, gastric duplications become symptomatic in nearly 2/3rd of patients during their first year of life [51]. Rarely, gastric duplications can remain asymptomatic throughout childhood and present later on in adult life. Gastric duplication cysts may present in many ways. The classical presentation in the infant is that of poor feeding and persistent non-bilious vomiting from a gastric outlet obstruction and a palpable epigastric mass which often mimic symptoms due to that of hypertrophic pyloric stenosis [52]. These symptoms can be more pronounced if the duplication involves the pylorus of the stomach [53,54]. Uncommonly, peptic ulceration of the gastric mucosa lining the duplication can cause hemetemesis and melena [13,27] in the presence of a communicating tract whereby the contents of the duplication are discharged into the normal stomach. Poor non-dependent drainage and pooling of the highly acidic secretions can cause severe local inflammation, perforation [18], acute gastro-intestinal haemorrhage [55] or free intra-peritoneal haemorrhage [56]. Ectopic sites of gastric duplications have been reported with the duplication cyst lined by gastric mucosa attached to the pancreas rather than to the stomach [57]. Recurrent pancreatitis can be precipitated by aberrant communications between the gastric duplication and the pancreatic duct which can make it difficult to clinically differentiate these duplications from congenital cysts, pancreatic pseudo cysts or malignant pancreatic cystic tumours [51,58].

Preoperative diagnosis of the duplication can often be difficult. Plain radiographs are usually non-specific. An upper GI contrast study may show evidence of an intramural filling defect indenting the gastric contour or an extrinsic compression along the greater curvature. In the presence of a communication between the cyst and the stomach, retention of the radio-opaque contrast in the duplication cyst may be seen long after the dye has cleared from the GI tract. Though a Tc [99] m pertechnetate scintigraphy can delineate the heterotrophic gastric mucosa, the uptake by the normal stomach lining may mask the delineation of the duplication [18]. The sensitivity for detecting ectopic gastric mucosa by this technique best approaches 85% with best results being seen after pre-treatment with cimetidine or glucagon [59]. In infants the normal gastric uptake of the tracer is low and the clearance of Tc [99] m pertechnetate from the blood can be prolonged due to renal immaturity. Hence, a combination of poor uptake by the gastric mucosa and a high background activity may cause these duplication cysts lined by heterotrophic gastric mucosa to appear photopaenic on initial images. However, a gradual reduction in the background activity due to the slow renal excretion of the tracer dye coupled with an increase in the secretory activity of the stomach may ultimately allow visualisation of the ectopic gastric mucosa on delayed images [13].

In the neonate, abdominal ultrasonography is the imaging modality of choice *(Figure 3).* The presence of a *gut signature sign* [60] or a *double wall sign* [61] caused by the hyper echoic inner mucosal layer and the relatively hypo echoic outer smooth muscle layer can help in identifying these duplications [62]. This is most easily seen in the dependent parts of the cyst [63]. The presence of peristaltic activity in the cyst may aid in the diagnosis [64].

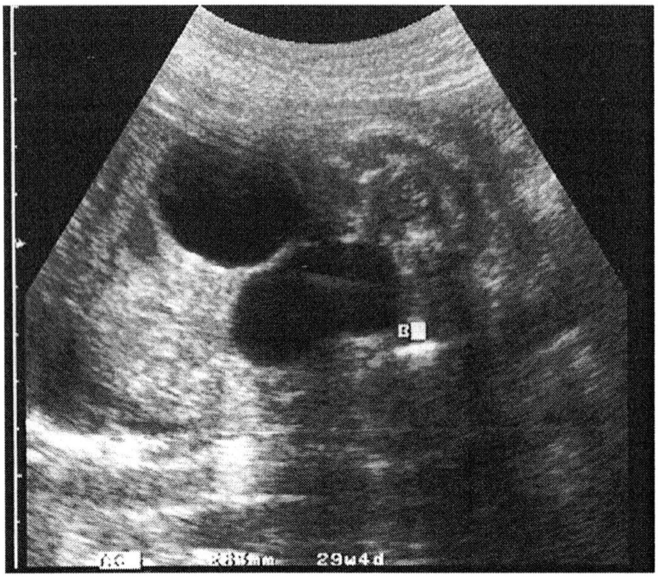

Figure 3. Ultrasonography demonstrating a gastric duplication cyst. An isolated gastric duplication cyst was confirmed and removed later by surgery.

Further use of imaging modalities can help to define the cyst. Endoscopic ultrasonography [65,66] though accurate in diagnosis of duplication cysts is invasive. Computed tomography (CT) scanning helps to delineate the separate wall of these cysts along with their configuration as to whether they are spherical, tubular or very rarely pedunculated [18]. MRI scanning holds promise for assessing duplications due to the high intensity signal generated due to the high water content of these duplication cysts [65] and also the possibility for precise localisation due to multi-planar imaging.

The immature epithelia lining the duplication cyst can, due to over expression of embryonic antigens, trigger the production of onco-fetal antigens. High concentrations of onco-fetal antigen *CA 19-9* alone [67] or in combination with carcino-embryonic antigen (*CEA)* [51] in the contents of gastric duplication cysts have been reported. This can serve to highlight the pre-cancerous potential of long standing gastric duplication cysts though a coexistent carcinoma arising from these cysts is rare with only 5 cases being reported so far [68].

Complications unrelated to the mass effect of the duplication include:

1) Bleeding - either within the lumen of the duplication or into the adjacent GI tract [13,27].
2) Perforation of the duplication [56].
3) Malignant transformation [68].

The most practical approach to the treatment of gastric duplications is a complete surgical excision especially in view of their propensity to produce complications. Surgical complications are related to the size and location of the duplication, communication with the parent gut, the presence of heterotrophic gastric mucosa and the level of involvement of the mesenteric vessels. The intended benefits should be carefully balanced against the peri-operative risks and the hazards of overzealous surgery before embarking on any surgical treatment.

Non-communicating gastric duplication cysts are classically managed by a complete excision. Violation of the gastric luminal cavity should be avoided but if required should be completed by a segmental gastric resection. If the duplication cyst is large and closely adherent to the native bowel, treatment options lie between a cyst excision combined with a gastrectomy or a more favoured partial excision of the duplication cyst along with mucosal stripping of the shared common wall. During surgery, care must be taken to recognize the presence of a common blood supply between the native bowel and the duplication cyst which if missed can potentially lead to major post-operative complications.

Internal drainage procedures of cysto-gastrostomy [13,27] or a Roux-en-Y cysto-jejenostomy [69] helps to avoid a gastrectomy but leaves behind potentially unstable mucosa and in the presence of heterotrophic gastric mucosa in the duplication cyst, increases the risk of secondary ulceration and haemorrhage [70]. Pyloric duplication cysts may be amenable to sub-mucosal excision of the cyst along with a pyloroantrectomy [53,47]. Laparoscopic resection of uncomplicated duplicated cysts has been successfully done [71,72].

Duodenal Duplications

Duodenal duplications are possibly the rarest of all intra-abdominal duplications with less than 100 cases being reported so far. The first case was described by *Sanger* in 1880. The close proximity of these cysts to the biliary and the pancreatic ductal systems makes any surgical intervention a challenge.

The majority of these duplications are cystic and do not communicate with the lumen of the native bowel [73]. However, these cysts are frequently associated with communicating channels extending to the biliary or the pancreatic ductal systems [21,74]. Though these duplications are usually fused to the postero-medial aspect of the second or the third part of the duodenum, they have been reported as extending into the liver or across the diaphragm or arising from the bile ducts or from the pancreas [75-77]. Classical symptoms can be due to a high intestinal obstruction or due to haemorrhage [73], which can be accompanied by pancreatitis or obstructive jaundice [78,79]. Up to fifteen percent of these duplications may contain heterotrophic gastric mucosa and this may predispose the patient to attacks of epigastric pain due to an underlying peptic ulceration or rarely a perforation [80].

In most cases extrinsic compression caused by the duplication on the duodenum is well highlighted by radiographic upper gastro-intestinal studies *(Figure 4)*. The role of ultrasonography as a diagnostic tool has gained importance especially in antenatal screening where a classical two layer pattern [81] may be picked up as early as 15 weeks gestation [82] *(Figure 5 a&b)*. However, in view of the possibility of type 3 choledochal cysts (choledochocoele), congenital pancreatic cysts or pancreatic pseudo cysts as differential diagnosis, it is an advantage to know the spatial orientation of the cyst in relation to the biliary and pancreatic ducts as well as the extent of their 'shared' wall with the duodenum. This is best demonstrated preoperatively by an ERCP [105] or MR cholangiography [77] or intra-operatively by cholangiography [13]. Intra-operative cholangiography or a direct cystogram goes further in helping to rule out aberrant communications between the cyst and the biliary or the pancreatic duct. Rarely a carcinoma can arise inside a duplication cyst and the presence of vegetations or mural nodules in these cysts on imaging should raise concern [83].

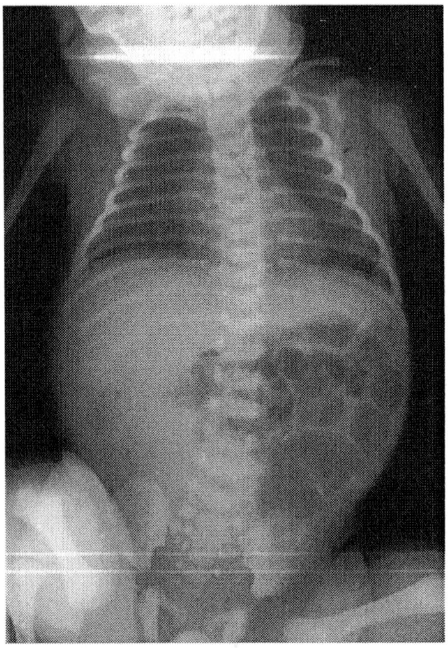

Figure 4. Radiograph of infant showing displacement of the bowel loops to the left by a soft tissue mass. A duodenal duplication cyst was later removed.

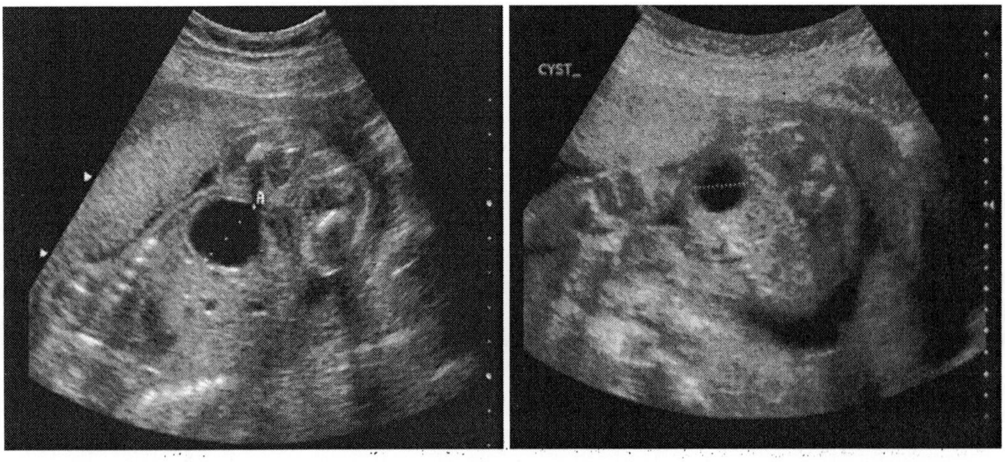

Figure 5 a, b: Second trimester antenatal ultrasonography (2 dimensional views) of a duodenal duplication cyst. Postpartum, the child developed features of intestinal obstruction. At surgery a duodenal duplication cyst was identified and removed.

Complete resection of these cysts remain the preferred treatment though this may not always be possible due to the complexity of the relation that these cysts have with the biliary and the pancreatic ductal systems. *Gardner* and *Hart* [84] in 1935 performed a cysto-duodenostomy for a duodenal duplication cyst, which was subsequently adopted as a standard surgical option for this type of lesion. This gradually evolved into marsupialisation of the cyst along with internal drainage procedures [13,27]. Endoscopic drainage of the cyst has been successfully attempted [85]. Though all these procedures are still done in managing large cysts or when the excision of the cyst could compromise the biliary tree, the detection of rests of ectopic gastric mucosa in these cysts and the recognition of the possible risk for malignant transformation in the cyst mucosa has made a complete or partial excision of the cyst along with a total stripping or excision of the mucosal lining the favoured treatment option [86].

Small Intestinal Duplications

Duplications occur most commonly in the small intestine with nearly 45% being localised to this region [6,13,16,87]. Though a few duplications have been reported in relation to the jejunum, the vast majority lie close to the ileum. Most of these duplications are cystic in nature though they can be tubular as well varying from a few centimetres in length to the entire length of the small bowel which may give the intestine an appearance of attempting to double itself.

These duplications lie on the mesenteric side of the native bowel and share a common source of blood supply with the adjacent bowel. Though the mucosa lining these cysts tends to mimic that of the adjacent intestine, heterotrophic gastric, pancreatic and colonic epithelia can occur, more so in tubular duplications [88]. Cystic duplications usually do not communicate with the lumen of the native intestine while tubular duplications may have communicating tracts with the enteric lumen, either proximally or distally.

Symptoms are caused by the duplication encroaching onto the normal bowel segment and are highly variable and depend on the type, size, location and the type of mucosa lining the duplication. The wide spectrum of symptoms and the presence of non-specific signs frequently simulate other conditions. Presentation can be with features of abdominal mass, distension, pain, vomiting, haemorrhage, melena or rarely perforation [6,27,37,70,89,90]. The incidence of peptic ulceration in small intestinal duplications, specially the tubular varieties, can be as high as 85%. Melena can occur in 20% to30% of the patients with small bowel duplications [6,70].

The perforations may occur either in the duplication itself or in the adjacent normal small intestine which has been exposed to the acid secreted by the heterotrophic gastric mucosa. The presence of communicating tracts, especially proximal ones can cause them to retain secretions. The accumulation of secretions within the closed lumen can cause distension and the weight of the 'loaded' duplication can precipitate mechanical obstruction of the adjacent bowel or rarely a volvulus. These duplications are often difficult to identify preoperatively because they can mimic the clinical symptomatology of acute appendicitis. In patients presenting acutely, the diagnosis of duplication is usually made at laparotomy. Uncommon presentations include intussusception [91] or volvulus [92] or a mobile right iliac fossa mass

[27], which can develop from small cystic duplications acting as lead points. Ileal duplications associated with urinary symptoms [93], with haemorrhagic pseudo-cyst formation [94], complete intestinal malrotation [95], co-existent ileal atresia [25] and tuberculosis of the mesenteric lymph nodes [96] have also been reported.

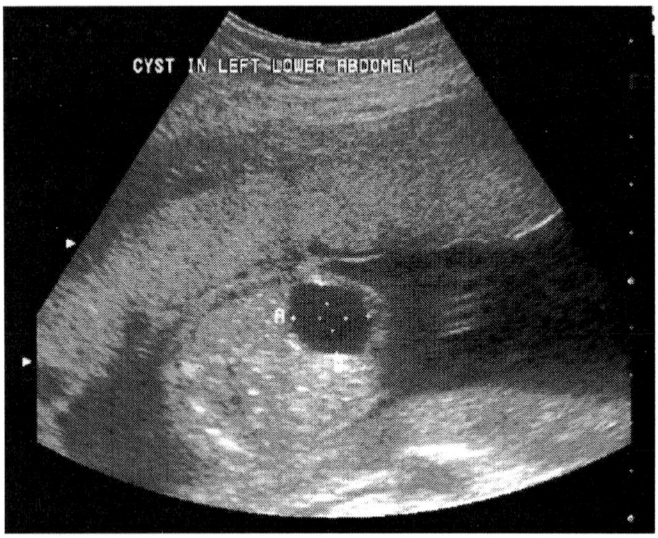

Figure 6. Antenatal ultrasonography showing suspected duplication cyst.

Abdominal radiography may show a non-specific soft-tissue mass within the abdominal cavity. Ultrasonography and barium studies are the most common imaging used to image duplication cysts. CT and MRI are used in difficult cases where a multi-planar approach is required. Ultrasonography is a practical, convenient and simple investigation, which can help to identify duplications *(Figure 6)*. Ultrasonography aids in the prenatal diagnosis and this condition can be suspected pre-natally if an intra-abdominal cystic mass is demonstrated in the second or third trimesters though diagnosis as early as 12 weeks has been reported [97]. Post-natally, Ultrasound scanning can help to differentiate a duplication cyst from a mesenteric cyst but may be of limited value in the presence of a co-existing perforation or bowel obstruction. At scanning, duplication cysts typically demonstrate a "*double layer sign*" which consists of an echogenic inner mucosal layer and a hyper echoic outer muscular layer. This appearance is usually not circumferential and the layers may vary in thickness but this classical feature is seen in over 50% of cases [62]. Radiographic contrast examination can show an extrinsic mass and in the presence of communicating tracts, contrast material may gain access and outline the duplication. A partially obstructed duplication cyst may simulate an intussusception on barium enema examination [98]. A Tc [99] m pertechnetate scintigraphy can be used preoperatively to identify the presence of ectopic gastric mucosa if a patient presents with melena but it may not help to distinguish between duplication and a *Meckel's* diverticulum, both of which may contain ectopic gastric mucosa. Intra-operatively, Tc [99] m pertechnetate scintigraphy can help to assess completeness of removal of all the involved mucosa [64].

Management depends on the type of these duplications. Total excision of the duplication without compromising the normal bowel, remains the treatment of choice. Cystic duplications are well demarcated and it may be possible for these to be enucleated or "shelled out"*(Figure 7)*. However, management of tubular duplications is more complicated due to sharing of a common blood supply with the adjacent bowel and due to their relatively long length.

Surgery for these duplications has evolved over the years. *Wrenn* [99] in1962 suggested a complete mucosal stripping through multiple sequential sero-muscular incisions in the wall of the duplication as a technique for managing long tubular duplications associated with heterotrophic gastric epithelium. Care must be taken to ensure that no residual mucosa is left behind as this could act as a source for the cyst to regenerate. *Schwartz* [100] in 1980 suggested that the presence of a plane of cleavage that occasionally exists between the duplication and the adjacent normal small intestine could be exploited to permit resection of the duplication without compromising the vascularity of the normal gut. *Norris et al* [101] in 1986 adopted the *Bianchi* [102] techniques used for lengthening the bowel in treating duplications. The two leaves of the mesentery were separated and the duplication was removed after carefully preserving the posterior arterial arcade to the normal gut. However it may be difficult to access the plane of cleavage or to separate the mesentery especially in the presence of a co-existent perforation or intestinal obstruction. When separation becomes difficult, techniques of mucosal stripping becomes useful in treating the duplication and at the same time eliminating the possibility of a subsequent peptic ulceration or a malignant degeneration of the epithelium.

A portion of the native bowel can be resected along with the duplication, especially if there is compromise of the vascular supply of the bowel with the resected ends being rejoined through a primary anastamosis [69]. However, if this would result in the major part of the small bowel being removed, which would lead onto a 'short bowel' syndrome in the patient, then a partial resection must be opted for [69]. Rarely, it may be possible for large ileal duplications to be dissected free from the adjacent small bowel without a combined intestinal resection anastamosis and without comprimising the viability of the bowel [95]. *Jewett et al* [103] performed a localised partial resection of an ulcerated segment of a long tubular duplication and completed the procedure by draining the closed distal end of the duplication into the stomach. This patient was reported to be asymptomatic after a 25-year follow up.

Duplications that cannot be resected can be drained into a Roux-en Y limb or into the adjacent intestine in the absence of heterotrophic epithelia. *Bishop* and *Koop* [69] described several such techniques for free drainage of the duplication by anastamosing the distal end of the duplication to the adjacent normal intestine.

Allowing the mucosa of the duplication to remain can pose the risk of developing complications of bleeding and peptic ulceration from undetected gastric epithelium or a gradual malignant degeneration of the unstable epithelium [104]. Malignancy developing in ileal duplication cysts is uncommon with adenocarcinomas forming the majority. Prognosis should remain guarded especially in the presence of involved lymph nodes.

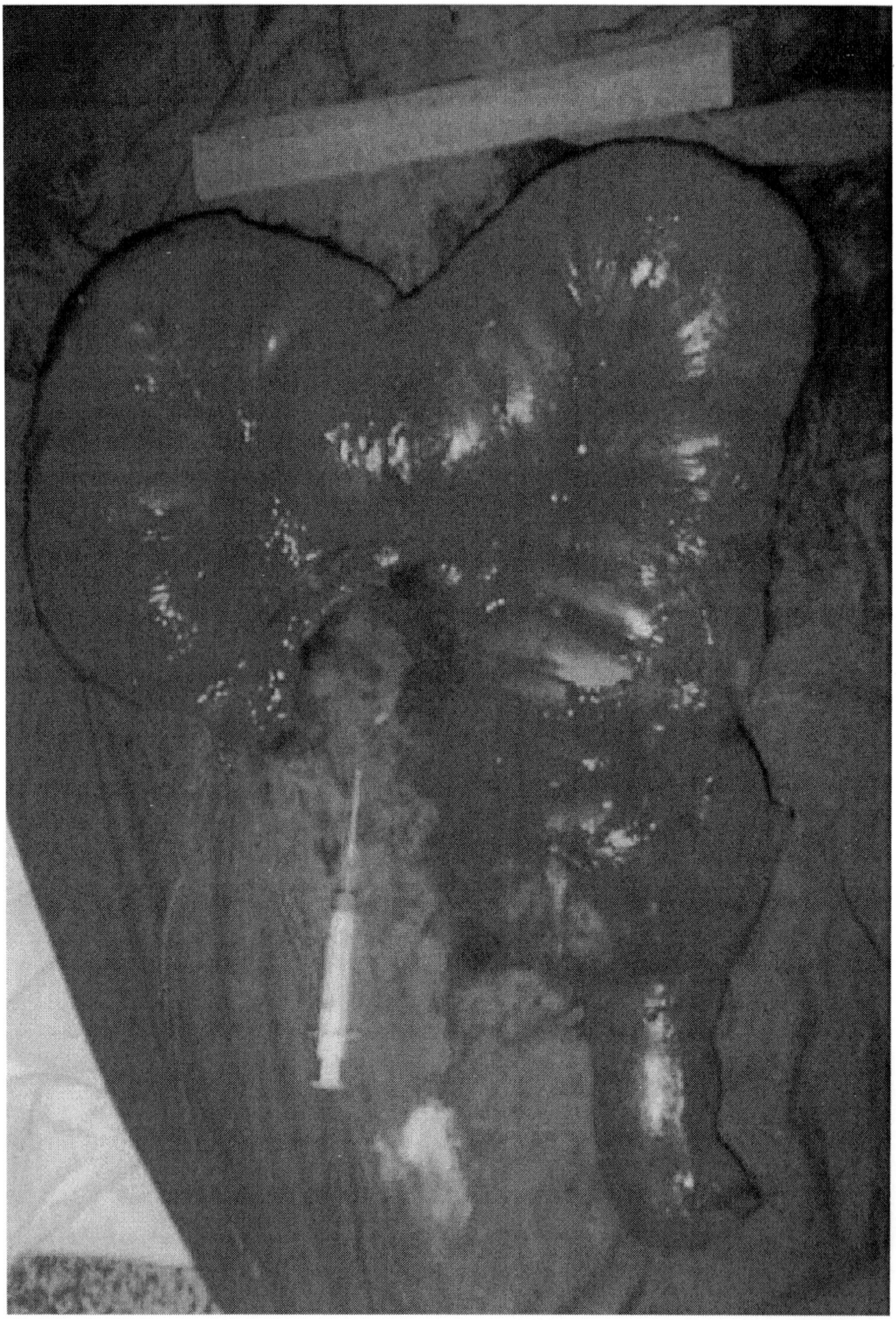

Figure 7. A complete duplication of the large bowel from the caecum (complete with its appendix) to the rectum- both blindly ending. The loop was distended with straw coloured fluid –which is seen aspirated in the syringe. The duplication was enucleated in-toto.

DUPLICATIONS OF THE APPENDIX

Duplication of the vermiform appendix is rare and occurs in 1 / 25,000 patients (0.004%) who are operated for acute appendicitis [106]. Appendiceal anomalies are of great practical importance and must be borne in mind at the time of surgery. Overlooking this condition can cause serious clinical and medico-legal issues [107] to be raised especially if at a later date, a second explorative laparotomy reveals a "previously removed" vermiform appendix.

The duplicated appendix can remain asymptomatic and may be picked up only incidentally during laparotomy performed for other reasons [108,109]. When appendiceal duplications are detected in childhood, the patients can have serious associated intestinal, genito-urinary or vertebral malformations. The appendiceal duplication can be associated with duplication of the colon, urinary system and external genitalia [110]. Rarely both the appendices can get inflamed [106] or the duplication can perforate and present with features of an acute abdomen111. Malignant foci can develop within a duplicated appendix [112].

The classification system for appendiceal duplications was first developed by *Cave* in 1936 [113], then modified by *Wallbridge* in 1962 [114] and finally by *Biermann* in 1993 [115].

Appendiceal duplications were classified into three types; A, B, and C:

Type A: occurs when both the appendices arise from a common base on the single caecum. This type is not usually associated with other congenital anomalies.

Type B: two separate appendices with distinct bases arising from common caecum.

Type C: two caecal structures, each with its own single appendix.

Types B and C can be associated with other gastrointestinal and genitourinary anomalies [107].

If the asymptomatic duplication is discovered when exploring for an acute appendicitis, it is advisable to remove both the appendices together so as to avoid diagnostic confusion that may arise if only the inflamed appendix is removed with the normal duplication being left behind in the abdomen. However, if the silent duplication is detected on investigation for another independent condition, the patient need not be subjected to an appendicectomy [116].

DUPLICATIONS OF THE COLON

Colonic duplications are among the least common of all GI duplications and form 15-18% of all the GI duplications [13,117]. Less than 100 cases have been reported so far in literature. Despite their rarity, these lesions tend to be the most complex and challenging. The colonic duplications most commonly involve the caecum and least commonly the transverse colon. Duplication of the hindgut, when discovered, should raise suspicion of a co-existent abnormality of the genitourinary (GU) tract. Rarely the patient may have a duplication of the entire urinary tract along with genital and bowel duplication [110].

These duplications can be either cystic or tubular. Cystic duplications can occur as isolated cysts or as cysts that communicate to the perineum through an external fistula, to the urinary tract through an internal fistula or to the adjacent colon [118,119].

Tubular duplications of the colon can occur as an isolated event but usually occur as a part of 'twinning' conditions with the patient having co-existent duplications of the anus, vagina and the penis [42,118]. The colons are usually fused and there may be the presence of two well developed penises in the male or two well developed vaginas each with an associated clitoris and labia in the female patient. Many of these patients have associated meningo-myeloceles and vertebral defects.

Kottra and *Dodds* [118] classified colonic duplications into 2 main groups *(Table 1 & Figure 8):*

Type 1 duplications are limited to the alimentary tract and localised to above the line of peritoneal reflection. These duplications can either be cystic (Type 1-a) or tubular (Type 1-b) or of a complex double-barrelled configuration with multiple tracts communicating with the adjacent normal colon (Type 1-c). This type of duplication can have associated ileal duplications or multiple duplications of the large bowel itself.

Type 2 duplications are associated with co-existent duplications of the genito-urinary tract, which can be quite complex in nature. This group of duplications include those with double genitalia and double urethra and bladder (Type II-a) or those with a fistula between the duplication and the genitor-urinary tract (Type II-b) or those duplications that present with an imperforate anus (Type II-c).

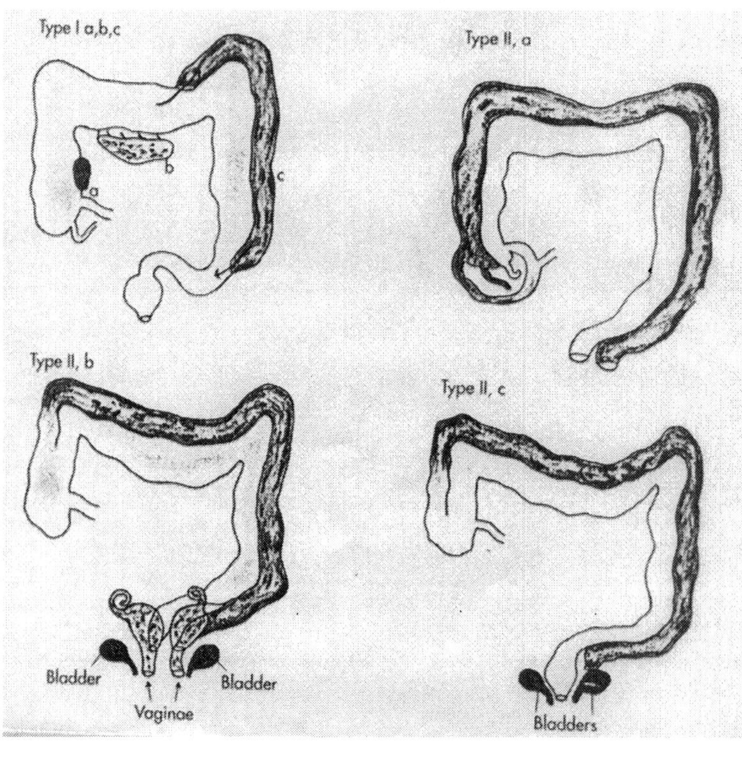

Figure 8.

Table 1.

CLASSIFICATION OF COLON DUPLICATIONS

Type I Duplication limited to alimentary tract (frequently asymptomatic)

a. Spherical(cystic)
b. Tubular
c. Double Barreled; one or more communications with colon

1. Limited to colon
2. Associated ileal duplication

d. Loop duplication;* separate mesentery and blood supply
e. Multiple duplications; combinations of a, b and c

Type II Colon duplication (usually double barreled) associated with duplications of the urinary or genital tracts (frequently symptomatic)

a. Two separate perineal Ani
1. Ani nearly always lie on either side of midline
2. Associated with double genitals and double urethra or bladder
3. Patients are continent and without symptoms, complaints limited to cosmetic disfiguration

b. Fistulas; the distal portion of one or both duplicates has a fistulous connection with another hollow viscus

1. Most with double genitals, some with lower urinary tract duplications
2. Symptoms related to the fistula or obstruction from inadequate drainage
3. Surgery usually successful

c. Imperforate anus; one or both rectums imperforate in the pelvis, no fistulas

1. All with duplications of the lower urinary tract, genitals usually single
2. Symptoms of obstruction
3. Operative results poor

* To date, reported only in the small bowel.

Clinical symptoms of hindgut duplications can be varied with a wide spectrum of symptoms both in type I and type II colonic duplications. They can remain asymptomatic for quite long periods of time [44,120]. Patients with type II duplications that are asymptomatic may present due to cosmetic problems.

Indications for surgical intervention arise when the patient becomes symptomatic or in the background of an acute setting. When symptomatic they can present with non-specific symptoms including vomiting, diarrhoea, constipation, melena or abdominal distension [93,119]. Specifically patients with a previously undetected duplication can present in the setting of an acute intestinal obstruction or bowel perforation or rarely gastrointestinal hemorrhage [44,93,121-123]. The incidence of heterotrophic mucosa in colonic duplications is much lower than in other locations and the colonic mucosa is inherently more resistant to acid erosion than mucosa in other locations [119]. Even if encountered incidentally, these lesions are better addressed surgically as they can cause complications at a future date including the rare possibility of a malignant degeneration of the colonic epithelium [13,104,124].

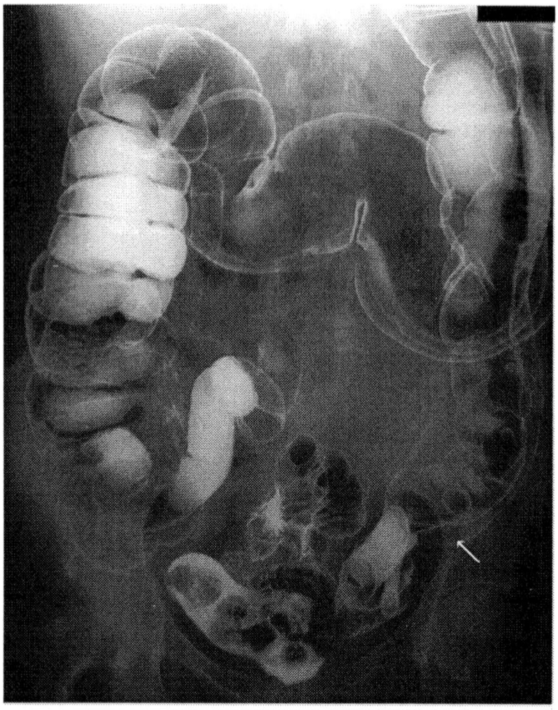

Figure 9. A type 1-c complete tubular duplication of the colon. Barium contrast enema shows the normal colon in the background of the duplicated segment. The duplicated segment stops short of the peritoneal reflection.

A preoperative diagnosis of colonic duplication is often difficult and in the presence of non-specific symptoms these duplications are often confused with other more common diagnoses. The complexity and the associations with malformations in other organ systems warrant a full investigation of both the gastro-intestinal and the genito-urinary tracts before embarking on any surgical treatment. Plain X-rays of the chest and abdomen because of the relative non-specificity may not provide sufficient evidence to reach a preoperative diagnosis. Barium enemas along with post-evacuation films may help in diagnosing colonic duplications pre-operatively. Radiologically the dilated colon may mimic a mega colon [125]. Contrast enemas can also help to demonstrate the presence of communications between the duplication and the normal colon [13,118]. Ultrasonography is a simple, practical and common investigation that may often help to establish a pre-operative diagnosis [126]. Computed tomography of the abdomen goes a step further in helping to identify and evaluate synchronous lesions once a single duplication has been identified [5,13]. About 40% of cystic colonic duplications involve the caecum and may show imaging features that resemble that of small bowel duplications.

Though the treatment can vary depending on the type of the duplication and the presenting symptoms, surgery remains essentially the treatment of choice in type I duplications. This usually includes complete resection of the duplication cyst along with a margin of the adjacent normal large bowel, the normal bowel being removed due to the intimate attachment or the sharing of a common wall between the two or due to the possibility of compromising the blood flow to the normal bowel following the isolated resection of the duplication1 [23,127]. In patients with long tubular duplications, the above procedure of cyst excision may cause the patient to develop a short bowel syndrome [13]. Colonic duplications found incidentally during routine checks can be managed conservatively if colonoscopy can demonstrate the presence of good communicating tracts to drain the duplication into the normal adjacent colon and the presence of normal colonic mucosa in the duplicated segment [120].

Small isolated cystic type I-a or I-b colonic duplications can be excised without an associated colonic resection [13]. In some cases of type I-c duplications (*Figure 9*), which feature both proximal and distal communications between the duplication and the normal colon, symptoms can be relieved non-operatively by a combination of stool softeners, enemas and dietary modifications [118]. If the symptoms persist, enlarging existing communicating tracts between the duplication and the normal colon [128] or excision of the common wall [69] may relieve symptoms by providing an internal drainage for the collected secretions. An alternative approach is to marsupialize the cyst by doing a partial cystectomy and combining this with a mucosal stripping of the remaining cyst wall [13,129].

Management of type II colonic duplications is more complex due to the nature of the multiple organ systems involved. Patients can be asymptomatic from the duplication and may present requiring treatment for cosmetic problems caused by the duplicated external genitalia [43]. The aim for surgery is to have both the colon and the duplicated segment draining through a single anal orifice. If the normal colon reaches the perineum, then the duplicated segment can be connected to the normal colon by dividing the septum to convert it into one large common colonic channel [130] or a side-to-side anastamosis between the colon and the duplication [128,131] .If the duplicated segment also reaches the perineum, the rectum belonging to the duplication can be transected with the proximal end being anastamosed to the normal colon. The distal end however, remains as a blind sac which can discharge small amounts of mucus through its ectopic opening into the vagina, urethra or as a peri-anal sinus [130]. If the volumes of secretions are large, they can be channelled into the normal rectum or anal canal by excising the in-between common septum. If neither the normal colon nor the duplication reaches the perineum then a formal pull-through procedure may be required. Though mucosal stripping of the duplication is ideal, it may not be necessary to excise the mucosa of the duplication if there is free drainage of the contents of the duplication into the normal colon [128]. Recto-vaginal or recto-urethral fistulas, which are typically seen in type II-b duplications can be closed using a vaginal approach [132] or by a peritoneal approach [133].

Treatment of the associated genitourinary anomalies has to be individualised with urinary and faecal continence being given priority [110]. Doubling of the genitalia can be corrected by excising the duplication primarily for cosmesis though reports of function of both vaginas and subsequent delivery through both, in a patient with double vagina has been reported [39].

ACKNOWLEDGEMENTS

Dr E Morris, Department of Radiology, Torbay DGH.

Dr P Stannard, Department of Obstetrics and Gynaecology, Torbay DGH.

Ms G Pandher, Department of Obstetrics and Gynaecology, Torbay DGH

REFERENCES

[1] Calder J: *Medical Essays Obser 1*:205,1733.

[2] Gross RE: Duplications of the alimentary tract. In *The surgery of infancy and childhood*. Philadelphia, 1953, W B Saunders.

[3] Ladd WE : Duplications of the alimentary tract. *South Med J.30*:363,1937.

[4] Ladd WE, Gross RE .Surgical treatment of duplications of the alimentary tract. *Surg Gynec Obstet*.1940; 70:295-307.

[5] O'Neil J, Rowe M. Duplications of the gastrointestinal tract. In: Essentials of Paediatric Surgery. St Louis, Mo. *Mosby Yearbook*.1995:520-5.

[6] Bower RJ, Sieber WK, Kiesewetter WB. Alimentary tract duplications in children. *Ann Surg*.1977; 188:669-74.

[7] Wrenn E. Alimentary tract duplications. In: Holder T, Ashcraft K, editors. *Paediatric Surgery*. Philadelphia: WB Saunders, 1992; 455-6 .

[8] Rios-Dalenz JC, Kress JW, Montgomery CG. Duplication of the small intestine with perforated ulcer in ectopic gastric mucosa. *Arch Surg*.1965; 91:863-8 .

[9] Newmar KH, Ching G, Halls G. Bleeding peptic ulcer caused by ectopic gastric mucosa in a duplicated segment of ileum. *Am J Gastroenterol*.1981; 75:158-62.

[10] Collins CD. Perforation of peptic ulceration in duplicated ileum. *Br J Surg*. 1972; 59:159-60.

[11] Kumar R, Tripathi M, Chandrasekhar N, Agarwala S, Kumar A, Malhotra A. Diagnosis of ectopic gastric mucosa using ^{99} Tc^{m}-pertechnetate:spectrum of scintigraphic findings. *Br J Radiol*. 2005; 78:714-20.

[12] Lecouffe P, Spyckerelle C, Venel H *et al*. Use of Tc 99 m –pertechnetate for abdominal scanning in localising an ileal duplication cyst: case report and review of literature. *Eur J Nucl Med*. 1992; 19:65-67.

[13] Holocomb GW III, Gheisser A,O"Neill J *et al* .Surgical management of alimentary tract duplications. *Ann Surg*. 1989; 209(2):167-174.

[14] Fortiadis C, Genetzakis M, Papandreou I *et al*. Colonic duplication in adults: report of two cases presenting with rectal bleeding. *World J Gastroenterol*. 2005; 11(32):5072-5074.

[15] Sieber WK. Alimentary tract duplication. *Arch Surg*. 1956; 73:383.

[16] Basu R, Forshall I, RickhamPP. Duplication of the alimentary tract. *Br J Surg*.1960; 47:477.

[17] Favara BE, Franciose RA, Akers DR. Enteric duplications: 37 cases- a vascular theory of pathogenisis. *Am J Dis Child*. 1971; 122:501.

[18] Kremer RM, Kepoff RB, Izant RJ. Duplication of the stomach. *J Pediatr Surg*. 1970; 5:360-4.

[19] Carachi R. The split notochord syndrome: a case report on a mixed spinal enterogenous cyst in a child with spina bifida cystica. *Z Kinder*. 1982; 35:32-34.

[20] Paddock RJ, Arensman RM. Polysplenic syndrome: spectrum of gastro-intestinal anomalies. *J Pediatr Surg*. 1982; 17:563-6.

[21] Luoma R, Raboei E. Duodenal duplication with pancreas bifidum-a case report. *Eur J Pediatr Surg*. 2001; 11(1):55-7.

[22] Lister J, Zachary RB. Cystic duplication of the tongue. *J Pediatr Surg*. 1968;3: 491-3.

[23] Swartz DL,Procaccino A, Becker M *et al.* Segmented colonic duplication presenting as a sigmoid volvulus.*Z Kinder*. 1983;38: 338-340.

[24] Wang Jun, Chengren S, Shiyao YU, Yan WU, Changui XU. A rare association of rectal and genitourinary duplication and ano-rectal malformation. *Chin Med J*. 2003; 116(12):1955-1957.

[25] Ratan SK, Rattan KN, Singh S, Marwah N. Ileal duplication cyst associated with type-3 ileal atresia: report of a case. *Surg Today*. 2004; 34(4):363-5.

[26] Galvez Y, Skaba R, Kalousova J, Rouskova B, Hribal Z, Znajdauf J. Alimentary tract duplications in children: high incidence of associated anomalies. *Eur J Pediatr Surg*. 2004; 14(2):79-84.

[27] Stringer MD, Spitz L, Abel R *et al.* Management of alimentary tract duplication in children. *Br J Surg*. 1995; 82:74-78.

[28] Potter EL. *Pathology of the foetus and newborn*. Chicago, 1961, Year Book Publishers.

[29] Keibel F. Zur Embyrologie des Menschen, der Affen und der halbaffen. *Anat Anz*. 27(suppl):39, 1905.

[30] Lewis F.T, Thyng F.W. The regular occurrence of intestinal diverticula in embryos of the pig, rabbit and man. *Am J Anat*. 7:505, 1907-1908.

[31] Bremer JL. Diverticula and duplications of the intestinal tract. *Arch Path*. 1944; 38:132-40.

[32] Sandler J. Zur Entwicklung des Menschilichen oudenums in Fruhen Embryonalstadium. *Morph J*. 1902; 29:187.

[33] Mellish RWP, Koop CE. Clinical manifestations of duplications of the bowel. *Pediatrics*. 1961; 27:397-407.1959; 25:209.

[34] Louw JH. Congenital atresia and stenosis in the newborn. *Ann Roy Coll Surg Engl*. 1959; 25:209.

[35] Saunders RL. Combined anterior and posterior spina bifida in a living neonatal human female. *Anat Rec*. 1943; 87:255-75.

[36] Bentley JFR, Smith JR. developmental posterior enteric remnants and spinal malformations. *Arch Dis Child*. 1960; 35: 76-86.

[37] Iyer CP, Mahour GH. Duplications of the alimentary tract in infants and children. *J Pediatr Surg*. 1995; 30:1267-70.

[38] Emura T, Hashizume K, Asashima M. Experimental study of the embryogenesis of gastrointestinal duplication and enteric cysts. *Pediatr Surg Int*. 2003; 19(3):147-51.

[39] Beach PD, Brascho J, Hein WR et al. Duplications of the primitive hindgut of the human being. *Surgery*. 1961; 49:779-85.

[40] Ravitch MM. Hindgut duplications; doubling of the colon and genital tracts. *Ann Surg*. 1953; 137:294.

[41] Surendran N, Mani Nainan K, Paulose MO. An unusual case of caudal duplication. *J Pediatr Surg* 1986; 21:924.

[42] O"Neill J A Jr, Holocomb GW III, Schnaufer L *et al.* Surgical experience with thirteen conjoint twins. *Am. Surg.* 1988; 208:299.

[43] Smith ED, Stephens FD. Duplication and vesico-intestinal fissure. *Birth defects: original article series.*1988; 24:551.

[44] George AT, S Varkey, A Kalam and N Surendran. Left over bowels: an unique complication in a surviving twin. *Post Grad Journal.* 2004; 80:736-7.

[45] Spitz L, Crabbe DC, Kiely EM. Seperation of thoraco-omphalopagus conjoint twins with complex hepato-biliary anatomy. *J Pediatr Surg.* 1997; 32:787– 9.

[46] Lobe TE, Oldham KT, Richardson CJ. Successful separation of a conjoined biliary tract in a set of omphalopagus twins. *J Pediatr Surg.* 1989; 24:930–2.

[47] Heiss K. Intestinal Duplications. In Oldham KT, Colombani PM and Foglia RP (eds): *Surgery of Infants and Children: Scientific Principles and Practice.* Philadelphia, PA, Lippincott-Raven, 1997, pp 1265-1274.

[48] Kremer RM, Kepoff RB, Izant RJ Jr. Duplication of the stomach. *J Pediatr Surg.* 1970; 5:360.

[49] Dudgeon DL. Lesions of the stomach. In: Ashcraft, Holder (Eds) *Paediatric Surgery,* 2nd ed. Chap 1993;24:295-7.

[50] Segal SR, Sherman NH, Rosenberg HK *et al.* Ultrasonographic features of gastrointestinal duplications. *J Ultrasound Med.* 1994; 13:863-870.

[51] Journo XBD, Moutardier V, Turrini O, Guiramand B *et al.* Gastric duplication in an adult mimicking mucinous cystadenoma of the pancreas. *J Clin Pathol.* 2004; 57:1215-18.

[52] Alschibaja T, Putram TC, Yabhin BA. Duplication of the stomach simulating hypertyrophic stenosis. *Am J Dis Child.* 1974; 127:120-2.

[53] Shah A, More B, Buick R. Pyloric duplication in a neonate: a rare entity. *Pediatr Surg Int.* 2005; 21(3):220-2.

[54] Patel MP, Meisheri IV, Waingankar VS *et al.* Duplication cyst of the pylorus- a rare cause of gastric outlet obstruction in the newborn. *J Postgrad Med.* 1997; 43:43-5.

[55] Barley DM, Wienberg G. Acute gastrointestinal hemorrhage in infancy from gastric duplication: imaging findings. *Emerg Radiol.* 2004; 10(4):204-6.

[56] Kleinhaus S, Boley SJ, Winslow P. Occult bleeding from a perforated gastric duplication in a infant. *Arch Surg.* 1981; 116:122.

[57] Soudarajan S, Subramaniam TK. Gastro-pancreatic duplications. *Pediatr Surg Int.* 1988; 3:288.

[58] Glaser C, Kuzinkovas V, Maurer C *et al.* A large duplication cyst of the stomach in an adult presenting as pancreatic pseudocyst. *Dig Surg.* 1998; 15:703-6.

[59] Seibert JJ, Williamson SL. Gastrointestinal scintigraphy, In Miller J, Gelfand M (eds): *Paediatric Nuclear Imaging*, Philadelphia, PA, Saunders, 1994, pp 157-194.

[60] Azzie G, Beasley S. Diagnosis and treatment of foregut duplications. *Seminars Pediatr Surg.* 2003; 12(1):46-54.

[61] Gupta AK, Guglani B. Imaging of congenital anomalies of the gastrointestinal tract. *Indian J Pediatr.* 2005; 72(5):403-414.

[62] Barr LL, Hayden CK, Stanberry SD *et al.* Enteric duplication cysts in children. Are their ultrasonographic wall characteristic diagnosis? *Pediatr Radiol.* 1990; 20:326-28.

[63] Khong PL, Cheung SCW, Leong LLY, Ooi CGC. Ultrasonography of intraabdominal cystic lesions in the newborn.*Clin Radiol.* 2003; 58:449-54.

[64] Dittrich JR, Spottswood SE, Jolles PR. Gastric duplication cyst. Scintigraphy and co-relative imaging. *Clin Nucl Med.* 1997; 22:93-96.

[65] Geller A, Wang KK, Dimango EP. Diagnosis of foregut duplication cysts by endoscopic ultrasonography. *Gastroenterol.* 1995; 109:838-42.

[66] Takahara T, Torigoe T, Haga H *et al.* Gastric duplication cyst. Evaluation by endoscopic ultrasonography and magnetic resonance imaging. *J Gastroenterol.* 1996; 31:420-24.

[67] Ikehata A, Sakuma T. Gastric duplication cyst with markedly elevated concentration of carbohydrate antigen 19-9. *Am J Gastroenterol.* 2000; 95:842-43.

[68] Kuraoka K, Nakayama H, Kagawa T *et al.* Adeno carcinoma arising from a gastric duplication cyst with invasion to the stomach: a case report with literature review. *J Clin Pathol.* 2004; 57:428-31.

[69] Bishop HC, Koop CE. Surgical management of duplications of the alimentary tract. *Am J Surg.* 1964; 107:434-42.

[70] Lldstad ST, Tollerud DJ, Weiss RG *et al.* Duplications of the alimentary tract. Clinical characteristics, preferred treatment and associated malformations. *Ann Surg.* 1988; 208:184-9.

[71] Tayar C, Brunetti F, Tantawi B *et al.* Laparoscopic resection of an adult gastric duplication cyst. *Ann Chir.* 2003; 128(2):105-8.

[72] Machado MA, Santos VR, Martino RB *et al.* Laparoscopic resection of gastric duplication: sucessful treatment of a are entity. *Surg Laparosc Endosc Percutan Tech.* 2003; 13(4): 268-70.

[73] Leenders EL, Osman MZ, Sakarochana K. Treatment of duodenal duplication with international review. *Am Surg.* 1970; 36:368.

[74] Prasad TR, Tan CE. Duodenal duplication cyst communicating with an aberrant pancreatic duct. *Pediatr Surg Int.* 2005; 21(4):320-2.

[75] Sonoda N, Takaya J, Okamoto K *et al.* Transdiaphragmatic duodenal duplication in a premature infant. *J Pediatr Surg.* 1987; 22:372.

[76] Akers DR, Favara BE, Franciosi RA *et al.* Duplications of the alimentary tract: report of three unusual cases associated with bile and pancreatic ducts.*Surgery.* 1972; 71:817.

[77] Okuyama H, MatsuoY, Fukui Y *et al.* Intrapancreatic duodenal duplication associated with pancreatic pseudocysts. *J Pediatr Surg.* 1992; 27:1573-4.

[78] Lavine JE, Harrison M, Heyman MB. Gastrointestinal duplication causing relapsing pancreatitis in children. *Gastroenterology.* 1989; 97:1556.

[79] Neihues R, Dietl KH, Betterdorf O *et al.* Duodenal duplication cyst mimicking pancreatic cyst in a patient with pancreatitis. *Gastrointest Endosc.* 2005; 62(1):190-92.

[80] Dickinson E, Weinberg SM, Vellios F. Perforating ulcer in a duodenal duplication. *Am J Surg.* 1971; 122:418.

[81] Deftereos S, Soultanidis H, Limas C *et al.* Duodenal duplication. Is Ultrasound appearance enough to confirm the diagnosis? *Rom J Gastroenterol.* 2004; 13(4):345-7.

[82] Borgnon J, Durand C, Gourlaouen D, Sagot P, Sapin E. Antenatal detection of a communicating duodenal duplication. *Eur J Pediatr Surg.* 2003; 13(2):130-3.

[83] Rice CA, Anderson TM, Sepahdari S. Computed Tomography and ultrasonography of carcinoma in duplication cysts. *J Comput Assist Tomogr*. 1986; 10:233-235.

[84] Gardner CE Jr, Hart D. Enterogenous cysts of the duodenum. *JAMA*. 1935;104:1809.

[85] Al Traif I, Khan MH. Endoscopic drainage of a duodenal duplication cyst. *Gastrointest Endosc*. 1992; 38(1):64-65.

[86] Raffensperger JG. Alimentary tract duplication. In: *Swenson's Paediatric Surgery*. 5th edn. CT: Appleton and Lange, 1990:579-85.

[87] Grosfeld JL, O"Neill JA, Clatworthy H W. Enteric duplications in infancy and childhood: an 18-year review. *Ann Surg*. 1970; 172:83.

[88] Wardell S, Vidican DE. Ileal duplication causing massive bleeding in a child.*J Clin Gastroenterol*. 1991; 12:681-4.

[89] Royle SG, Doig CM. Perforation of the jejunum secondary to a duplication cyst lined by ectopic gastric mucosa. *J Pediatr Surg*. 1988; 23:1025-6.

[90] Castro-Castaneda S, Chavez-Delgado ME, Cerda-Camacho F. Severe hemorrhage intestinal in a child with ileal duplication and brief entity review. *Cir Pediatr*.2005; 18(3):142-7.

[91] Daniss RK, Graviss ER. Jejunal intraluminal diverticular duplication with recurrent intussusception. *J Pediatr Surg*. 1982; 17:84-5.

[92] Howanietz C, Lachmann D, Remes I. Volvulus as a rare complication of enterogenous cyst in newborns.*Z Kinderchir*. 1969; 6:48.

[93] Otter MI, Marks CG, Cook MG. An unusual presentation of intestinal duplication with a literature review. *Dig Dis Sci*. 1996; 41(3):627-9.

[94] Hwang IK, Namkung S, Kim BS *et al*. Perforated ileal duplication cyst with haemorrhagic pseudocyst formation. *Pediatr Radiol*. 2003; 33(7):489-91.

[95] Balen EM, Hernandez-Lizoain JL, Pardo F *et al*. Giant jejuno-ileal duplication: prenatal diagnosis and complete excision without intestinal resection. *J Pediatr Surg*. 1993; 28(12):1586-8.

[96] Punjani RM. An unusual case of intestinal duplication. *Indian J Surg*. 2003; 65:187-9.

[97] Chen M, Lam YH, Lin CH *et al*. Sonographic features of ileal duplication duplication cyst at 12 weeks. *Prenat Diagn*. 2002; 22(12):1067-70.

[98] Sonoda N, Matsuzaki S, Ono A *et al*. Duplication of the caecum in a neonate simulating intussusception. *Pediatr Radiol*. 1985; 15:427-428.

[99] Wrenn EL. Tubular duplications of the small intestine.*Surgery*. 1962; 52:494.

[100] Schwartz DL *et al*. Tubular duplication with autonomous blood supply: resection with preservation of adjacent bowel. *J Pediatr Surg*. 1980; 15:341.

[101] Norris RW, Brereton RJ, Wright VM *et al*. A new surgical approach to duplications of the small intestine. *J Pediatr Surg*. 1986; 21(2):167-70.

[102] Bianchi A: Intestinal loop lengthening- a technique for increasing small intestinal length. *J Pediatr Surg*. 1980; 15:145.

[103] Jewett TC, Walker AB, Cooney DR. A long term follow-up on a duplication of the entire small intestine treated by gastro duplication. *J Pediatr Surg*. 1983; 18:185.

[104] Orr MM, Edwards AJ. Neoplastic change in duplications of the alimentary tract. *Br J Surg*. 1975; 62:269-74.

[105] Filston HC, McLeod ME, Bolman RM *et al.* Improved management of pancreatic lesions in children aided by ERCP. *J Pediatr Surg.* 1980; 15:121-28.

[106] Chew DK, Borromeo JR, Gabriel YA *et al.* Duplication of the vermiform appendix. *J Pediatr Surg.* 2000; 35:617- 8.

[107] Mitchell IC, Nicholls JC. Duplication of the vermiform appendix. Report of a case: review of the classification and medico-legal aspects. *Med Sci Law.* 1990; 30(2).124-26.

[108] Sobhian B, Mostegel M, Kunc C *et al.* Appendix vermiformis duplex—a rare surprise. *Wien Klin Wochenschr.* 2005; 117(13-14):492-4.

[109] Kothari AA, Yagnik KR, Hathila VP. Duplication of the vermiform appendix. *J Postgrad Med.* 2004; 50:285-6.

[110] Jianhong L, Xuewu J, Xianliang H. An exceptional combined malformation: duplication of the urinary and intestinal tracts and the vulva. *J Pediatr Surg.* 2005; 40(3):E5-9.

[111] Yanar H, Ertekin C, Unal ES *et al.* The case of acute appendicitis and appendiceal duplication. *Acta Chir Belg.* 2004; 104(6):736-8.

[112] Sington JD, Warren BF, Manek S. Reduplication cyst of appendix with mucinous carcinoma and Mullerian metaplasia: a case report. *J Clin Pathol.* 2002; 55(7):551-3.

[113] Cave AJE. Appendix vermiformis duplex. *Journal of Anatomy.* 1936; 70:283-92.

[114] Wallbridge PH. Double appendix.*Br J Surg.* 1962; 50:346-7.

[115] Biermann R. Appendix duplex. *Eine Pathologische Raritat.* 1993; 64:1059-61.

[116] Lin BC, Chen RJ, Fang JF *et al.* Duplication of the vermiform appendix. *Eur J Surg.* 1996; 162:589-91.

[117] Puligandla PS, Nguyen LT, Flageole H *et al.* Gastrointestinal duplications. *J Pediatr Surg.* 2003; 38:740-744.

[118] Kottra JJ, Dodds WJ. Duplication of the large bowel. *Am J Roentgenol.* 1971; 113:310.

[119] Yousefzadeh DK. Tubular colonic duplication- review of 1876 to 1981 literature. *Pediatr Radiol.* 1983; 13:65.

[120] Kim YW, Kim J, Lee KY *et al.* A symptomatic tubular duplication of the transverse colon in an adult. *Yonsei Med J.* 2005; 46(1): 189-191.

[121] Correia-Pinto J, Romero R, Carvalho JL *et al.*.Neonatal perforation of a Y-shaped sigmoid duplicationl. *J Pediatr Surgl.* 2001; 36(9):1422-4.

[122] Piolat C, N"die J, Andrini P *et al.* Perforated tubular duplication of the transverse colon: a rare cause of meconium peritonitis with prenatal diagnosis. *Pediatr Surg Int.* 2005; 21(2):110-112.

[123] Frittelli P, Coasta G, Zanella L *et al.* Intestinal duplication in an adult. A case report of colonic duplication and a review of literature. *Chir Ital.* 2002; 54:721-728.

[124] Horie H, Iwasuki I, Takahashi H. Carcinoid in a gastrointestinal duplication. *J Pediatr Surg.* 1986; 21:902-904.

[125] Hsu CF, Huang FC, Ko SF *et al.* Duplication of the transverse colon: report on one case. *Acta Paediatr Taiwan.* 2003; 44(1): 47-9.

[126] Hayden CK Jr. Ultrasonography of the gastrointestinal tract in infants and children*Abdom Imag.* 1996; 21:9-20.

[127] Robert J, Ambrosetti P, Widgren S *et al.* Perforated tubular duplication of the sigmoid colon in adults. *Gastroenterol Clin Biol.* 1990; 14:776-779.

[128] Soper RT: Tubular duplication of the colon and the distal ileum. *Surgery.* 1968; 63:998.

[129] Cooksey G, Wagget J. Tubular duplication of the rectum treated by mucosal resection. *J Pediatr Surg.* 1984; 19:318-320.

[130] Ravitch MM. Duplication of the gastrointestinal tract. In Ravitch MM, Welch KJ, Bandolph JG (Eds). *Pediatric Surgery.* Chicago: Year Book of Medicine; 1986:911-920.

[131] Lister J. Duplication of the alimentary tract. In Lister J Irving I (eds). *Neonatal Surgery (eds 3).* London: Butterworth; 1990:474-484.

[132] Yucesan S, Zorludemir U, Olcay I. Complete duplication of the colon. *J Pediatr Surg.* 1986; 21:962-963.

[133] Li L, Zhang J, Wang Y, Chen R *et al.* Complete duplication of the colon: definitive management by resection of the duplication without the normal bowel. *Chin Med J.* 2002; 115(5):779-781.

In: New Developments in Birth Defects Research
Editor: Nelson A. Gaslem, pp. 137-149

ISBN 1-60021-400-2

Chapter 5

NON-INVASIVE PRENATAL DIAGNOSIS OF CYSTIC FIBROSIS USING FETAL DNA IN MATERNAL PLASMA

M. C. González-González*, M. García-Hoyos, M. J. Trujillo Tiebas, I. Lorda, M Rodríguez de Alba, F. Infantes, J. Gallego, C. Ayuso and C. Ramos

Fundación Jiménez Díaz Avda. Reyes Católicos 2, 28040 Madrid, Spain.

ABSTRACT

Cystic fibrosis (CF) is the most common autosomal recessively inherited disorders in Caucasian population. Prenatal diagnosis of CF is very frequently required and is performed by molecular analysis of the mutations that the fetus could have inherited of the parents. This procedure is carried out at 10-13 weeks of gestation using DNA from chorion villus sample (CVS) and includes 2% risk of abortion. During the last years, much attention has been paid to the possibility of developing non-invasive methods for prenatal diagnosis without any risk for the fetus. Recently, the discovery of fetal DNA in maternal plasma is offering a new strategy to study some conditions of the fetus in a safer way. Because of the presence of maternal DNA in plasma, these approaches are limited to paternally inherited disorders or present "de novo" in the fetus. Up to now, the studies carried out have mainly shown fetal sex detection, fetal RhD and quantitative variations in gestations at risk of pre-eclampsia or fetal chromosomal anomalies. As a prenatal diagnosis unit, these reports have prompted us to investigate the possibilities of using fetal DNA in maternal plasma as a possible alternative tool in the prenatal diagnosis routine.

We have evaluated our experience on the CF prenatal diagnosis field in 13 families. We have also tested the possibility of performing a prenatal diagnosis of a paternally

* Correspondence concerning this article should be addressed to M. C. González-González, Fundación Jiménez Díaz Avda. Reyes Católicos 2, 28040 Madrid, Spain. E-mail: cgonzalezggen@yahoo.es.

inherited CF mutation using fetal DNA present in maternal plasma. Different diagnosis techniques and strategies were used depending on the mutation found in the families that participated in the present study. We show the results from parental and CVS DNA analyses and we comment the obtained results of these conventional CF prenatal diagnoses. On the other hand, we used maternal blood in order to detect and analyze fetal DNA in one of the families that participate in the study. This non-invasive diagnosis was performed at 13 weeks of gestation using DNA extracted from maternal plasma. We used a single PCR amplification of the paternal mutation (Q890X) and posterior restriction analysis of the PCR product. We successfully detected the presence of the mutation and thus, the fetal condition of being a carrier of the paternal mutation. We conclude that the use of fetal DNA for the diagnosis of cystic fibrosis could be a reliable technique that can substantially reduce invasive test.

Keywords: fetal DNA, maternal plasma, Cystic Fibrosis, prenatal diagnosis, non-invasive

Introduction

Cystic fibrosis (CF) is the most common autosomal recessive disorder among Caucasian population with a carrier prevalence of 1/25. Due to the severity of this disorder, affected families with CF may require a prenatal diagnosis to consider terminating pregnancy when the fetus is affected. There are many studies that have evaluated the benefit of CF screening in risk population and neonatal screening as the only way to decrease the disease frequency giving reproductive choices about future pregnancies (Scotet et al., 2003, Richards CS et al., 2004). Recently, hyperechogenic fetal bowel at routine ultrasound in the second trimester has been recognized to be associated with CF (Casaccia G et al., 2003), this finding could also lead to investigate for parent CFTR mutations screening and to offer a prenatal diagnosis if the parents are carriers.

In many molecular laboratories it is routine to determine the genotype of individuals with CF and then, relatives can be tested for the mutation known to be in the family. The partner of someone with a family history of the disease could undergo testing for the most common mutations (comprising near 90% of CF mutations) and a genetic counseling and prenatal diagnosis could be offered. However, many couples at risk have been identified through a first affected newborn.

It is important to take into account that there is the possibility of residual risk of an unknown heterozygous state given the large number of mutated alleles not covered entirely by routine genetic test and the heterogeneity of the population. Casals T et al. (1997) published a study of 640 Spanish CF families showing the most common mutations in Spanish population and seven novel CFTR mutations (G85V, T582R, R851L, F1074L, E692X, Q1281X, 711+3A→T, 406-112 A/T, 3850-129T/C, 741 C/T) were identified. Some of these mutations are severe and could be responsible for a pancreatic sufficiency/insufficiency variable phenotype. This data proves the high molecular heterogeneity in CF mutations, indication that a wide mutation screening is necessary to characterize the frequency of CF mutations in each particular population. After testing, some couples have problems with reproductive decision-making, but the majority of the affected pregnancies are terminated (JC Polnay, 2002). Nevertheless, it remains the risk related to sample taking (chorion villus sample or amniocentesis) that very often discourages some couples from having an invasive procedure.

There is increasing interest in the use of alternative methods such as preimplantation genetic diagnosis (PGD) for those parents afraid of having a baby with a particular disorder. Although there has been high development of PDG in the last years, this technique requires very high-qualified professional, and it is only available in certain health's centers.

The development of noninvasive prenatal diagnostic methods that do not carry any fetal risk has been a goal for researchers in the last years. Few years ago, the possibility of detecting and analyzing fetal cells in maternal peripheral blood was widely investigated (Bianchi et al., 1990, Rodriguez de Alba et al., 2001). However, the low amount of fetal cells found in maternal blood does not permit a routine implementation of these techniques yet. The high degree of maternal cell contamination makes the identification and analysis of single fetal cells quite difficult and time-consuming, although by now it appears to be the only strategy to be able to detect fetal aneuploidies in a non-invasive way. Nowadays, new techniques to isolate and analyze fetal cells in maternal plasma are being investigated (Al-Mufty et al., 2004, Bischoff et al., 2003).

The discovery of fetal DNA in maternal plasma and serum is opening new strategies for non-invasive prenatal diagnosis. This finding suggested that maternal plasma fetal DNA would be very valuable material for no-invasive prenatal diagnosis. To date, fetal DNA detection have been mainly used to diagnose fetal gender (Pertl et al., 2001, Sekizawa et al., 2001) and RhD condition (Bischoff et al., 1999). Using maternal plasma authors such as Amicucci et al. (2000) have diagnosed a paternally inherited myotonic dystrophy, Saito et al. (2000) have detected an achondroplasia mutation and Chen et al. (2000) have carried out a study of a paternally inherited aneuploidy. As we comment in this chapter, our group was able to detect a cystic fibrosis mutation in a fetus using DNA from maternal plasma (González-González, 2002). We also have diagnosed a non-carrier Huntington disease fetus and an affected Hungtinton disease fetus (González- González et al., 2003 González-González et al., 2003b).

In the last few years, it has been also described some characteristic regarding the behavior of this fetal DNA. The concentration of fetal DNA in maternal plasma/serum has been found to increase with gestacional age (Lo YMD, 1998) and after delivery to be cleared rapidly (Lo YMD, 1999). Quantitative variations have been observed in gestations at risk of pre-clampsia or fetal chromosomal anomalies (Zhong XY, 2001, Lo et al., 1999). It has been also postulated that the presence of two-way trafficking of free DNA between the mother and fetus may have potential implications for the development of certain autoinmunes diseases. Tan et al. (1987) was the first author to describe the presence of high levels of circulating DNA in patients with systemic lupus erythematosus.

These observations suggest that maternal plasma could be a useful tool for the non-invasive prenatal diagnosis of certain fetal conditions. As a prenatal diagnosis unit, we feel strongly that the use of the procedures based in the analysis of fetal DNA in maternal plasma has an enormous potential as alternative to conventional methods to diagnose fetal disorders.

The diagnosis of inherited disorders is routinely performed in our laboratory and the fetal DNA analysis in maternal plasma would be very useful in such cases. There are many

Mendelian disorders in which affected families require a prenatal diagnosis and cystic fibrosis is one of the most common.

Conventional prenatal analysis of CF involves the extraction of DNA from chorion villus sample (CVS) at 10 to 13 weeks of gestation or amniocentesis at 15 to 17 weeks of gestation to detect the presence of any parental mutation. As the disease (CF) is caused by many different mutations, there are several molecular approaches to diagnose this disorder according to the mutation: INNO-LiPA CFTR typing strip (Innogenetics) for the most frequent mutation, PCR and restriction analysis, SSCP, microsatellite haplotypes, direct sequencing, etc. These technologies afford quite an efficient screening for a large set of mutation that are very valuable for prenatal diagnosis.

We had previously performed a study of fetal DNA in serum and plasma using QF-PCR to detect fetal sex. We also searched the blood fraction in which more fetal DNA could be detected and the earliest gestational age to detect fetal DNA. Our study in 196 samples (gestacional ages from 10th weeks to 22nd weeks), showed that plasma was the best blood fraction: 88% of the cases were correctly diagnosed in plasma in contrast to the 82% of the cases in serum. Best results obtained in plasma could be due to fact that the coagulation process in serum involves a higher release of free maternal DNA that could interfere with the fetal DNA analysis (Emmanuel and Pestka, 1993). The earliest week of gestation to detect fetal DNA was the 10th.

Due to the promising obtained results in our first study, we explored the possibility of using the analysis of fetal DNA in maternal plasma for prenatal diagnosis of monogenic disorders such CF. Recently, thirteen couples have attended our unit for prenatal diagnosis of CF. In all the cases, a molecular study of the parents was performed and a CVS was carried out at 10-13th weeks of gestation. In one of these families we carried out the analysis of fetal DNA in maternal plasma for the CF prenatal diagnosis of the paternal mutation at 13th weeks of gestation (data published by Prenat. Diagn. 2002:22; 946-948). The low amount of fetal DNA in maternal plasma limits the use of DNA and makes necessary a specific design of the diagnosis methodology. It is also important the fact that the overriding presence of maternal DNA does not permit to distinguish it from the fetal one. The analysis of fetal DNA could be very useful to look for the presence or absence of the paternal mutation to determine the fetal condition of being carrier or non-carrier of paternal mutation.

Patients

We studied 13 couples attended to our prenatal diagnosis unit for a prenatal diagnosis of cystic fibrosis. 10 ml of peripheral blood was taken to each patient. At 11-13th week of gestation, a chorion villus sample was performed in every case.

For the analysis of fetal DNA in maternal plasma, We collected 10 ml of maternal blood of a pregnant woman at the 13th week of gestation, previous of the invasive procedure and under informed consent.

Methods for Conventional Diagnosis of CF

DNA extraction: DNA from whole blood was extracted by using the QIAmp DNA Blood mini Kit (QIAGEN Inc, Hilden, Germany). DNA from CVS was extracted by using the QIAmp DNA Tissue Kit (QIAGEN Inc, Hilden, Germany).

PCR: for the detection of the most common CF mutations the INNO-LiPA CFTR12/CFTR17+Tn kit (Innogenetics) was used.

The rare mutation R347 was detected by the amplification of exon 7 as described (Zielenski et al., 1991). Cycling parameter were 10 min denaturation at 95°C followed by 30 cycles of 95°C 30 sec, 58°C 30 sec 72°C 1 min. Fluorescent dideoxy chain termination method was used to perform sequencing using an internal primer located 3′to Ex7i-3: 5′GCAAACTTCATTAGAACTGAC 3′. The resultant single stranded DNA was purified after PCR. Capillary electrophoresis was performed to visualize the results (ABIprism 310).

PCR and restriction analysis was used for the Q890X mutation using *Mse* I restriction enzyme (as described in "methods of the analysis of fetal DNA in maternal plasma").

Methods for the Analysis of Fetal DNA in Maternal Plasma

We studied a family whose first son was diagnosed of having CF. A molecular study of the son confirmed two different mutations of CF. Using the INNO-LiPA CFTR12/CFTR17+Tn kit (Innogenetics) a G542X mutation was discovered and then, PCR and restriction analysis showed a Q890X mutation. We performed a molecular analysis of the parents and we discover the mother was a heterozygous carrier of G542X mutation and the father was a heterozygous carrier of the Q890X. A CVS was performed in a second pregnancy showing a healthy male.

At the second pregnancy 15 ml of peripheral maternal blood in EDTA was taken for fetal DNA analysis, under informed consent and previous to the invasive procedure (CVS). The blood sample was processed 1-3h after blood collection to avoid DNA degradation, and it was centrifuged at 3000 rpm for 10 min. The plasma was removed very carefully so as not to disturb the buffy coat or blood cot to avoid maternal contamination and it was transferred to a fresh polypropylene tube. Subsequently, the plasma obtained was re-centrifuged at 3000 rpm for 10 min and then it was aliquoted and frozen at –20°C.

For DNA extraction, 2 ml of plasma was processed with the QIAmp DNA Blood mini Kit (QIAGEN Inc, Hilden, Germany) with a final volume elution of 100μl in the supplied buffer.

From the plasma extracted DNA, 20μl and 30μl were used as template for PCR, we also use DNA from peripheral whole blood from relatives and water as negative PCR control. For the Q890X locus, 15pmol of each primer F: 5′GGTGCATGCTCTTCTAATG 3′, R: 5′ AAGGCACATGCCTCTGTGC 3′ we used in a 50μl reaction along with 1,5mM $MgCl_2$, PCR 10X buffer (Roche, Manhein, Germany) 0,2 mM of each dNTP (Amersham Pharmacia Biotech Inc, USA) and 1,5 U of Fast Start DNA polimerase (Roche, Manhein, Germany). Cycling conditions were 94°C 5min and 48 cycles of 94°C 1min, 56°C 1 min, 72°C 1,5 min. The Q890X mutation consists of an A to G substitutions which creates a *Mse* I restriction site that is used to detect the mutation. The PCR product (15μl) was incubated at 65°C for 3h with 20U of *Mse*I ADN 3,5μl of buffer R (MBE Fermentas) and water up to a total volume of 35μl. Obtained fragments were visualized after 2h electrophoresis in a 3% agarose gel and in a 6% polyacrilamide gel stained with ethidium bromide.

Strict precautions against exogenous DNA contamination were used: sterile and separated areas to DNA extraction and post PCR handling, sterile pipettes, filter tips.

Table 1. Obtained results from the conventional study of Cystic fibrosis. Data shows parental mutations and results from prenatal diagnosis.

case	Maternal mutation	Paternal mutation	CVS results
1	ΔF508	ΔF508	Het-ΔF508
2	ΔF508	711+5G	711+5G
3	ΔF508	ΔF508	ΔF508
4	G542X	Q890X	Q890X/G542
5	G542X	Q890X	Q890X
6	ΔF508	ΔF508	ΔF508
7	ΔF508	ΔF508	ΔF508
8	ΔF508	ΔF508	ΔF508/ΔF508
9	1609 del CA	R334W	R334W
10	1092 Tyr-Cys	ΔF508	healthy
11	G542X	ΔF508	ΔF508/G542X
12	ΔF508	R347H	ΔF508
13	ΔF508	ΔF508	ΔF508

RESULTS

Analysis by Conventional Methods

The study of the parents DNA showed that the most frequent mutation was ΔF508 (61,5%), followed by G542X (11,5%) and Q890X (7,6%%), then, we found other mutations: 1092 Tyr-Cys, R334W, 1609 del CA, R347H, 711+5G (3,9% frequency each one). In the study, 6 out of the 13 couples were both carriers of the same mutation (ΔF508). Table 1 shows results from every family study. Results from the analysis of CVS showed only one healthy fetus non carrier or any CF mutation. The study showed six healthy fetus carrier of ΔF508 mutation in heterocygosis. 5 out of this 6 fetuses had parents carriers of the same mutation (ΔF508) the other one had only inherited the maternal ΔF508 mutation.

In those cases in which parents were carrier of different CF mutation, three healthy fetuses were only carrier of paternal mutation, one healthy fetus was carrier of maternal mutation and two fetuses were carrier of both parental mutation (affected fetuses).

Analysis of Fetal DNA in Maternal Plasma

In the detection of Q890X mutation of CF, a 485 band is expected in normal homozygous patient in an acrylamide/agarose gel. The mutation introduces a new restriction enzyme site and thus, the heterozygote carrier pattern is expected to show three fragments of 485, 350 and 135 bp. Figure 1 shows the obtained results in the polyacrylamide gel. Lane 1 shows (20μl of DNA from maternal plasma) a 485bp and a 350 bp bands (135 bp band is absent because of long electrophoresis), corresponding to the paternally inherited mutation Q890X. In lane 2 (30μl of DNA from maternal plasma) we were not able to amplify neither maternal DNA nor fetal DNA, it could be due a PCR failure. The presence of the mutation in the fetus was confirmed by molecular analysis of the chorion biopsy. The results in agarose gel showed extremely faint bands.

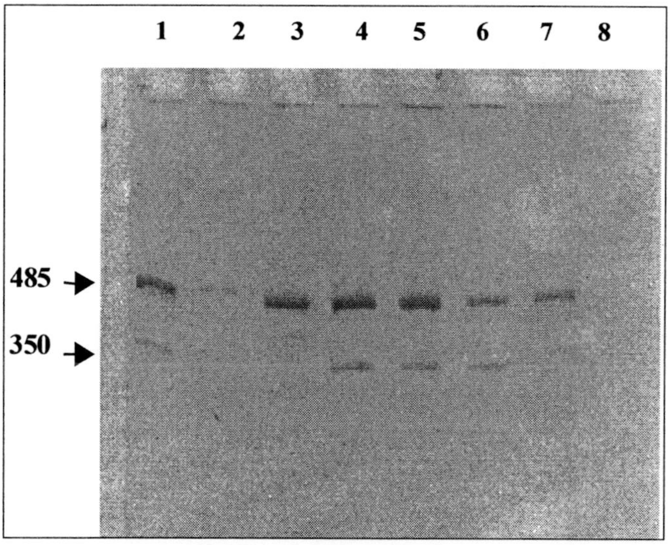

Figure 1. Results obtained in the non-invasive CF study. Lane 1 and 2 : amplification of maternal plasma (20 and 30μl of DNA from maternal plasma respectively). Lane 3: mother, lane 4: father, lane 5: affected son, lane 6: brother of the father, 7: healthy son, lane 8: negative PCR control.(González-González et al., Prenat. Diagn. 2002; 22: 946-948, Copyright © John Wiley & sons, reproduced with permission)

Our results in the prenatal diagnosis of CF in CVS showed 6 cases in which both parent were carrier or different mutations. In all those cases, the diagnosis of paternal mutation using fetal DNA in maternal plasma could have been possible and very valuable as first pre-test in early gestation. The absence of paternal mutation would mean that the fetus could be only carrier of the maternal mutation, therefore to allow the diagnosis of a healthy fetus. The parental study of cystic fibrosis mutations is always essential in the non-invasive procedure to use an adequate diagnosis technique that allows us manage every particular case.

We successfully detected a paternal CF mutation in a non-invasive way using fetal DNA from maternal plasma in a very early gestacional age. The volume of plasma DNA used for PCR was an important fact due to the low amount of fetal DNA in the total amount of DNA present in maternal plasma. Due to the early pregnancy condition we processed 3 ml of plasma to ensure enough fetal DNA for a successful amplification. When we used 20μl of DNA obtained from maternal plasma as a template to PCR it was sufficient for amplification, however, PCR failed when we used 30μl. It could be due to an unexpected PCR error or an inhibition PCR for an excessive amount of total DNA. Results from electrophoresis in the agarose gel were not conclusive for the fetal DNA analysis because bands were extremely faint compared to the ones obtained in the acrylamide gel.

Although this technique does not have high sensibility it has high specificity as the presence of the paternal pattern band in the maternal plasma only could be due to the amplification of the fetal DNA. The present case could not avoid the invasive procedure, but it was a very interesting assay to confirm the possibility of detecting an inherited paternal mutation for the non-invasive diagnosis of monogenic disorders. Other CF mutation detection could require different diagnosis techniques and we are now working with more advances techniques such as QF-PCR or real time PCR, as extremely sensitive techniques. Previously, we had used QF-PCR technique for detection of fetal DNA along gestation. Because we know it was a female fetus, we selected primers for the HPTR gene (located in the X chromosome) The different size of mother and father alleles allowed us to distinguish the fetus paternally inherited allele from maternal alleles. The fetal DNA follow-up along gestation assay showed that we could detect it from the 10th week of gestation and no longer than 24 hours after delivery. We could also observe that the fetal DNA peak area seen in QF-PCR was greater as the gestation advanced, confirming that fetal DNA amount increases with the advance of gestation (figures 2,3). This technique could allow performing microsatellite haplotypes for indirect diagnosis of CF using maternal plasma.

Recently, Nasis et al. (2004) have used allele-specific PCR to improve the sensitivity in the detection of a CF mutation for fetal DNA in maternal plasma. This method permits a reliable detection of a paternally inherited mutation (D1152H) detecting 5 copies of de CF D1152H mutant allele in the presence of up to 100 000 copies of the wild-type allele.

The most important benefit of these techniques is the applicability for the detection of a wide range of inherited diseases without risk for the fetus and in a gestacional age similar to conventional procedures (CVS or amniocentesis). It is always essential to perform a previous analysis of parental mutation. When parents are both carrier of the same mutation it is impossible the analysis of fetal DNA because we can not distinguish whether the fetus has inherited the paternal mutation or we have been analyzing the corresponding maternal sequence. However, this approach would be applicable as an alternative method that might permit the parents to pursue a first trimester prenatal test when parental mutations are different. We would be only able to detect the fetal condition of being a carrier or non-carrier of the paternal mutation. This information would be very important for parents discouraged from having an invasive method now that if the fetus is not carrier of the paternal mutation we are determining that the fetus will be healthy or healthy carrier of the maternal mutation.

The technical parameters affecting the reliability of the detection of fetal DNA in maternal plasma need to be taken into account for its use as a routine prenatal diagnosis procedure. In our experience, after venepucture it is necessary to centrifuge the whole blood to obtain the plasma as soon as possible and then, aliquot, and freeze it until DNA extraction. We carried out this process in no more than 24 hours. Few samples were processed after this time (48 and 72 hours) and using these samples we were able to detect maternal DNA but not fetal DNA. Previous studies indicate that fetal DNA in maternal plasma is stable even 24 hours after collection (Angert et al., 2003). The time a sample spends in the tube before processing could not only affect the amount of total DNA by releasing DNA due to apoptosis of maternal cells, but also affect the stability of free-cell fetal DNA. These data need to be deeply studied to establish protocols for the transmission of samples from distant places.

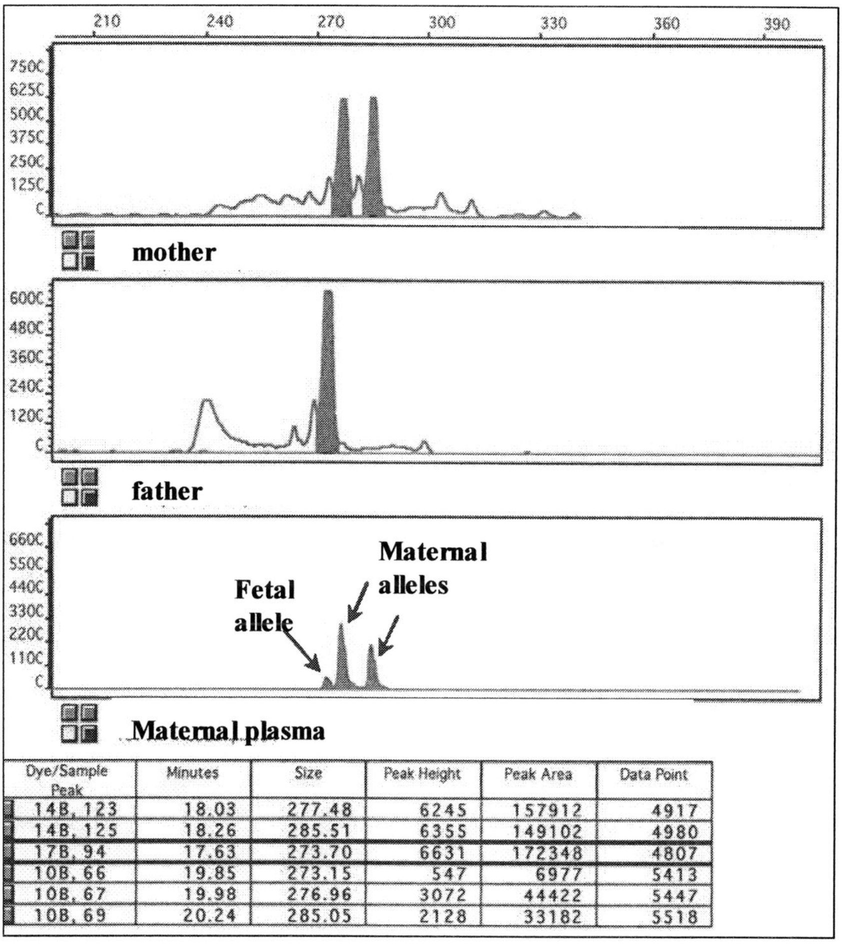

Dye/Sample Peak	Minutes	Size	Peak Height	Peak Area	Data Point
14B, 123	18.03	277.48	6245	157912	4917
14B, 125	18.26	285.51	6355	149102	4980
17B, 94	17.63	273.70	6631	172348	4807
10B, 66	19.85	273.15	547	6977	5413
10B, 67	19.98	276.96	3072	44422	5447
10B, 69	20.24	285.05	2128	33182	5518

Figure 2. Results obtained from parental DNA amplification of the HPTR gene and maternal plasma at 10th week of gestation.

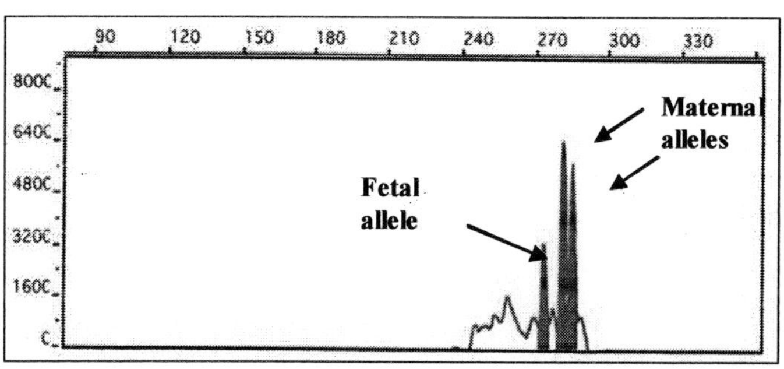

Figure 3. Results obtained from maternal plasma at 32+4 weeks of gestation.

A great limiting factor is the fact that free fetal DNA exists in the maternal circulation at low amount, mean percentage of free fetal DNA is around 3- 6 % in early and advanced gestation respectively (Lo et al.,1998). Any method that could increase this percentage would make easier to detect fetal DNA and therefore, to perform a more reliable diagnosis. Dhallan et al., (2004) using formaldehyde to reduce cell lysis proved an increase of the relative percentage of free fetal DNA up to 25% versus 6% obtained by other groups.

A further complication is the possibility of false positive results that also limits of the use of fetal DNA PCR for diagnostics. Sample handling could be the reason of this artifact. We feel strongly that it is essential to avoid any risk of exogenous DNA contamination, which includes sterile pipettes, filter tips, and separated sterile areas for DNA extraction and PCR handling. New technologies to detect fetal DNA such as Real-time PCR offers to date the highest level of safety and represents the most secure amplification procedure.

Gestacional age is an important fact to consider. The sensitivity of the techniques increases substantially as the pregnancy progress due to the increase of fetal DNA with the gestation. In a very early week of gestation false negative results may occur, therefore, in case of negative results it would be essential to repeat the technique collecting new blood sample in few days to confirm our results.

We consider that fetal DNA analysis would be very also very useful to apply in the prenatal diagnosis of a paternally inherited dominant mutation and we evaluated the possibility of studying fetal DNA for Huntington disease (HD) prenatal diagnosis. We used QF-PCR technology for its high sensibility in detecting small amounts of fetal DNA in maternal plasma even in early gestation, reducing experimental time and the possibility of contamination with exogenous DNA. We carried out two prenatal diagnosis of HD and we successfully diagnosed an affected fetus and a healthy one in the 13th week of gestation (González-González 2003 a and 2003b).

Fetal sex detection in maternal plasma would be also very valuable in cases of X-linked disorders. In those cases, the number of invasive prenatal test could be dramatically reduced. It would be possible to perform a protocol in which maternal plasma would be collected an early week of gestation to detect fetal sex and then, these results would be confirmed by ultrasound.

These techniques would be only applicable when the involved target is in the fetus but absent in the mother. Nowadays, the main purpose of the prenatal diagnosis is the detection of fetal aneuploidies. However, due to the overriding presence of maternal DNA we were only able to detect fetal sequences of paternal origin in maternal plasma, and most of the aneuploides such as 21 trisomy (Down Syndrome) are maternally inherited. Previous research of our group has been dealing with the analysis of fetal cells in maternal blood (Rodríguez de Alba, 2001). The high degree of maternal cell contamination makes the identification and analysis of single fetal cells difficult and time-consuming, but by now, it appears to be the only strategy to detect fetal aneuploides in a non-invasive way. Lately Poon et al. (2002) have focused on the biology of epigenetic phenomena (DNA methylation) reasoning that using DNA methylation differences between the mother and fetus it could be possible to overcome this limitation. This epigenetic analysis has many applications to disorders associated with genomic imprinting such as Prader-Willi and Angelman syndromes, it could be also useful to certain aneuploides that may be associated with methylation abnormalities

(Yu J et al., 1997, Kuromitsu J, 1997). Advances in the research of the fetal epigenetic markers are necessary to demonstrate the value of these findings.

A number of investigators have shown that fetal RNA is present in the maternal plasma in addition to fetal DNA, The inherent liability of RNA has made these observations rather surprising. Ng EK et al. (2003) have demonstrated this fetal RNA to be of placental origin. The development of placental mRNA markers that can be detected in maternal plasma will open many new investigations.

Fetal DNA analysis from maternal plasma is a promising technique that could be shortly applicable in clinical practice to the diagnosis of the most common Mendelian disorders such as CF. Further approaches should focus on the study of a large number of patients and different techniques to define the sensitivity and specificity of these diagnostic approaches.

On the basis of our current experience with fetal DNA in maternal plasma it is obvious that new technology will shortly increase the possibilities for non-invasive prenatal diagnosis.

ACKNOWLEDGEMENT

Comunidad de Madrid (08.6/0028/2000 3) and FIS (PI040218) supported this project. We thank Fundacion Conchita Rábago for their support to Cristina González-González.

REFERENCES

Al-Mufti R, Hambley H, Farzaneh F, Nicolaides KH. Assessment of efficacy of cell separation techniques used in the enrichment of foetal erythroblasts from maternal blood: triple density gradient vs. single density gradient. *Clin Lab Haematol.* 2004; 26(2):123-8

Amicucci P, Gennarelli M, Novelli G, Dallapiccola B. Prenatal diagnosis of myotonic dystrophy using fetal DNA obtained from maternal plasma. *Clin Chem.* 2000; 46(2):301-2.

Angert RM, LeShane ES, Lo YM, Chan LY, Delli-Bovi LC, Bianchi DW. Fetal cell-free plasma DNA concentrations in maternal blood are stable 24 hours after collection: analysis of first- and third-trimester samples. *Clin Chem* 2003; 49(1):195-8.

Bianchi DW, Flint AF, Pizzimenti MF, Knoll JH, Latt SA. Isolation of fetal DNA from nucleated erythrocytes in maternal blood.Proc Natl Acad Sci U S A. 1990; 87(9):3279-83.

Bischoff FZ, Marquez-Do DA, Martinez DI, Dang D, Horne C, Lewis D, Simpson JL. Intact fetal cell isolation from maternal blood: improved isolation using a simple whole blood progenitor cell enrichment approach (RosetteSep). *Clin Genet.* 2003; 63(6):483-9.

Bischoff FZ, Nguyen DD, Marquez-Do D, Moise KJ Jr, Simpson JL, Elias S. *J Soc Gynecol Investig.* Noninvasive determination of fetal RhD status using fetal DNA in maternal serum and PCR.1999; 6(2):64-9.

Casaccia G, Trucchi A, Nahom A, Aite L, Lucidi V, Giorlandino C, Bagolan P. The impact of cystic fibrosis on neonatal intestinal obstruction: the need for prenatal/neonatal screening. *Pediatr Surg Int.* 2003; 19(1-2):75-8. 2003.

Chen CP, Chern SR, Wang W. Fetal DNA in maternal plasma: the prenatal detection of a paternally inherited fetal aneuploidy. *Prenat Diagn.* 2000; 20(4):355-7.

Dhallan R, Au WC, Mattagajasingh S, Emche S, Bayliss P, Damewood M, Cronin M, Chou V, Mohr M. Methods to increase the percentage of free fetal DNA recovered from the maternal circulation. *JAMA.* 2004 3; 291(9):1114-9.

Emanuel SL, Pestka S. Amplification of specific gene products from human serum. *Genet Anal Tech appl.* 1993; 10, 144-146.

Gonzalez-Gonzalez MC, Garcia-Hoyos M, Trujillo MJ, Rodriguez de Alba M, Lorda-Sanchez I, Diaz-Recasens J, Gallardo E, Ayuso C, Ramos C. Prenatal detection of a cystic fibrosis mutation in fetal DNA from maternal plasma. *Prenat Diagn* 2002; 22:946-8.

Gonzalez-Gonzalez MC, Trujillo MJ, Rodriguez de Alba M, Garcia-Hoyos M, Lorda-Sanchez I, Diaz-Recasens J, Ayuso C, Ramos C (2003a) Huntington disease-unaffected fetus diagnosed from maternal plasma using QF-PCR. *Prenat Diagn* 2003 a; 23:232-4.

Gonzalez-Gonzalez MC, Trujillo MJ, Rodriguez de Alba M, Ramos C. Early Huntington disease prenatal diagnosis by maternal semiquantitative fluorescent-PCR. *Neurology* 2003b; 60;1214-5.

Kuromitsu J, Yamashita H, Kataoka H, Takahara T, Muramatsu M, Sekine T. A unique dowregulation of h2-calponin gene expression in Down syndrome: a possible attenuation mechanism for fetal survival by methylation at the CpG island in the trisomic chromosome 21. *Mol Cell Biol* 1997; 17:707-712.

Lo YM, Tein MS, Lau TK, Haines CJ, Leung TN, Poon PM, Wainscoat JS, Johnson PJ, Chang AM, Hjelm NM Quantitative analysis of fetal DNA in maternal plasma and serum: implications for noninvasive prenatal diagnosis. *Am J Hum Genet* 1998; 62; 768-75 .

Lo YMD, Zhang J, Leung TN, Lau TK, Chang AM, Hjelm NM. Rapid clearance of fetal DNA from maternal plasma. *Am J Hum Genet* 1999; 64: 218-224.

Nasis O, Thompson S, Hong T, Sherwood M, Radcliffe S, Jackson L, Otevrel T. Improvement in sensitivity of allele-specific PCR facilitates reliable noninvasive prenatal detection of cystic fibrosis. *Clin Chem.* 2004; 50(4):694-701.

Ng EK, Tsui NB, Lau TK, Leung TN, Chiu RW, Panesar NS, Lit LC, Chan KW, Lo YM. mRNA of placental origin is readily detectable in maternal plasma. *Proc Natl Acad Sci U S A.* 2003; 15;100(8):4748-53.

Pertl B, Bianchi DW. Fetal DNA in maternal plasma: emerging clinical applications. *Obstet Gynecol* 2001;98(3):483-90.

Polnay JC, Davidge A, Lyn U C, Smyth AR. Parental attitudes: antenatal diagnosis of cystic fibrosis. *Arch Dis Child.* 2002; 87(4):284-6.

Poon LL, Leung TN, Lau TK, Chow KC, Lo YM.Differential DNA methylation between fetus and mother as a strategy for detecting fetal DNA in maternal plasma. *Clin Chem.* 2002; 48(1):35-41.

Richards CS, Grody WW. Prenatal screening for cystic fibrosis: past, present and future. *Expert Rev Mol Diagn.* 2004; 4(1):49-62.

Rodriguez de Alba M, Palomino P, Gonzalez-Gonzalez C, Lorda-Sanchez I, Ibanez MA, Sanz R, Fernandez-Moya JM, Ayuso C, Diaz-Recasens J, Ramos C (2001) Prenatal diagnosis on fetal cells from maternal blood: practical comparative evaluation of the first and second trimesters. *Prenat Diagn* 21; 165-70.

Saito H, Sekizawa A, Morimoto T, Suzuki M, Yanaihara T .Prenatal DNA diagnosis of a single-gene disorder from maternal plasma. *Lancet* 2000; 30; 1170.

Scotet V, Audrezet MP, Roussey M, Rault G, Blayau M, De Braekeleer M, Ferec C. Impact of public health strategies on the birth prevalence of cystic fibrosis in Brittany, France. *Hum Genet.* 2003; 113(3):280-5.

Sekizawa A, Kondo T, Iwasaki M, Watanabe A, Jimbo M, Saito H, Okai T. Accuracy of fetal gender determination by analysis of DNA in maternal plasma. *Clin Chem.* 2001; 47(10):1856-8.

Tan CK, Sullivan K, Li XY, Tan EM, Downey KM, So AG.Autoantibody to the proliferating cell nuclear antigen neutralizes the activity of the auxiliary protein for DNA polymerase delta. *Nucleic Acids Res.* 1987; 25;15(22):9299-308.

Yu J, Tong S, Shen Y, Kao FT. Gene identification and DNA sequence analysis in the GC-poor 20 megabse region of human chromosome 21. *Proc Natl Acad Sci. USA* 1997; 94:6862-6867.

Zhong XY, Holzgreve W, Hahn S (2001) Circulatory fetal and maternal DNA in pregnancies at risk and those affected by preeclampsia. *Ann N Y Acad Sci.* 2001; 945;138-40.

Zielenski J, Rozmahel R, Bozon D, Kerem B, Grzelczak Z, Riordan JR, Rommens J, Tsui LC. Genomic DNA sequence of the cystic fibrosis transmembrane conductance regulator (CFTR) gene. *Genomics.* 1991; 10(1):214-28.

In: New Developments in Birth Defects Research
Editor: Nelson A. Gaslem, pp. 151-176

ISBN 1-60021-400-2

Chapter 6

SCREENING FOR CYSTIC FIBROSIS MUTATIONS IN SOUTHERN EUROPEAN COUNTRIES: METHODS FOR MOLECULAR DIAGNOSIS, PRENATAL DIAGNOSIS AND CARRIER IDENTIFICATION AMONGST HIGH-RISK INDIVIDUALS- THE GREEK EXPERIENCE

Emmanuel Kanavakis* and Maria Tzetis
Dept. of Medical Genetics, University of Athens, St. Sophia's Children's Hospital, Athens, 11527, Greece.

ABSTRACT

Cystic fibrosis (CF) mutation analysis on 500 CF patients, characterized 83 different mutations (20 so far specific to our population) accounting for 92% of CF genes and generating 111 different genotypes. Seven mutations were common [p.F508del (54.5%), c.621+1G>T (6.3%), p.G542X (3.9%), p.N1303K (2.3%), c.2789+5G>A (2.0%), c.2183AA>G (1.5%), p.E822X (1.8%)], 16 showed frequencies between 0.4% and 1.1%, while the remaining (60) were very rare (1 to 3 alleles). Denaturing gradient gel electrophoresis (DGGE) screening of 15 exons (3, 4, 7, 9, 10, 11, 12, 13, 14b, 16, 17b, 19, 20, 21, and 23) detected 86% of CF alleles. Haplotypes for eight diallelic and three microsatellite markers have been characterized for the common, a few rare and novel Greek mutations. In order to test the contribution of the CFTR gene in male infertility, we carried out mutation testing on subjects suffering from the monosymptomatic form of CFTR. Mutation testing was carried out on 134 male infertility subjects including 88

* Correspondence concerning this article should be addressed to Emmanuel Kanavakiș, Maria Tzetis, Dept. of Medical Genetics, University of Athens, St. Sophia's Children's Hospital, Athens, 11527, Greece. Fax: +30210 7795553; Email: ekanavak@cc.uoa.gr. mtzeti@cc.uoa.gr.

suffering from azoospermia (Congenital bilateral absence of vas deferens-CBAVD and Obstructive azoospermia-OA) and 46 with severe oligospermia. The results showed that 56.2% of CBAVD males carried one mutation/variant in the CFTR gene while 27.1% were compound heterozygotes for one mild (belonging to class IV or V) and one severe mutation. Of the OA males, 27.5% had at least 1 CF allele while only 13% of the severe oligospermia males were carriers. Carrier screening was initiated, with emphasis on individuals and couples in high-risk groups –with a family history of CF, one partner with CF, and couples with male infertility seeking in vitro fertilization (IVF). Mutation analysis on 900 individuals (175 couples, 91 unaffected CF siblings, 285 CF family relatives and 174 general population subjects), identified a total of 188 heterozygotes the majority amongst siblings and relatives of index cases. Of the 175 couples, 23 had advanced ongoing pregnancies upon request for CF screening. In total six couples were found requiring prenatal diagnosis.

Results of 167 prenatal diagnoses (including 110 due to bowel echogenicity), testing a total of 57 different parental genotypes, are reported. One hundred and sixty-seven prenatal tests resulted in 41 affected, 80 heterozygous, 46 normal fetuses and one incomplete diagnosis. Of the echogenic bowel fetuses, 15 had one detectable mutation and in 4 cases homozygosity with severe mutations was detected.

Keywords: Cystic Fibrosis/ mutation screening/ CBAVD/ obstructive azoospermia/ oligospermia/ ICP/ prenatal diagnosis/ echogenic bowel

Introduction

Cystic fibrosis (CF; OMIM 219700, CFTR; OMIM 602421) is a severe autosomal recessive genetic disease, affecting 1 in 2500 Caucasians with 4% being asymptomatic carriers of mutations in the gene [Welsh et al., 2001; Kerem et al., 1989; Riordan et al., 1989; Rommens et al., 1989]. The median age of diagnosis is 7 months with more than 60% of the affected individuals diagnosed by 1 year of age. Without treatment, CF is typically a fatal disorder in infancy and childhood. The concentration of salt in the sweat of CF patients is usually elevated (>60mEq/l) and it is used as a diagnostic test. With currently improved treatment the median age of survival has increased to more than 30 years. However patients continue to have a considerable burden of illness and die prematurely due to chronic pulmonary damage from excessive inflammation and chronic infection [Welsh et al., 2001]. There is substantial variability in the clinical expression of the disease, with patients symptomatic at birth, while others not presenting symptoms for months or even years. More than 96% of men with CF have anomalies in the Wolffian structures causing obstructive azoospermia and infertility with the body and tail of the epididymis and seminal vesicles atrophic or absent. In approximately 85% of CF patients, the exocrine pancreas is affected (PI, pancreatic insufficiency). In the remaining 15% of patients, the exocrine pancreas is functionally adequate (PS, pancreatic sufficiency). The gene which was characterized in 1989 [Kerem et al., 1989; Riordan et al., 1989; Rommens et al., 1989], is located on chromosome 7q31.2, encoding a glycosylated transmembrane protein. The 1480 amino acid transmembrane protein has a symmetrical structure of two repeats composed of a transmembrane region (TMD) containing six transmembrane helices (TM) and a nucleotide binding domain (NBD), separated by a large hydrophilic regulatory (R) domain. These features are characteristic of a large family of ATP-Binding Cassette Transporters (ABC transporters) found in prokaryotes and eukaryotes. The difference is that the R domain is unique to the CFTR protein [Vankeerberghen et al., 2002]. The CFTR protein is a chloride ion channel, regulating salt and water transport and is expressed in the apical membrane of epithelial exocrine cells. Besides its function as a chloride channel, CFTR regulates other apical membrane conductance pathways. Activity of the epithelial sodium channel is inversely related to CFTR activity. CFTR is thought to regulate the outwardly rectifying chloride channel (ORCC) by facilitating cellular release of ATP. CFTR might also transport HCO_3 or regulate its transport through epithelial cell membranes. CFTR contributes to normal pancreatic secretion by diluting and alkalinizing the pancreatic juice to prevent obstruction of the smaller pancreatic ducts with proteinaceous plugs, therefore reduced CFTR function might also contribute to ductal plugging in pancreatic disease other than CFTR [Cohn 2005].

Since the initial characterization of the predominant mutation in the Caucasian population, F508del [Kerem et al., 1989], more than 1000 mutations have been reported to the Cystic Fibrosis Genetic Analysis Consortium [CFGAC: http://www.genet.sickkids.on.ca/cftr/], most of which are presumed to be pathogenic. These mutations express their effects through a variety of molecular mechanisms that include either the failure of production of CFTR protein or the production of a mutant protein with no or variable residual function and are thus subdivided into six classes: [Zielenski, 2000; Vankeerberghen et al., 2002]. Class I includes nonsense, frameshift and splice site mutations, giving rise to the formation of premature termination signals. Such proteins are often unstable and are expected to be degraded resulting in minimal or no functional CFTR chloride activity in the affected epithelia. Class II contains missense and amino acid deletion mutations including F508del, and is associated with improper maturation of the corresponding CFTR proteins. These immature mutant proteins will remain associated with molecular chaperones and will ultimately be degraded and as a result will not appear at the cell surface. Class III are missense mutations, mostly located in the nucleotide binding domains. They affect the regulation of the CFTR channel by interfering with the phosphorylation of the R domain and binding and hydrolysis of ATP at both nucleotide binding domains. They result in a decrease of the net chloride transport activity of the channel. Class IV mutations are also missense located in the pore of the channel and give rise to a CFTR channel with defective conductive properties. Class V are missense and alternate splicing mutations mostly causing reduced CFTR synthesis. Especially with splice-site mutations, normal splicing can still occur in a small proportion of these transcripts and a small amount of functional CFTR protein will be produced resulting in a mild phenotype. Class VI are mutations that affect CFTR protein regulation of other channels or decrease the apical stability of the protein. Class I-III and VI mutations are characterized as severe and are associated with pancreatic insufficiency since no functional CFTR is present at the apical membrane, whereas patients with rarer class IV-V mutations with some residual function are mostly pancreatic sufficient and characterized as mild. Although classic CF is diagnosed in infancy or early childhood, atypical cases of CF may be diagnosed in adults with mild monosymptomatic diseases such as congenital bilateral absence of the vas deferens (CBAVD, CAVD), idiopathic chronic or acute and recurrent pancreatitis (ICP and ARP), sinusitis, diffuse bronchiectasis, chronic obstructive pulmonary disease or asthma [Kanavakis et al., 1998; Tzetis et al., 2001a; Noone and Knowles, 2001; Casals et al., 2004; Claustres, 2005; Ahmed et al., 2003]. Individuals with atypical CF phenotypes have normal or borderline sweat chloride tests and are often compound heterozygotes carrying one severe and one mild mutation/variant (class IV and V mutations), or are homozygous for the IVS8-5T variant. Near the 3' region of intron 8 in the splice acceptor site, there is a tract of 5, 7, or 9 thymidine residues. Usually 7 or 9 thymidines are present, which allows normal gene splicing and CFTR production. When 5 thymidine residues are present-the IVS8-5T variant-abnormal splicing occurs, which leads to the skipping of exon 9 and the presence of approximately only 5-10% of the normal CFTR messenger RNA. The CFTR mRNA deleted for exon 9 maintains an open reading frame and would encode a CFTR isoform that is missing amino acids 404-464 of the first nucleotide binding domain (NBD1). This protein is not properly processed and is not capable of generating Cl^- conductance in response to cAMP [Strong et al., 1993]. The 5T variant is present on about 5% of the alleles in the general population and is associated with male infertility and/or mild pulmonary symptoms. This allele shows incomplete penetrance which limits its prognostic or diagnostic value for individual patients [Groman et al., 2004].

CF is an autosomal recessive disorder and affected individuals typically inherit one mutated allele from each parent. Therefore couples who have had one affected offspring are likely to be CF carriers with a 25% recurrence risk in each future pregnancy. Healthy siblings of an affected person have a two-thirds chance of being CF carriers. Second- and third-degree relatives of affected individuals have a 50% and 25% risk of being carriers, respectively. Complex alleles, in which more than one mutation is present in cis, have been observed [Zielenski and Tsui 1995]. F508del shows a higher frequency in northern European in comparison to southern European populations [Welsh et al., 2001], where the percentage of non-F508del chromosomes associated with CF is high. The frequencies and types of mutations found in populations vary according to the geographic and ethnic origin of the population studied. In populations with high heterogeneity, mutation analysis can be facilitated by association between haplotypes for diallelic and microsatellite polymorphisms for each CF mutation. Several highly polymorphic microsatellite and diallelic markers have been described within the CFTR gene and have been used in association analysis with CF mutations in other populations [Dork et al., 1992; Claustres et al., 1996]. Accurate knowledge of CF mutations in a specific population provides information for CF prevention programs applicable through heterozygote screening and prenatal diagnosis.

The aim of genetic screening for CF is to aid the process of reproductive decision making. This is principally achieved by identifying carrier couples who can have prenatal diagnosis and selective termination of pregnancy. Because it is not feasible to determine the carrier status of all persons of reproductive age in the population, selective screening by focusing on the relatives of the index case can be used as an alternative approach. This has the advantage of detecting a higher ratio of carriers and restriction of assays to the mutant alleles in the index case at least for first degree relatives. CF carrier testing should also be offered to males with a family history of unilateral or bilateral absence of vas deferens and their partners. Prenatal diagnosis for CF is additionally offered to pregnancies diagnosed with echogenicity of the fetal bowel. Fetal echogenic bowel, with a prevalence of 0.6-1.8% in second trimester pregnancies, is defined as echogenicity of the fetal bowel approaching that of the surrounding bone. It is described as a normal variant but also in association with chromosomal abnormalities (~9%), cystic fibrosis (~2%), intrauterine growth restriction (~8%), intestinal obstruction, congenital infection (~3%), and intra-amniotic bleeding [Monaghan et al., 1999]. In pregnancies with a 25% risk of cystic fibrosis the echogenic bowel may represent meconium impaction and solidification in the small bowel. Procedure for CF screening in these pregnancies is to test for 85-90% of CF alleles found in the specific population. Screening is done within limited time constraints due to advanced age of pregnancy.

This study aims to offer a strategy for CFTR mutation screening for populations with high molecular heterogeneity using the Greek population as one such example. We report results of the molecular analysis of 500 Greek classic CF patients, including haplotype information, and CF mutation screening for atypical CF on 134 male subjects suffering from infertility (CBAVD, OA and Oligospermia). A total of 152 prenatal diagnoses for pregnancies at a 1 in 4 risk, 15 for couples with male infertility problems and 110 due to fetal bowel echogenicity are reported. The outcome of carrier detection offered to relatives of CF patients and their partners, couples with male infertility seeking IVF and members of the general population (total of 900 individuals) is also discussed.

MATERIALS AND METHODS

Molecular Characterization and Haplotype Analysis

A total of 500 unrelated CF patients of Greek origin (1000 chromosomes), the majority of who attend the Cystic Fibrosis Unit of the St. Sophia's Children's Hospital and children and adults from other Cystic Fibrosis units in Greece, were included in this study. Diagnostic criteria involved positive sweat tests and typical clinical findings of pulmonary and gastrointestinal disease. The 27 exons and neighboring intronic regions of the CFTR gene were assessed by denaturing gradient gel electrophoresis (DGGE). Haplotype analysis for the diallelic sites –XV2c-KM19-D9-J44-M470V-T854-TUB20– was conducted on 261 p.F508del, 116 non-p.F508del and 51 normal chromosomes. For the three microsatellite loci, IVS8CA-IVS17BTA-IVS17BCA, analysis was performed on 146 p.F508del, 85 non-p.F508del and 136 normal alleles.

Monosymptomatic CFTR Screening

Male Infertility Congenital Bilateral Absence of vas Deferens (CBAVD) - Obstructive Azoospermia (OA) - oligospermia

Male subjects (n=134) suffering from infertility with azoospermia (48 CBAVD and 40 OA) or severe oligospermia (46) were studied. The patients were referred to us from various infertility clinics. The diagnosis of CBAVD was based on the small volume of ejaculate and complete absence of spermatozoa, and the typical biochemical changes found in vas deferens agenesis [Kanavakis et al., 1998]. The presence of the vas deferens in the 40 males with OA was confirmed by clinical examination. Renal ultrasound was not performed on the CBAVD patients in order to exclude renal agenesis as the cause of CBAVD. Analysis included DGGE screening of 15 exons, and sequencing if the mutation(s) did not present with a known pattern.

None of the monosymptomatic disease patients had any of the classic symptoms of CF including serious pulmonary involvement.

Heterozygote Screening

Carrier identification through DGGE screening of 15 exons (for 86% of detectable CF alleles) was completed for 900 individuals. These included 175 couples (350 individuals) belonging to a high-risk group with a family history of CF or seeking in vitro Fertilization (IVF) due to male infertility, 91 unaffected CF siblings, 285 CF family relatives (not married therefore not part of couple screening) and 174 general population subjects.

Prenatal Diagnosis

Prenatal diagnosis (PND) was offered to 150 families (152 diagnoses), the majority of which had at least 1 affected child and to seven couples (15 prenatal diagnoses), with male infertility problems. Chorionic villus (CVS) biopsy was the study material in 139 cases and amniotic fluid (AF) in 28 cases. Six cases involved twin pregnancies, four from IVF couples and one triplet. Pre-implantation Genetic Diagnosis (PGD) [Vrettou et al., 2002] was performed in two IVF couples followed by 1 triplet pregnancy and one singleton. The PGD results were confirmed by PND. In two cases we observed parental alleles carrying two mutations in cis, and four cases involving compound heterozygous parents, two asymptomatic and two CBAVD.

A combination of DGGE-CFTR mutation screening and polymerase chain reaction–mediated site-directed mutagenesis (PMS) [Friedman et al., 1991; Tzetis et al., 1997] for the confirmation of the mutation(s) was used for each diagnosis. Each prenatal diagnosis included re-testing of sample DNA from parents and healthy and/or affected child. The three microsatellite markers (IVS8CA, IVS17BTA and IVS17BCA) used for indirect analysis of CF mutation(s), confirmation of paternity and possible maternal contamination of the fetal DNA sample were amplified for all the family members.

Prenatal Diagnosis due to Fetal Bowel Hyperechogenicity

A total of 74 amniotic fluid samples (including parental DNA in 37 cases) and 36 couples were tested for CF mutations. None of the couples had a prior medical history of CF.

The cases were referred from different maternity hospitals and gynecologists (performing the ultrasound) to the Department of Medical Genetics of the University of Athens between 1999 -2005. The grade of echogenicity and criteria for sonographic diagnosis used by these centers was heterogeneous and often did not accompany the sample to be tested for CF. When amniocentesis for prenatal karyotyping to exclude aneuploidy was performed- CF testing included parental and fetal DNA to avoid false negative results due to non paternity. If the parents wanted to avoid an invasive procedure, parental carrier status was initially determined and amniocentesis offered to couples with both members CF carriers.

The average gestational age at amniocentesis was 20.5 weeks (range 20–23 weeks) for the 74 cases of fetal bowel hyperechogenicity and amniotic fluid was the study material. DNA from both or one of the parents when possible was incorporated in the analysis which included DGGE screening of 15 exons, confirmation with PMS or sequencing if the mutation(s) did not present with a known pattern. The three microsatellite markers (IVS8CA, IVS17BTA and IVS17BCA) were used for confirmation of paternity and possible maternal contamination of the fetal DNA sample.

The study was approved by the hospital's review board and all participants provided informed consent.

DNA Mutation Analysis

Genomic DNA was extracted from white blood cells, CVS and AF samples by standard isolation procedures using QIAamp DNA blood mini kit (Qiagen, Hilden, Germany) [Kanavakis et al., 2003]. The presence of mutations in the 27 exons of the CFTR gene and neighbouring intronic regions of the CFTR gene was assessed by denaturing gradient gel electrophoresis (DGGE) after simple or multiplex PCR of patient DNA [Fanen et al., 1992]. The intron 8 poly (T) variants of the CFTR gene were analyzed as described [Friedman et al., 1997]. All DNA samples showing a shift in DGGE mobility and not presenting a pattern of a known mutation were re-amplified from genomic DNA. Direct sequencing was performed using the VISGEN Long Read Tower system-V3.1 and the Cy5/Cy5.5 Dye primer bi-directional sequencing kit according to the manufacturer's instructions (Visible Genetics Inc., Toronto, Canada). All sequencing primers for the generation of the PCR products additionally contained universal 5' M13 sequences [Forward: 5'-GTAAAACGACGGCCAGT-3'; Reverse: 5'-CAGGAAACAGCTATGAC-3']. PCR primers for the CFTR gene exons were as previously described [Zielenski et al., 1991]. Common mutations in prenatal diagnoses were confirmed with the PMS methodology [Friedman et al., 1991; Tzetis et al., 1997].

Haplotype Analysis

For the diallelic sites, the PCR conditions and primers used are as described [Dork et al., 1992]. For haplotype analysis, restriction digests of the RFLP-PCR products were separated by agarose gel electrophoresis. Allele 1 represents the absence of a restriction site while allele 2 its presence. The GATT polymorphism was detected by the difference in mobility of the PCR product on 10% polyacrylamide gels. Allele 1 denotes 7 repeats, allele 2 six and allele 3 eight repeats. Microsatellites IVS8CA, IVS17BTA and IVS17BCA were analysed in a multiplex fluorescent PCR using the conditions reported previously [Morral et al., 1992]. All forward primers were fluorescently Cy5.5 labeled (Proligo LLC, Boulder, CO, USA). An aliquot of the reaction was mixed with a loading dye and 100 bp and 350 bp size markers (VISGEN Long Read Tower system-V3.1, Visible Genetics, Inc., Toronto, Canada), heated at 95°C for 5 min and cooled on ice. It was subsequently separated on a 6% denaturing polyacrylamide gel. Allele fragment sizes were determined in comparison with external size markers by an automated DNA sequencer and analyzed using the Fragment Analysis Software (Visible Genetics, Inc., Toronto, Canada).

Haplotypes were assigned where phase could be established, by typing of both parents and affected child in each CF pedigree.

Table 1. Frequencies of CFTR mutations identified in 500 Greek patients with cystic fibrosis, diagnosed on a clinical basis.

Mutation	Location Exon/intron	No. of chromosomes (Frequency %)	Microsatellite haplotype[b]	Ethnic prevalence[c]
p.F508del	10	545 (54.5)	25-31/32-13	Pan-European
c.621+1G>T	intron 4	63 (6.3)	23-32-13	Welsh
p.G542X	11	39 (3.9)	25-33/34-13	Mediterranean
p.N1303K	21	23 (2.3)	25/26-32-13	Mediterranean
c.2789+5G>A	intron 14b	20 (2.0)	8-18/28-18	Mediterranean
p.E822X[a]	13	18 (1.8)	17-30-13	Greek
c.21833AA>G	13	15 (1.5)	17-29/31-13	Hispanic
p.R1158X	19	11 (1.1)	25-34-13	Mediterranean
p.G85E	3	9 (0.9)	18-8/24-18/13	
p.R334W	7	8 (0.8)		Multi-ethnic
c.574delA	4	8 (0.8)		
p.W1282X	20	8 (0.8)	18-8-17	Ashkenazi Jewish
c.1677delTA	10	7 (0.7)		Russian
c.3120+1G>A	intron 16	7 (0.7)		African-American/Arabian
p.W496X	10	7 (0.7)	18-32-13	
c.3272-26A>G	intron 17a	7 (0.7)	18-8-18	Mediterranean
p.I507del	10	6 (0.6)	26-32-13	Hispanic
c.711+3A>G	intron 5	6 (0.6)		Mediterranean
c.621+3A>G[b]	intron 4	6 (0.6)		Mediterranean
p.R1070Q	17b	5 (0.5)		Bulgarian
p.R1070Q+S466X	17b and 10	4 (0.4)		Bulgarian
c.1525-1G>A	intron 9	4 (0.4)		Mediterranean
p.L137P[a]	4	4 (0.4)		Greek
p.A46D[a]	2	3 (0.3)	25-33-13	Greek
c.3120+1kbdel8.5kb	intron 16	3 (0.3)		Arabian
c.2184insA	13	3 (0.3)		
p.G551D	11	3 (0.3)		Celtic
p.D110H	4	3 (0.3)		Mediterranean
p.C276X	6b	3 (0.3)		
p.R117C	4	3 (0.3)		
CFTRdel2,3(21kb)	Deletion of exons 2 and 3	3 (0.3)		Eastern Slavic
p.C524X	10	2 (0.2)		
p.R553X	11	2 (0.2)		Swiss

Table 1. Frequencies of CFTR mutations identified in 500 Greek patients with cystic fibrosis, diagnosed on a clinical basis. (Continued)

Mutation	Location Exon/intron	No. of chromosomes (Frequency %)	Microsatellite haplotype[b]	Ethnic prevalence[c]
c.3152delT[a]	17a	2 (0.2)	18-34-13 & 17-49-18	Greek
p.D110E[a]	4	2 (0.2)		Greek
c.4382delA	24	2 (0.2)		Mediterranean
c.1898+1G>A	intron 12	2 (0.2)		Welsh
c.2790-1G>C	intron 14b	2 (0.2)		
p.M348K	7	2 (0.2)		Mediterranean
p.E831X	13	2 (0.2)		Syrian
p.L1065F[a]	17b	2 (0.2)		Greek
p.A46D+c.3272-4A>G[a]	2 and intron 17a	1 (0.1)		Greek
c.1898+1G>T	intron 12	1 (0.1)	19-8-13	East Asian
p.D1445N[a]	24	1 (0.1)		Greek
p.D1152H	18	1 (0.1)		
c.296+1G>C[a]	intron 2	1 (0.1)		Greek
p.R75L	3	1 (0.1)		
c.3849+4A>G	intron 19	1 (0.1)		
p.R1162X	19	1 (0.1)		Multi-ethnic
p.G1069R	17b	1 (0.1)		
p.E725K[a]	13	1 (0.1)		Greek
p.F1052V	17b	1 (0.1)		
c.525delT	4	1 (0.1)		Yugoslavian
p.R347P	7	1 (0.1)		
p.R347H	7	1 (0.1)		
p.L732X	13	1 (0.1)		
p.D836Y	14a	1 (0.1)		
c.2751+2T>A[a]	intron 14a	1 (0.1)	18-32-13	Greek
p.F1074L	17b	1 (0.1)		
c.1497delGG[a]	intron 9	1 (0.1)	18-30-17	Greek
p.S813P[a]	13	1 (0.1)		Greek
c.1571delG	10	1 (0.1)		Slavic
c.2118del4	13	1 (0.1)		
c.547insTA	4	1 (0.1)		
p.G1244V	20	1 (0.1)		
p.Q2X; p.R3W	1	1 (0.1)		
p.R75X	3	1 (0.1)		Hispanic
c.1716+1G>A[a]	intron 10	1 (0.1)		Greek
c.441delA	4	1 (0.1)		
p.D565G[a]	12	1 (0.1)		Greek
p.R352W	7	1 (0.1)		
p.Y247X[a]	6a	1 (0.1)	17-34-13	Greek
p.S945L	15	1 (0.1)		
p.P1021A[a]	17a	1 (0.1)		Greek
p.S997F	16	1 (0.1)		
pE823X[a]	13	1 (0.1)		Greek
c.4040delA	21	1 (0.1)		
c.2752-26A>G[a]	intron 14a	1 (0.1)	17-25-13	Greek
p.L1093P	17b	1 (0.1)		
c.406-6T>C	intron 3	1 (0.1)		Mediterranean
c.457TAT>G	4	1 (0.1)		Mediterranean
c.3849+10kbC>T	intron 19	1 (0.1)		Ashkenazi Jewish
c.2418GG>T[a]	13	1 (0.1)		Greek

Table 1. Frequencies of CFTR mutations identified in 500 Greek patients with cystic fibrosis, diagnosed on a clinical basis. (Continued)

Mutation	Location Exon/intron	No. of chromosomes (Frequency %)	Microsatellite haplotype[b]	Ethnic prevalence[c]
Unknown		79 (7.9)		
TOTAL		100		

[a]Mutations described for the first time by our group. [b]Most common haplotype in the Greek population. [c]Bobadilla et al., 2002; Estivill et al., 1997; CFGAC database. Variants are described using DNA and protein designation: intronic changes, deletions, insertions and frameshifts are reported at the cDNA level (c.) and amino acid changes at the protein level (p.)

RESULTS

Molecular Characterization

In the sample of 500 Greek CF patients 83 different mutations were detected including three complex alleles, and 20 mutations so far only identified in the Greek population (table 1). These 83 mutations account for 92% of CF genes generating 111 different genotypes, including 10 different homozygote genotypes with the following mutations: p.F508del, c.621+1G>T, p.G542X, p.R1158X, p.I507del, p.W496X, p.E822X, c.2789+5G>A, p.G85E and p.R1070Q. Seven mutations were quite common belonging (except for p.E822X) to a group that are common worldwide with p.F508del accounting for 54.5%. Sixteen show frequencies between 0.4% and 1.1% while the remaining 60 were very rare found in 1–3 chromosomes.

Haplotype Analysis

The phase of the diallelic and microsatellite haplotypes was determined by family studies (typing of both parents and affected CF child). For the normal alleles a total of 27 different diallelic [most common 11117212 (16%)] and 69 microsatellite [most common 17-29/30/31-13 (19.1%) and 18-31/32-13 (15.4%)] haplotypes were found. A total of 16 diallelic and 18 microsatellite haplotypes were found for p.F508del. Haplotype 12216112 (65.2%) was the most common (in accordance with other European populations) while 25-31/32-13 (40.4%), 26-32/33-13 (15.7%) and 17/19-31-13 (8.9%) were the most common p.F508del microsatellite haplotypes. 25-31-13 may have arisen by slippage from the most common European 23-31-13 haplotype, which has a frequency of only 6.5% in the Greek population. The non-p.F508del alleles were associated with 22 diallelic (most common 12216112 – 25.7%, 11127212 – 3.7%) and 31 microsatellite haplotypes. The most common haplotype for c.621+1G>T was 23-32-13, for p.G542X 25-33/34-13, for p.N1303K 25-32-13 and for p.E822X 17-30-13 (tables 2–4).

Male Infertility: CBAVD, Obstructive Azoospermia (OA) and Oligospermia

In the 48 males with CBAVD, a total of 22 different molecular defects were observed, with 56.2% carrying some type of molecular defect in the CFTR gene, and 27.1% being compound heterozygotes of two mutations or a mutation and the IVS8-5T allele. As expected a high frequency of p.F508del (20.8%) was found. Some of the mutations were common with CF patients (p.W496X, c.621+1G>T, c.4010delTAT, p.R1158X), while the rest except for p.L932X were missense or splicing with high residual levels of functional CFTR (p.M1I, p.R352W, c.711+3A>G, p.F1052V, p.R117C, p.D110E, p.D110H, p.D565G, c.3272-26A>G, p.I521F, p.P1021A, p.G817V, p.M952I). The presence of genomic variants with variable penetrance (p.F508C, p.R668C, p.R75Q, p.R1162L) was also noted, as well as a high frequency (11/48, 22.9%) of IVS8-5T exon 9 mis-splicing variant, compared to 3% in the controls.

Table 2. CFTR haplotypes for Diallelic and Microsatellite markers for 217 p.F508del Greek chromosomes.

XV2C-KM19-D9-J44-GATT-M470V-T854T-TUB20	**8CA-17BTA-17BCA**
1-2-2-1-6-1-1-2 (135)	**25-31-13(26), 25-32-13(15)**, 25-33-13(2), 25-27-13(1), 25-49-13(1), 25-7-13(1), 25-35-13(2), **26-32-13(10), 26-33-13(7)**, 26-31-13(2), 26-34-13(2), **23-31-13(3)**, 23-28-13(2), 23-32-13 (1), **24-31-13(3)**, 24-33-13(2), 19-31-13(2), 19-29-13(1), **19-32-13(2)**, 19-34-13(1), **17-31-13(4)**, 17-30-13(2), **18-32-13(3)**, 18-31-13(1), 18-29-13(1)
1-1-2-1-6-1-1-2 (20)	**25-31-13(6), 25-32-13(1)**, 25-30-13(1), **26-32-13(2)**, 26-31-13(1), 17-30-13(1)
1-2-1-1-6-1-1-2 (14)	**25-31-13(2), 25-32-13(1), 17-31-13(2), 19-31-13(1)**
1-2-2-1-6-1-2-2 (8)	**25-31-13(1), 25-32-13(1)**, 26-34-13(1), 19-34-13(2)
2-2-2-1-6-1-1-2 (8)	**18-32-13(2), 19-31-13(2)**
1-1-1-1-6-1-1-2 (5)	**25-32-13(2), 26-32-13(1)**
1-2-2-1-6-1-1-1 (5)	**26-33-13(1)**, 18-29-13(1), 23-31-13(1), 25-27-23(1)
2-1-1-1-6-1-1-2 (2)	**25-31-13(2)**, 24-32-13 (1)
2-2-1-1-6-1-1-2 (2)	**25-31-13(1)**
2-1-1-2-6-1-1-2 (2)	17-24-13(1), 17-34-13(1)
2-1-2-1-6-1-1-2 (1)	**19-31-13(1)**
1-1-2-2-6-1-1-2 (1)	17-32-13 (1)
2-1-2-2-6-1-1-2 (1)	17-32-13(1)
2-2-2-1-6-1-2-2 (1)	**26-33-13(1), 19-31-13(1), 18-32-13 (2), 24-31-13(1)**
2-2-2-1-6-1-1-1 (1) 1-2-2-2-6-1-1-2 (1)	**25-31-13(1)**

Allele 1 denotes the absence of the restriction site, whereas Allele 2 denotes its presence. Numbers for microsatellites GATT, IVS8CA, IVS17BTA, and IVS17BCA are the number of repeats. Numbers in parentheses denote the number of chromosomes for the specific haplotype in p.F508del chromosomes. Most common diallelic and microsatellite haplotypes are in bold letters. Most common microsatellite haplotypes are: 25-31-13(39), 25-32-13(20), 26-32-13(15), 26-33-13 (8), 19-31-13(7), 17-31-13(6), 18-32-13(5), 24-31-13(4), 17-30-13(3), 23-31-13(3).

Of the 40 OA males 27.5% had at least 1 CF allele, and 3 carried a severe mutation (p.F508del, p.W496X, and p.W1282X) and the IVS8-5T allele in trans or genomic variants with variable penetrance. Of the 46 males with severe oligospermia, 13% were found to be carriers of a CFTR mutation/variant and 2.2% carriers of the IVS8-5T allele (table 5).

Table 3. Haplotypes for diallelic and microsatellite DNA markers for CFTR mutations in Greek CF patients.

Mutation	XV2C-KM19-D9-J44-GATT-M470V-T854T-TUB20	8CA-17BTA-17BCA
c.621+1G>T (26)	**1-2-2-1-6-1-1-2 (20),** 1-1-2-1-6-1-1-2 (3), 2-2-2-1-6-1-1-2(2)	**23-32-13(7)**, 24-32-13(4), 23-31-13(4), 24-33-13(2), 24-8-17(1), 22-8-13(1), 18-8-17(1)
p.G542X (19)	**1-2-2-1-6-1-1-2 (10),** 2-2-2-1-6-1-1-2 (3), 1-1-1-6-1-1-2 (2), 2-2-1-1-6-1-1-2 (1), 1-2-1-1-6-1-1-2 (2), 1-1-1-2-1-6-1-1-2 (1)	**25-34-13(3), 24-33-13(3)**, 25-31-13(1), 19-35-13(1), 26-32-13(1), 17-31-13(1)
p.N1303K (14)	**1-2-2-1-6-1-1-2 (5), 1-1-2-1-6-1-1-2 (5)**, 2-2-2-1-6-1-1-2 (2), 1-1-1-2-7-1-1-2(1), 1-2-1-1-6-1-1-2 (1)	26-32-13(2), 25-32-13(2), 26-33-13(1), 25-7-13(1), 17-8-13(1), 25-28-13(1)
c.2183AA>G (7)	**2-2-2-1-7-1-1-2 (3)**, 1-2-2-1-6-1-1-2 (2), 2-2-1-1-7-1-1-2(1)	17-29-13(2), 17-31-13(1)
p.E822X (10)	**1-1-1-2-7-2-1-2 (5)**, 1-1-1-1-7-2-1-2 (2), 2-1-1-2-7-2-2-2 (1)	**17-30-13(7)**, 17-32-13(2), 17-7-18(1)
c.2789+5G>A (3)	1-1-1-1-8-2-1-2 (1), 2-1-2-1-8-1-2-1 (1), 1-2-2-1-7-1-1-2(1)	18-8-18 (1), 18-28-18(1)
p.R1158X (6)	**2-2-2-1-6-1-1-1 (3)**, 2-1-1-2-6-1-1-2 (1), 1-2-1-1-6-1-1-2(1), 2-1-1-1-7-2-1-2 (1)	**25-34-13(3)**, 25-33-13(1), 17-28-13(1)
p.R1070Q (3)	1-1-2-1-6-1-1-2 (2), 1-1-1-2-7-1-1-2(1)	18-35-13(1), 19-32-13(1), 17-31-13(1)
p.G85E (5)	2-2-2-1-8-2-2-1 (2), 1-2-2-1-8-2-2-1(1), 1-1-1-2-8-2-1-2(1)	**18-8-18(3),** 18-24-13(1)
c.3272-26A>G (4)	2-2-2-1-?-1-2-1(2), 1-1-1-?-2-2-1 (1)	**18-8-18(3)**
p.I507del (4)	1-2-2-1-6-1-1-2 (1), 2-2-2-1-6-1-1-2 (2), 1-2-1-1-6-1-1-2(1)	26-32-13(1), 20-32-13(1), 24-31-13(1), 18-31-13(1)
p.W1282X (2)	1-2-2-1-6-1-2-1(2)	18-8-17(1)
p.C276X (1)	1-2-1-1-?-?-1-2	18-47-13
c.1898+1G>T (1)	1-1-1-2-?-?-1-2	19-8-13
c.3849+10kbC>T (1)	1-2-2-1-7-1-1-2	17-31-13
p.W496X (1)	2-2-2-2-?-1-1-2	18-32-13
p.A46D (1)	1-2-2-1-7-1-1-2	25-33-13
c.3152delT (2)	2-1-1-2-7-1-1-2 (1), 2-2-2-1-7-1-2-2 (1)	18-34-13, 17-49-18
c.2752-26A>G (1)		17-25-13
p.Y247X (1)	2-1-1-2-6-1-1-2	17-34-13
c.1497delGG (1)	1-2-2-1-7-1-2-1	18-30-17
p.L1065F (1)	1-2-2-2-6-2-1-2	
p.K162E (1)		18-30-13
c.2751+2T>A (1)	1-1-1-2-7-2-1-2	18-32-13

Allele 1 denotes absence of restriction site, whereas allele 2 denotes its presence. Numbers for microsatellites GATT, IVS8CA, IVS17BTA and IVS17BTA are the number of repeats. Numbers in parentheses denote the number of chromosomes with the specific haplotype. Haplotypes in bold denote the most common haplotype for the mutation. DNA and protein designation: intronic changes, deletions, insertions and frameshifts are reported at the cDNA level (c.) and amino acid changes at the protein level (p.)

Heterozygote Screening

Mutation analysis on 900 individuals identified a total of 188 heterozygotes. More specifically 58/91 heterozygotes (63.7%) were identified amongst the siblings of CF index cases, 115/285 (40.4%) amongst the CF family relatives (R) and 15/174 (8.6%) amongst the general population individuals (GP). Amongst the 175 couples screened, 14 had a CF partner (GP/CF), 106 had a partner with family history of CF (GP/R), 23 had a male partner with infertility (GP/CBAVD) and in 32 couples both were general population subjects (GP/GP). Of the 175 couples, 23 were already pregnant upon request for CFTR screening, and six were found requiring prenatal diagnosis [1 GP/R (0.9%), 2 GP/GP (6.25%), 2 GP/CBAVD (8.7%) and 1 GP/CF (7.1%)].

Table 4. Allele Frequencies for the intron 8 CA repeat in normal and CF chromosomes.

		FREQUENCY OF													
No of repeats		**Normal (n=136)**		**p.F508del (n=146)**		**c.621+1G>T (n=20)**		**p.G542X (n=10)**		**p.N1303K (n=8)**		**p.E822X (n=10)**		**p.R1158X (n=5)**	
8CA	17BTA	8CA	17BTA	8CA	17BTA	8CA	17BTA	8CA	17BTA	8CA	17BTA	8CA	17BTA	8CA	17BTA
13	7	0.007	0.015		0.007						0.125		0.1		
16	***8***	0.022	***0.11***				0.2				0.125				
17	9	**0.294**	0.074	0.089				0.1		0.125		1		0.2	
18	18	**0.397**	0.007	0.068		0.05									
19	20	0.132	0.007	0.089				0.1							
20	22	0.015	0.007												
22	23	0.015	0.007			0.05									
23	24	0.007		0.048	0.007	***0.55***									
24	25	0.044	0.007	0.048		***0.35***		***0.3***							
25	26	0.029	0.007	**0.466**				**0.4**		**0.5**				0.8	
26	27	0.007		**0.192**	0.014			0.1		**0.375**					
	28		0.015		0.014						0.125				0.2
	29		0.081		0.02										
	30		***0.103***		0.027								***0.7***		
	31		**0.22**		**0.438**		**0.2**		0.2						
	32		**0.147**		**0.315**		**0.55**		0.1		**0.5**		0.2		
	33		0.066		0.089		0.2		***0.3***		0.125				0.2
	34		0.029		0.048				***0.3***						***0.6***
	35		0.015		0.014				0.1						
	36		0.015												
	38		0.015												
	45		0.029												
	47		0.007												
	48		0.007												
	49				0.007										
	55		0.007												

Note- numbers of chromosomes studied appear in parentheses; numbers in bold: most common haplotypes. DNA and protein designation: intronic changes, deletions, insertions and frameshifts are reported at the cDNA level (c.) and amino acid changes at the protein level (p.)

Prenatal Diagnosis

For the 167 prenatal diagnoses performed a total of 57 different genotypes (of which 13 from the IVF couples), were assessed. Direct analysis was possible in all but four cases for which only one parental mutation was known. In these cases microsatellite analysis in addition to testing for the one parental mutation was conclusive for three and not possible for one. This fetus was diagnosed as having the one parental allele through mutation analysis, and the microsatellite sites were not informative. In 46 prenatal diagnoses the fetuses were diagnosed as normal, in 80 as heterozygotes and 41 as affected. The results are in agreement with those expected for an autosomal recessive disease. The outcome of all cases that were diagnosed as being unaffected by CF was a normal child. In two cases where one of the parents had two mutations in cis, p.R1070Q+p.S466X and p.Q2X+p.R3W, respectively, fetal DNA was tested for one of the mutations of the complex allele (p.R1070Q and p.Q2X, respectively). Similarly in four couples with one parent compound heterozygote but asymptomatic (Genotypes: p.F508del/p.K162E and p.R1158X/p.R1070Q) and two mono-symptomatic CBAVD parents (Genotypes: p.F1052V/p.F1052V and p.F508del/p.M952I), fetal DNA was tested for 3 parental mutations. If the embryo combined one severe and one mild parental mutation, genetic counselling on the clinical phenotype is difficult. Such a case arose in two prenatal diagnoses involving IVF couples. The fetuses were diagnosed as homozygous with genotypes p.F1052V/p.M348K and p.G565G/p.406-6T>C respectively. Both couples were counselled on the expected mildness of the phenotype, and both decided to carry the pregnancies to term.

Table 5. Summary of CFTR mutation screening on male infertility patients

CBAVD Patients (n=48)		**Obstructive Azoospermia(n=40)**	**Oligospermia (n=46)**
2 mutations	**1 mutation AND/OR IVS8-5T**		
p.F508del/p.M1I & IVS8-5T	p.F508del(4), & IVS8-5T(3)	p.W496X/p.I506V(1)	p.F508del(2)
p.F508del/c.711+3A>G	p.D565G(3)	p.F508del & IVS8-5T(1)	p.G542X(1)
p.F508del/p.F508C	c.3272-26A>G(1)	c.2790-8C>G(1)	p.C491S(1)
p.F508del/p.D110E	p.L932X & IVS8-5T(1)	p.S549N(1)	p.F1052V(1)
p.F508del/p.R352W	c.711+3A>G & IVS8-5T(1)	p.W1282X & IVS8-5T(1)	c.2752-6T>C(1)
p.F508del/p.M952I	c.4010delTAT(1)	p.F1052V(1)	IVS8-5T(1)
c.621+1G>T/p.R117C	p.I521F(1)	p.D110H(1)	
p.F1052V/p.F1052V	p.R1158X(1)	c.406-6T>C(1)	
	p.P1021A(1)	p.R75Q(2)	

Table 5. Summary of CFTR mutation screening on male infertility patients (Continued)

CBAVD Patients (n=48)		**Obstructive Azoospermia(n=40)**	**Oligospermia (n=46)**
	p.D110H(1)	IVS8-5T(1)	
	p.G817V(1)		
	c.3659delC(1)		
	IVS8-5T(3)		
Total: 8	**Total: 20**	**Total:11**	**Total: 7**

Numbers in parentheses denote number of chromosomes. DNA and protein designation: intronic changes, deletions, insertions and frameshifts are reported at the cDNA level (c.) and amino acid changes at the protein level (p.)

Prenatal Diagnosis due to Fetal Bowel Echogenicity

Seventy-four AF samples were tested for CF mutations due to bowel hyperechogenicity in the fetus, detected during a routine second trimester ultrasound examination. Homozygosity was detected in 4 cases (3.6%), with the following severe disease indicating genotypes: p.F508del/p.L732X, p.F508del/c.574delA, p.F508del/p.F508del, and p.F508del/p.G542X. Fifteen of the (13.6%) had one detectable mutation, 10 with p.F508del, and 1 each for c.621+1G>T, p.I148T, c.2789+5G>A, p.R297Q, p.E822X. An additional finding was the presence of particular polymorphisms: 5/110 instances of 1716G/A (p.E528E), 2 of c.2752-15G/C, 2 of p.R1162L and 1 of c.4029A/G. The significance of these findings can not be readily explained (table 6).

Table 6. Summary of echogenic bowel families tested and CF genotype results.

Both parents and/or fetus negative	24	
One parent carrier- fetus negative	2	p.I148T, p.F508del
One parent carrier- fetus not tested	5	c.621+3A>G, p.R75Q and 3 with p.F508del
One parent carrier- fetus carrier	7	c.621+1G>T, p.I148T and 5 with p.F508del
Both parents carriers- fetus affected	4	p.F508del/p.L732X, p.F508del/c.574delA, p.F508del/p.F508del, p.F508del/p.G542X
Fetus only tested- negative	29	
Fetus only tested- carrier	8	p.E822X; c.2789+5G>A; p.R297Q; and 5 p.F508del
Couple only tested–both negative	31	
TOTAL	110	4 homozygotes AND 15 with 1 detectable mutation

Conclusion

Molecular Heterogeneity of CF in Greece

The most common CFTR mutations worldwide, showing frequencies >1%, are the following: p.F508del, p.G542X, p.N1303K, p.G551D and p.W1282X. Another 19 mutations are found in 0.1–1% of cases showing considerable variation for different populations, with the majority being restricted to particular geographic areas. Mutation p.F508del shows a North-to-South Europe decreasing frequency gradient (30–90%) while the percentage of non-p.F508del chromosomes associated with CF increases [CFGAC: http://www.genet.sickkids.on.ca/cftr; Estivill et al., 1997; Bobadilla et al., 2002]. The Mediterranean area has the highest CFTR heterogeneity, making genetic diagnosis by mutation analysis especially difficult [Claustres et al., 1996; Chillon et al., 1994; Casals et al., 1996; Kanavakis et al., 2003; Mendes et al., 2003; Castaldo et al., 2004; des Georges et al., 2004; Radivojevic et al., 2004]. For the Spanish CF patients, 73 different mutations have been identified accounting for 87% of CF alleles with only 10 of them having a frequency higher than 1% and for the French population 105 mutations account for 86% of CF chromosomes [Casals et al., 1996; Gasparini et al., 1993; des Georges et al., 2004]. Studies of North-eastern Italian CF patients identified 62 mutations accounting for 73.8% of detectable CF alleles while for the Celtic population from Brittany, France, 19 mutations account for 98% of CF chromosomes [Gasparini et al., 1993; Ferec et al., 1992; Des Georges et al., 2004].

DGGE analysis of the 27 exons and neighboring intronic regions of the CFTR gene revealed the presence of 83 different mutations covering 92% of CF alleles, proving that the Greek population has one of the highest rates of CFTR mutation heterogeneity. Twenty of the characterized mutations are apparently specific to the Greek population and the majority are found in one or two alleles with the exception of p.E822X which has achieved a high frequency in Central Greece. The list of mutations found in our population is shown in table 1. Three of these (p.F508del, p.G542X and p.N1303K) are common worldwide, the rest with the exception of p.E822X, are common in the Mediterranean area, some achieving relatively high frequencies in wide geographic areas and others being common in small regions [CFGAC: http://www.genet.sickkids.on.ca/cftr; Estivill et al., 1997; Bobadilla et al., 2002]. The wide distribution of p.F508del, p.G542X and p.N1303K suggests an ancient origin for these mutations [Morral et al., 1994]. Mutation p.G542X is common in the Mediterranean, with a mean frequency of 4.3%, while p.N1303K is found in most of the western Mediterranean countries with highest frequency in Tunisia (17.2%). The other common mutations such as c.621+1G>T, considered a Celtic mutation, c.2789+5G>A and c.2183AA>G, considered Southern European, have achieved relatively high frequencies in the south-eastern Mediterranean region. Mutation p.R1158X is very rare and is found in southern Italy with comparable frequencies to those found in Greece with only two alleles described in France and one in Spain; therefore, it must have an origin and diffusion in the specific European region [Claustres et al., 1996; Tzetis et al., 1997; Castaldo et al., 1999; Castaldo et al., 2004; Chillon et al., 1994]. Mutation p.E822X has only been found in the Greek population and is confined to a specific region of Central Greece. Sixteen mutations show frequencies between 0.4 and 1.1% (table 1). Of these c.1677delTA and p.R1070Q have reached high frequencies in Bulgaria and Turkey, c.3272-26A>G in Portugal, France and Belgium (with frequencies ranging from 1% to 2.8%) and c.3120+1G>A is considered an African mutation, reaching high frequencies amongst the African–Americans (13.9%) [Dork et al., 1998; Bobadilla et al., 2002]. Mutation p.R334W is common in the Eastern Mediterranean, reaching a very high frequency in Crete. p.W1282X has the highest frequency in Israel, being the most common mutation and c.621+3A>G also found in the French population, initially reported as a polymorphism was later proven to be a splicing mutation [CFGAC database http://www.genet.sickkids.on.ca/cftr; Estivill et al., 1997; Amaral et al., 2001; Dork et al., 1998; Tzetis et al., 2001b].

Haplotype Analysis

The normal chromosomes were found associated with a total of 11 alleles for the IVS8CA site (17 and 18 being the commonest) and 23 for the IVS17BTA site (30, 31 and 32 being the commonest). The IVS17BCA site showed the lowest variability with only six alleles of which 13 and 17 had the highest frequency. Mutation p.F508del associated with seven alleles for the IVS8CA site (25 and 26 most common), 12 IVS17BTA alleles (31 and 32 most common) and only allele 13 for the IVS17BCA site. The other common mutations showed lower allele variability for both the IVS8CA and IVS17BTA sites (tables 2–4). Strong linkage disequilibrium was observed for p.F508del and one diallelic haplotype (12216112 –65.2%), which accounts for only 0.02% of normal Greek chromosomes. The other two most frequent disease causing mutations such as c.621+1G>T, p.G542X and p.N1303K also reside on the typical p.F508del haplotype. This specific diallelic haplotype is commonly associated with p.F508del and common mutations in other populations supporting the theory of an ancient origin of these mutations [Dork et al., 1992; Morral et al., 1993; 1994; 1996]. Microsatellite haplotype 25-31-13, which may have arisen by slippage from the most common European haplotype 23-31-13, was found most commonly associated with p.F508del, while p.G542X (25-33/34-13) and p.N1303K (25-32-13) have the 8CA-25 repeat allele in common with p.F508del. The most common haplotype for mutation c.621+1G>T was 23-32-13 (tables 2 and 3). The observed higher heterogeneity for the p.F508del diallelic haplotype background and the difference in the major microsatellite haplotype from Northern European populations supports the theory of a longer history of p.F508del in Southern Europe which would have allowed time for recombination with other haplotypes [Claustres et al., 1996; Morral et al., 1994]. Mutation p.R1158X, which is specific to the Southern Mediterranean region, is on a different diallelic and microsatellite framework than that observed for Italy and France, suggesting a recurrent origin or several recombination events [Castaldo et al., 1999]. The microsatellite haplotype was 16-7-17 for Italian CF chromosomes and 16-7/45-17/13 for the two French alleles being different from the Greek 25/17-28/33/34-13 (25-34-13; 3 alleles). The mutation could have been introduced to Southern Italy from ancient Greeks. The rare and specific Greek mutations are each associated with specific diallelic and microsatellite markers, which agrees with the theory that these mutations have a fairly recent origin. This especially applies to mutation p.E822X which is exclusively associated with a microsatellite framework (17-30-13) which is common in the normal chromosomes and with the commonest diallelic haplotype (11117212) for the normal alleles. The analysis of haplotypes and mutations in the Greek population adds to the information on CFTR gene mutations in Europe. This study also confirms that polymorphism analysis is a valid procedure to asses the genetic heterogeneity of a population and to evaluate the origin of a mutation. The high mutational heterogeneity and haplotypic variability shown in the Greek population is consistent with an earlier appearance of CFTR mutations in southern Europe, which would have allowed time for haplotypic recombination and slippage at microsatellites to occur [Claustres et al., 1996; Morral et al., 1996; Bertrapetit et al., 1996; Angelicheva et al., 1997].

Monosymtomatic CFTR

Male infertility: CBAVD, Obstructive Azoospermia (OA) and Oligospermia

CF-related infertility in men is primarily due to obstruction or absence of the vas deferens [Welsh et al., 2001] though a defect in spermatogenesis may be a contributing factor, as decreased numbers of mature spermatids and the presence of many malformed late spermatids are also found in CF [Trezise et al., 1993].

The relationship between CBAVD and CF gene mutations has previously been demonstrated [Chillon et al., 1995; Costes et al., 1995; Kanavakis et al., 1998; Claustres et al., 2000; Claustres, 2004]. In the majority of cases two CFTR mutations (including the IVS8-5T allele) were present in approximately 47% and one mutation in 24% of CBAVD patients. The IVS8-5T allele is the most commonly found CFTR defect in CBAVD males [Chillon et al., 1995; Estivill et al., 1996; Kanavakis et al., 1998; Claustres et al., 2000; Groman et al., 2004]. Generally one "severe" allele is combined with one "mild" or variant allele, such that the mild allele appears to dominate and cause a milder phenotype. These milder alleles may produce CFTR protein with low levels of expression (8-10% of normal) and thus cause disease in the vas deferens tissue and not in other organs affected by cystic fibrosis. Increased frequency of CF mutations in healthy men with reduced sperm quality and also in men with obstructive azoospermia with the presence of the vas deferens has also been reported [Van der Ven et al., 1996; Meschede et al., 1997; Kanavakis et al., 1998].

Our results show that of the 48 CBAVD males, 27.1% were compound heterozygotes, the majority with p.F508del (20.8% vs 54.5% for classic CF patients) and a mild mutation/variant in trans including the IVS8-5T allele, while 25% had only one mutation. The frequency of the IVS8-5T allele among CBAVD males was 22.9% compared to 3% in the general population. In this group of patients a total of 22 different defects were observed with the majority of mutations except for p.R352W, p.M952I, p.L932X, c.4010delTAT, p.G817V, c.3659delC, c.2790-8C>G, p.S549N, p.C491S, c.2752-6T>C and p.M1I also found in our cohort of CF patients (tables 1 and 5). In only four of the eight compound heterozygote CBAVD patients the sweat test was >60mEq/l. Furthermore three of the 48 CBAVD men also presented with recurrent bronchitis or chronic cough.

Of the 40 men with OA, 27.5% had at least one CF allele and three carried a severe mutation also found in our cohort of CF patients (p.F508del, p.W496X, p.W1282X) and the IVS8-5T allele in trans or genomic variants with variable penetrance. The frequency of the

IVS8-5T allele was 7.5%. The sweat test was borderline positive (40-60mEq/l) in three patients. The high frequency of CFTR mutations in males with OA (27.5%) suggests that the CFTR protein may play a critical role in spermatogenesis or sperm maturation that is independent of its function in the development of epithelial ducts such as the vas deferens [Trezise et al., 1993; Van der ven et al., 1996; Meschende et al., 1997].

Of the 46 males with severe oligospermia, 13% were found to be carriers of a CFTR mutation/variant and 2.2% carriers of the IVS8-5T allele (table 5).

In conclusion CFTR mutations may represent one of the most common abnormalities associated with male infertility, especially with CBAVD (CFTR mutation frequency 56.2%) but also in OA (27.5%). These results are relevant for couples treated by in-vitro fertilization (IVF) and intracytoplasmic sperm injection (ICSI). Patients with male infertility and their partners should be extensively tested by scanning techniques such as DGGE covering exons that harbour at least 85% of CFTR mutations of the specific ethnic group. Because of the incomplete penetrance of mild mutations for some combinations of CFTR genes in these couples (rare missense and severe mutation), counselling on the phenotypic consequences for their children is very difficult. We have encountered such combinations in two couples (with the following genotypes: p.F1052V/p.M384K and p.G565G/c.406T>C), which are discussed further below in this chapter. Finally, patients with CBAVD who have a positive sweat test and are compound heterozygotes for two CFTR mutations or one mutation/and the IVS8-5T allele probably warrant further clinical follow-up for potential late complications of CF, especially advice on persistent pulmonary symptoms.

Heterozygote Screening

For recessive conditions such as CF the goal of genetic screening is to recognize asymptomatic heterozygous carriers and to aid the process of reproductive decision making. Two distinct types of genetic screening strategy have been proposed. One offers testing to the population at large; the other targets high-risk groups identified through a family history or a specific clinical phenotype [Super et al., 1994; Brock 1995; Mennuti 2001; Palomaki et al., 2004]. Carrier screening for the population at large is not currently possible, we therefore concentrated on testing individuals belonging to a high-risk group including siblings of index cases, CF family relatives (R) and their partners (when available) and both members of couples seeking IVF due to male infertility. A common reason for performing IVF and intracytoplasmic sperm injection (ICSI) is congenital bilateral absence of vas deferens (CBAVD). Because of the high frequency of CFTR mutations found in infertile males with CBAVD [Kanavakis et al., 1998; and results in this chapter], the male partner needs to be screened and couple screening is recommend in such cases. The remaining carrier risk, after negative screening for 85% of detectable CF alleles, is 1/161. Couples in which one partner is a definite carrier and the other has a negative mutation analysis have their risk of having an affected child reduced to 1/644 from 1/100, and in cases when neither partner tests positive the risk is 1/103324. For most couples this could be reassuring information. Through such a screening program on 900 individuals a total of 188 heterozygotes were identified. As expected a high number of heterozygotes were found amongst the 91 siblings of CF index cases (63.7%) and amongst the CF family relatives (R) (40.4%). The carrier frequency amongst the general population individuals was 8.6% (15/174). Six couples where both members were carriers were identified amongst the 175 couples screened [1GP/R (0.9%), 2GP/GP (6.25%), 2GP/CBAVD (8.7%) and 1GP/CF (7.1%)]. Prenatal diagnosis was performed in these cases including two twin pregnancies conceived through ICSI, because the male partner had CBAVD. The results of the pregnancies were one homozygous, four heterozygous and three normal infants. While diagnostic methods are not automatic and robust enough for heterogeneous CF populations, the diagnostic strategy of DGGE screening of 15 CFTR exons (accounting for 86% of CF alleles) in combination with haplotype association of certain mutations is presently an appropriate tool for screening the Greek population. This strategy also provides rapid, accurate and reliable prenatal diagnosis for the majority of couples.

Prenatal Diagnosis

The characterization of mutations and their frequencies in a specific population is a prerequisite for setting up screening and prenatal diagnosis programs. For the highly heterogeneous Greek population a strategy of DGGE and sequencing resulted in the characterization of 92% of CF alleles. In the case of families with a one in four risk, if the causative mutation(s) have been identified in both parents before pregnancy, DGGE analysis permits the determination of presence or absence of the mutation(s) in the chorionic villus or amniotic fluid sample within 2 days. The additional use of the polymorphic microsatellite markers permits prenatal diagnosis in cases where only one parental mutation is known and also checks for maternal contamination and confirms paternity of the fetal DNA sample. For the 176 prenatal diagnoses performed a combination of direct mutation and microsatellite analysis was conclusive in all but one case. Microsatellite analysis is performed even in those cases where the causative mutation(s) have been identified in a given family. The extremely sensitive technique of fluorescent PCR will reveal the presence of even minute quantities of maternal contamination in the fetal sample. We have not observed any cases of maternal contamination in any of the fetal samples we have so far tested. A factor that complicates CFTR mutation screening and prenatal diagnosis is the presence of complex alleles. We observed two such cases in which parental alleles had two mutations in cis (p.R1070Q+p.S446X and p.Q2X+p.R3W, respectively). In such cases careful analysis must precede the prenatal diagnosis for the confirmation of the cis positioning of the two alleles. In the course of genotyping our CF patient population we observed two cases where one parent, without clinical symptoms of CF, is a compound heterozygotes for two CF mutations (p.F508del/p.K162E and p.R1158X/p.R1070Q). In such cases the fetal DNA must be tested for three parental mutations. In the course of screening for male infertility we identified two couples requiring prenatal diagnosis where the CBAVD males were compound heterozygotes (p.F1052V/p.F1052V and p.F508del/p.M952I). In these cases fetal DNA was also tested for three parental mutations. When the genotype of the embryo combines one parental severe mutation and one mild mutation, genetic counselling on the clinical phenotype of the embryo is difficult. In two IVF couples the fetuses were diagnosed with the following genotypes:

p.F1052V/p.M384K and p.G565G/c.406T>C. The couples after being counselled on the expected mildness of the phenotype, decided to carry the pregnancies to term. These cases should be elucidated when modifying factors (possibly other genes) affecting the clinical phenotype are identified.

Prenatal Diagnosis due to Echogenic Bowel

For pregnancies presented with echogenic bowel (EB) we have tested both parental and fetal DNA in the majority of cases. A negative screening of about 62 mutations (86% of detectable CF alleles) reduces the probability of CF diagnosis when both parents have been excluded as carriers. According to the currently available literature when no CF mutations are identified the risk that the fetus is affected with CF is between 1/453 and 1/1516, while a fetus with one CF mutation has a 21–47% probability of being affected with CF. Direct fetal studies should be performed to additionally avoid cases of non-paternity which could lead to false–negative diagnosis and testing for chromosomal abnormalities [Bosco et al., 1999; Monaghan et al., 1999; Strocker et al., 2000; Sepuvelda et al., 2000]. We identified four homozygous fetuses (3.6%) and fifteen (13.6%) with a single CF mutation (table 6). Our data indicated that the prior risk of CF in a fetus with echogenic bowel for our population is 3.6% (1/28 births, ~90 times higher than prevalence in the general population) and the remaining risk of a heterozygous fetus having CF is 17.23% [Bosco et al., 1999]. The 4 couples with affected fetuses opted for pregnancy termination. Parents were given genetic consultation of ~17% remaining risk of CF for the 15/110 fetuses with one detected mutation. Thirteen continued to term and resulted in apparently healthy infants after clinical assessment. One family opted for pregnancy termination and one pregnancy is still ongoing.

Fetal echogenic bowel is an ultrasound marker associated with various fetal complications one of which is Cystic Fibrosis. A difficult situation arises when the fetus carries one identifiable CF mutation. Assuming a prior risk of CF in EB of 3.6% as calculated from our cohort of cases, the residual risk for the fetus being affected can be calculated to be ~17%. This is an important finding that will help in the correct counseling of these couples.

The expanded research into the CFTR gene and classic and monosymptomatic forms of CF adds to the challenges of appropriate testing. Knowledge of certain CFTR mutations may indicate a severe or mild phenotype, however predicting the severity of the disease from the genotype will not be possible until additional factors affecting disease severity (environmental and genetic) are elucidated. Information that will emerge during the next years will most probably open new ways for the development of mutation specific therapies. Finally there is now great hope for an ultimate cure through gene replacement therapy although important technical hurdles need to be overcome before its application on a routine basis.

Acknowledgements

The authors wish to thank Konstantina Pouliou for technical assistance. This work was partially funded by the Research Institute for the Study of Genetic and Malignant Disorders in Childhood.

References

Ahmed N, Corey M, Forstner G et al. molecular consequences of cystic fibrosis tramsmembrane regulator (CFTR) gene mutations in the exocrine pancreas. *Gut* 2003: 52: 1159-1164.

Amaral MD, Pancheco P, Beck S et al. Cystic fibrosis patients with the 3272–26A>G splicing mutation have milder disease than F508del homozygotes: a large European study. *J Med Genet* 2001: 38: 777–782.

Angelicheva D, Calafell F, Savov A et al. Cystic fibrosis mutations and associated haplotypes in Bulgaria – a comparative population genetic study. *Hum Genet* 1997: 99: 513–520.

Bobadilla JL, Macek MJr, Fine JP, Farrell PM. Cystic Fibrosis: A Worldwide analysis of CFTR mutations- Correlation with incidence data and application to screening. *Hum Mutat* 2002: 19: 575-606.

Bonizzato A, Bisceglia L, Marigo C et al. Analysis of the complete coding region of the CFTR gene in a cohort of CF patients from north-eastern Italy: Identification of 90% of the mutations. *Hum Genet* 1995: 95: 397–402.

Bertrapetit J, Calafell F. Genetic and geographical variabilityin cystic fibrosis: evolutionary considerations. *Ciba Found Symp* 1996: 197: 97–118.

Bosco AF, Norton ME, Lieberman E. Predicting the risk of cystic fibrosis with echogenic fetal bowel and one cystic fibrosis mutation. *Obstet Gynecol* 1999: 94: 1020–1023.

Brock DJH. Heterozygote screening for cystic fibrosis. *Eur J Hum Genet* 1995: 3: 2–13.

Castaldo G, Fuccio A, Cazeneuve C et al. Detection of five rare cystic fibrosis mutations peculiar to southern Italy. Implications in screening for the disease and phenotype characterization for patients with homozygote mutations. *Clin Chem* 1999: 47: 929–931.

Castaldo G, Polizzi A, Tomaiuolo R et al. Comprehensive Cystic Fibrosis mutation epidemiology and haplotype characterization in a Southern Italian Population. *Ann Hum Genet* 2004: 69: 15-24.

Casals T, Gimenez J, Ramos M, Nunes V, Estivill X. Prenatal diagnosis of cystic fibrosis in a highly heterogeneous population. *Prenat Diagn* 1996: 16: 215–222.

Casals T, De-Gracia J, Gallego M et al. Bronchiectais in adult patients: an expression of heterozygosity for CFTR gene mutations? *Clin Genet* 2004: 65: 490-495.

Chevalier-Porst F, Bonardot AM, Gilly R, Chazalette JP, Mathieu M, Bozon D. Mutation analysis in 600 French cystic fibrosis patients. *J Med Genet* 1994: 31: 541–544.

Chillon M, Casals T, Gimenez J, Nunes V, Estivill X. Analysis of the CFTR gene confirms the high genetic heterogeneity of the Spanish population: 43 mutations account for only 78% of CF chromosomes. *Hum Genet* 1994: 93: 447–451.

Chillon M, Casals T, Gimenez J, Nunes V, Estivill X. Analysis of the CFTR gene in the Spanish population: SSCP screening for 60 known mutations and identification of four new mutations (Q30X, A120T, 1812–1G>A, and 3667del4). *Hum Mutat* 1994: 3: 223–230.

Chillon M, Casals T, Mercier B et al. Mutations in the cystic fibrosis gene in patients with congenital absence of the vas deferens. *N Engl J Med* 1995: 332: 1475-1480.

Claustres M, Desgeorge M, Moine P, Morral N, Estivill X. CFTR haplotypic variability for normal and mutant genes in cystic fibrosis families from southern France. *Hum Genet* 1996: 98: 336–344.

Claustres M, Guittard C, Bozon D et al. Spectrum of CFTR mutations in cystic fibrosis and in congenital absence of the vas deferens in France. *Hum Mut* 2000: 16: 143-156.

Claustres M. Symposium: Genetic aspects of male (in)fertility. Molecular pathology of the CFTR locus in male infertility. *Reprod BioMedicine Online* 2005: 10: 14-41.

Cohn JA. Reduced CFTR function and the pathobiology of Idiopathic Pancreatitis. *J Clin Gastroenterol* 2005: S70-S77.

Costes B, Fanen P, Goossens M, Ghanem N. A rapid, efficient, and sensitive assay for simultaneous detection of multiple cystic fibrosis mutations. *Hum Mutat* 1993: 2: 185–191.

Costes B, Girodon E, Ghanem N et al. Frequent occurrence of the CFTR intron 8 (TG)n5T allele in men with congenital bilateral absence of the vas deferens. *Eur J Hum Genet* 1995: 3: 285-293.

Cystic Fibrosis Genetic Analysis Consortium- CFGAC. The CFTR mutation database http://www.genet.sickkids.on.ca/cftr.

Des Georges M, Guittard C, Altieri JP, Templin C, Sarles J, Sarda P, Claustres M. High heterogeneity of CFTR mutations and unexpected low incidence of cystic fibrosis in the Mediterranean France. *J Cyst Fibros* 2004: 3: 265-272.

Dork T, Neumann T, Wulbrand U et al. Intra- and extragenic marker haplotypes of CFTR mutation in cystic fibrosis families. *Hum Genet* 1992: 88: 417–425.

Dork T, El-Harith EH, Struhrmann M et al. Evidence for a common ethnic origin of cystic fibrosis mutation 3120+1G>A in diverse populations. *Am J Hum Genet* 1998: 63: 652–662.

Estivill X. Complexity in monogenic disease. *Nat Genet* 1996:12: 348-350.

Estivill X, Bancells C, Ramos C. Geographic distribution and regional origin of 272 cystic fibrosis mutations in European populations. The Biomed CF Mutation Analysis Consortium. *Hum Mutat* 1997: 10: 135–154.

Fanen P, Ghanem N, Vidaud M et al. Molecular characterization of cystic fibrosis: 16 novel mutations identified by analysis of the whole cystic fibrosis transmembrane conductance regulator (CFTR) coding regions and splice site junctions. *Genomics* 1992: 13: 770–776.

Feldman GL, Monaghan KG. Prenatal diagnosis of cystic fibrosis. In: Milunski A, ed. *Genetic Disorders and the Fetus. Diagnosis, Prevention and Treatment,* 4th edn. Baltimore: The John Hopkins University Press, 1998: 506–528.

Ferec C, Audrezet MP, Mercier B et al. Detection of over 98% cystic fibrosis mutations in a Celtic population. *Nat Genet* 1992: 3: 188–191.

Friedman KJ, Highsmith WEJr, Silverman LM. Detecting multiple cystic fibrosis mutations by polymerase chain reaction-mediated site-directed mutagenesis. *Clin Chem* 1991:37:753-5.

Friedman KJ, Heim R, Knowles MR, Silverman LM. Rapid characterization of the variable length polythymidine tract in the cystic fibrosis (CFTR) gene: Association of the 5Tallele with selected CFTR mutations and its incidence in atypical sinopulmonary disease. *Hum Mutat* 1997: 10: 108–115.

Gasparini P, Marigo C, Bisceglia G et al. Screening of 62 mutations in a cohort of cystic fibrosis patients from north eastern Italy: their incidence and clinical features of defined genotypes. *Hum Mutat* 1993: 2: 389–394.

Groman JD, hefferon TW, Casals T et al. Variation in a repeat sequence determines whether a common variant of the Cystic Fibrosis Transmembrane Conductance Regulator gene is pathogenic or benign. *Am J Hum Genet* 2004: 74: 176-179.

Kanavakis E, Tzetis M, Antoniadi Th, Pistofidis G, Milligos S, Kattamis C. Cystic fibrosis mutation screening in CBAVD patients and men with obstructive azoospermia or severe oligospermia. *Mol Hum Reprod* 1998: 4: 333–337.

Kanavakis E, Efthymiadou A, Strofalis S, Doudounakis S, Traeger-Synodinos J, Tzetis M. Cystic Fibrosis in Greece: molecular diagnosis, haplotypes, prenatal diagnosis and carrier identification amongst high-risk individuals. *Clin Genet* 2003: 63: 400-409.

Kerem B, Rommens JM, Buchanan JA et al. Identification of the cystic fibrosis gene: genetic analysis. Science 1989: 245: 1073–1080.

Mendes F, Rosa M, Dragomir A, et al. Unusually common cystic fibrosis mutation in Portugal encodes a misprocessed protein. *Biochem Biophys Res Commun* 2003: 311:665-71.

Mennuti MT. Lights! Camera! Action! *Obstet Gynecol* 2001: 98: 539–541.

Meschende D, Dworniczak B, Behre HM et al. CFTR gene mutations in men with bilateral ejaculatory-duct obstruction and anomalies of the seminal vesicles. *Am J Hum Genet* 1997: 61: 1200-1202.

Monaghan KG, Feldman GL. The risk of prenatal diagnosis with prenatally detected echogenic bowel in an ethnically and racially diverse North American Population. *Prenat Diagn* 1999: 19: 604–609.

Morral N, Estivill X. Multiplex PCR amplification of three microsatellites within the CFTR gene. *Genomics* 1992: 13: 1362–1364.

Morral N, Nunes V, Casals Tet al. Microsatellite haplotypes for cystic fibrosis: mutation frameworks and evolutionary tracers. *Hum Mol Genet* 1993: 2: 1015–1022.

Morral N, Bertranpetit J, Estivill X et al. The origin of the major cystic fibrosis mutation (DF508) in European populations. *Nat Genet* 1994: 7: 169–175.

Morral N, Dork T, Llevadot R et al. Haplotype analysis of 94 cystic fibrosis mutations with seven polymorphic CFTR DNA markers. *Hum Mutat* 1996: 8: 149–159.

Noone PG, Knowles MR. "CFTR-opathies": disease phenotypes associated with cystic fibrosis transmembrane regulator gene mutations. *Respir Res* 2001: 2: 328-332.

Palomaki GE, FitzSimmons SC, Haddow JE. Clinical sensitivity of prenatal screening for cystic fibrosis via CFTR carrier testing in a United States panethnic population. *Genet Med* 2004: 6: 405-414.

Radivojevic D, Djurisic M, Lalic T et al. Spectrum of cystic fibrosis mutations in Serbia and Montenegro and strategy for prenatal diagnosis. *Genet Test* 2004: 8:276-80.

Riordan JR, Rommens JM, Kerem B et al. Identification of the cystic fibrosis gene: cloning and characterization of complemantary DNA. *Science* 1989: 245: 1066–1073.

Rommens JM, Iannuzzi MC, Kerem B et al. Identification of the cystic fibrosis gene. chromosome walking and jumping. *Science* 1989: 245: 1059–1065.

Sepuvelda W, Sebine NJ. Fetal echogenic bowel: a complex scenario. *Ultrasound Obstet Gynecol* 2000: 16: 510–514.

Strocker AM, Snijders RJ, Carlson DE et al. Fetal echogenic bowel: parameters to be considered in differential diagnosis. *Ultrasound Obstet Gynecol* 2000: 16: 519–523.

Strong TV, Wilkinson DJ, Mansoura MK et al. Expression of an abundant alternatively spliced form of the cystic fibrosis transmembrane conductance regulator (CFTR) gene is not associated with a cAMP-activated chloride conductance. *Hum Mol Genet* 1993: 2: 225-230.

Super M, Schwarz MJ, Malone G, Roberts T, Howorth A, Dermody G. Active cascade testing for carriers of cystic fibrosis gene. *Br Med J* 1994: 308: 1462–1468.

Trezise AEO, Linder CC, Grieger D et al. CFTR expression is regulated during both the cycle of semineferous epithelium and the oestrous cycle of redents. *Nat Genet* 1993: 3: 157-164.

Tzetis M, Kanavakis E, Antoniadi Th, Doudounakis S, Adam G, Kattamis C. Characterization of more than 85% of cystic fibrosis alleles in the Greek population, including five novel mutations. *Hum Genet* 1997: 99: 121–125.

Tzetis M, Efthymiadou A, Strofalis S et al. CFTR gene mutations- including three novel nucleotide substitutions- and haplotype background in patients with asthma, disseminated bronchiectasis and chronic obstructive pulmonary disease. *Hum Genet* 2001a: 108: 216-211.

Tzetis M, Efthymiadou A, Doudounakis S, Kanavakis E. Qualitative and quantitative analysis of mRNA associated with four putative splicing mutations (621+3A>G, 2751+2T>A, 296+1G>C, 1717–9T>C-D565G) and one nonsense mutation (E822X) in the CFTR gene. *Hum Genet* 2001b: 109: 592–601.

Van der Ven K, Tsui LC, Boat TF et al. Cystic Fibrosis mutation screening in healthy men with reduced sperm quality. *Hum Reprod* 1996: 11: 513-517.

Vankeerbergerghen A, Cuppens H, Cassiman JJ. The Cystic Fibrosis transmembrane conductance regulator: an intriguing protein with pleiotropic functions. *J Cystic Fibrosis* 2002: 1: 13-29.

Vrettou C, Tzetis M, Traeger-Synodinos J, Palmer G, kanavakis E. Multiplex sequence variation detection throughout the CFTR gene appropriate for preimplantation genetic diagnosis in populations with heterogeneity of cystic fibrosis mutations. *Mol Hum Reprod* 2002: 8: 880-886.

Welsh MJ, Ramsey BW, Accurso F, Cutting GR. Cystic Fibrosis. In: Sly WS, Valle D, eds. *The Metabolic and Molecular Bases of Inherited Disease*, 8th edn, Vol. 3. New York: McGraw-Hill 2001, pp. 5121–5188.

Zielenski J, Rozmahel R, Bozon D et al. Genomic DNA sequence of the cystic fibrosis transmembrane conductance regulator (CFTR) gene. *Genomics* 1991: 10: 214-228.

Zielenski J, Tsui LC. Cystic Fibrosis: genotypic and phenotypic variations. *Annu Rev Genet* 1995: 29: 777–807.

Zielenski J. Genotype and Phenotype in cystic fibrosis. *Respiration* 2000: 67: 117–133.

In: New Developments in Birth Defects Research
Editor: Nelson A. Gaslem, pp. 174-205
ISBN 1-60021-400-2

Chapter 7

CYSTIC FIBROSIS: THE FIRST IDENTIFED GLUTATHIONE TRANSPORT DISEASE

Valerie M. Hudson
Brigham Young University, UT USA

ABSTRACT

Cystic fibrosis (CF) is a genetic disease at once tragic and theoretically puzzling. Predominantly found in Caucasian and Semitic populations, its incidence in the United States is 1 in approximately 3000 births. The global population of cystic fibrosis sufferers has been estimated to be about a quarter of a million persons, many of whom will never be accurately diagnosed during their lifetime. Average life expectancy in the United States has risen to about 32 years of age, but the median age at death for the most common mutation pair, delF508/delF508, remains about 23 years of age even with the most advanced care. The life expectancy of females with cystic fibrosis tends to be a few years shorter than the life expectancy of males. Proximate cause of death in about 95% of cases is respiratory failure [1].

In this essay, we will examine recent research findings and clinical trial results that offer a new specification of the linkage between genetics and disease in the case of CF: a linkage involving the transport of reduced glutathione (GSH).

Cystic fibrosis (CF) is a genetic disease at once tragic and theoretically puzzling. Predominantly found in Caucasian and Semitic populations, its incidence in the United States is 1 in approximately 3000 births. The global population of cystic fibrosis sufferers has been estimated to be about a quarter of a million persons, many of whom will never be accurately diagnosed during their lifetime. Average life expectancy in the United States has risen to about 32 years of age, but the median age at death for the most common mutation pair, delF508/delF508, remains about 23 years of age even with the most advanced care. The life expectancy of females with cystic fibrosis tends to be a few years shorter than the life expectancy of males. Proximate cause of death in about 95% of cases is respiratory failure [1].

The very real tragedy of CF does not belie the theoretical puzzlement it causes researchers. How, exactly, do CF mutations (one thousand and counting), give rise to the unique pathophysiology of CF? It has been known since 1989 that CF mutations cause the anion efflux channel created by the CFTR protein in the cell membrane to be missing or defective. What is the relationship of that channel dysfunction to the three hallmarks of CF disease: thickened mucus, chronic and exuberant inflammation, and ineffective pathogen clearance by the immune system? Theories abound, but the mechanism remains notably underspecified.

In this essay, we will examine recent research findings and clinical trial results that offer a new specification of the linkage between genetics and disease in the case of CF: a linkage involving the transport of reduced glutathione (GSH).

Not Just a Chloride Channel

The CFTR channel has a long-standing nickname: "the chloride channel." Indeed, much CF research and theorizing revolves around the efflux, or lack of efflux of the chloride anion from CF cells. Theories relating chloride, sodium, and water movements are central to the current understanding of CF [2].

However, it is possible that this emphasis on chloride has been less than helpful. Pharmaceutical modification of chloride or sodium concentrations, such as through the use of amiloride, has not been shown to reverse CF symptoms [3]. There is more to the theoretical picture than chloride alone.

New research demonstrates that there are other anions of possible clinical relevance whose efflux is affected by CFTR mutation. Two that are receiving attention at this point in time are bicarbonate and reduced glutathione (GSH). Though we will concentrate on glutathione in this essay, bicarbonate's importance in regulation of pH has attracted the attention of several research teams whose work will undoubtedly be tracked with care by CF clinicians and patients [4,5].

It was the work of two Canadian researchers, Paul Linsdell and John Hanrahan, that first brought to the attention of the CF research community in 1998 that cellular efflux of GSH was significantly reduced by dysfunction of the CFTR channel [6]. In the subsequent five and a half years, other research teams have moved swiftly to confirm and extend those findings. Using cell lines of CF lung epithelia, Gao et al. were also able to demonstrate significantly reduced efflux of GSH [7]. Ilana Kogan and colleagues found this same diminished GSH efflux with a variety of CFTR mutants, including G551D, R347D, K464A, and K1250A [8,9], and through the use of sophisticated tests were able to confirm that purified CFTR protein alone directly mediates nucelotide-dependent GSH flux and not via other associated chloride transport proteins. Brian Day and colleagues also found a 50% reduction in lung epithelial lining fluid (ELF) GSH levels in uninfected CFTR knockout mice [10]. Finder et al. have uncovered a 49% reduction of GSH in in bronchoalveolar lavage fluid from CF patients [11].

In short, these research teams discovered that CF mutations cause a primary and profound glutathione transport malfunction. Would such a significant decrease in GSH efflux cause disease? The answer is yes.

GSH, GSH Transport, and Health

Unless one is actually working in the field of glutathione research, it is not uncommon to find oneself relatively uninformed about its several pivotal roles in health and disease. But even a cursory glance at the over 60,000 abstracts on glutathione or GSH compiled on PubMed can serve to propel the uninitiated into a broader understanding of this ubiquitous and physiologically essential tripeptide.

GSH is synthesized by the cells of the body from the amino acids glutamine, glycine, and cysteine, with cysteine serving as the rate-limiting component. Meister states that an adult human male will synthesize approximately 10 grams of GSH per day [12]. In addition to synthesis, glutathione is available in small amounts in the human diet, and there exist specific co-transporters of intact glutathione in the mammalian jejunum [13,14-17].

Organ systems, and even cell types, differ according to the *level of total glutathione* (GSH+GSSG, the latter being glutathione disulfide) and the *glutathione redox ratio* (GSH:GSSG) found therein. In systems openly exposed to oxidants, such as the lung or cornea, or devoted to detoxification, such as the liver, the level of total glutathione may be quite high, and the redox ratio also quite high [18]. But even within such systems, differences may be found between various cell types; for example, monocytes have, in general, higher levels of total glutathione than neutrophils [19].

Let us now turn to a discussion of glutathione's functions. We will divide this discussion into four parts: 1) glutathione as an antioxidant; 2) glutathione's role in mucus viscosity; 3) glutathione as an immune system modulator; and 4) glutathione's relationship to the NO system of the body.

Glutathione as an Antioxidant

Glutathione's sulfur-hydrogen, or thiol, group is a potent reducing agent, and GSH can be considered the one of the body's most important water-soluble antioxidants. Antioxidant defenses in humans are comprised of both enzymatic and non-enzymatic defenses; some defenses operate intracellularly and others have additional extracellular functions. The antioxidant enzymes are glutathione peroxidase, superoxide dismutase, and catalase. There are two types of non-enzymatic antioxidants, the water soluble and the fat soluble. The water soluble antioxidants are reduced glutathione and ascorbic acid; the fat soluble are alpha-tocopherol and the carotenoids. The enzymatic antioxidants are lodged within the cellular membranes (though there is a free plasma glutathione peroxidase [348]); in contrast the water soluble antioxidants (as free molecules) are present in the cytosol of the cells, though some, including GSH, are also present in the extracellular environment. The fat soluble antioxidants are found within the lipid membranes. Each antioxidant defense system protects the cells from oxidative damage in its own sphere of action, and a deficiency in any category puts the cell at risk for oxidative damage. It should be noted that GSH is a precursor for the function of glutathione peroxidase. In addition to its cellular functions, GSH is also present in extracellular epithelial fluids, such as the epithelial lining fluid (ELF) of the lung, blood plasma, semen, saliva, and so forth, where antioxidant action is similarly useful.

GSH provides powerful antioxidant protection to body systems heavily exposed to reactive oxygen species (ROS), such as the lung [20,21]. For example, the normal level of extracellular GSH in the lung epithelial lining fluid (ELF) is 140 times the normal level of extracellular GSH in blood plasma, and it is probable that the lung, under oxidative stress, becomes a net importer of circulating GSH [22]. In addition, under conditions of oxidative or nitrosative stress, vulnerable proteins may undergo s-glutathiolation, wherein GSSG binds to protein, thus protecting it, and also allowing for that binding to be reversed when the stress has passed [23]. However, it would be wrong to view GSH only or even most importantly in terms of its antioxidant properties when considering its importance in lung defense.

Glutathione and Maintenance of Proper Mucus Viscosity

A second property of reduced glutathione that should not be overlooked is its promotion of mucolysis. Because of its chemistry, GSH, like N-acetylcysteine (NAC), is able to cleave disulfide bonds, which serves to reduce the viscoelasticity of mucus when the glutathione system is functioning normally [24,25]. Furthermore, reduced glutathione plays a role in establishing the volume of periciliary fluid, and also affects mucus hydration through its indirect relationship with epithelial sodium channels (ENaC), topics we will explore in a later section.

Glutathione and Immune Function

A third property of reduced glutathione is to regulate inflammation and immune response. This regulation is carried out in a number of ways, which will be discussed below. Generally speaking, however, the main mechanism of regulation is by redox potential. Since GSH is synthesized by virtually every cell in the body, a redox equilibrium is established within each of these cells, and the efflux of GSH from the cells establishes an extracellular redox equilibrium as well. Both intracellular and extracellular redox equilibria vary: extracellularly, the equilibrium varies by bodily system, as noted above; and intracellularly, the equilibrium varies by cell type. As noted previously, the intracellular GSH level of monocytes is three times that of neutrophils [19]. The redox potential, expressed by the ratio GSH:GSSG influences many sensitive cellular systems and functions. Indeed, as we shall see, inflammation, immune response, and cell viability, among other things, are intimately tied to this ratio. If, as we will hypothesize in a later section, CF leukocytes and lymphocytes (along with other cells possessing anion channels redundant to the CFTR) are prone to chronic alteration of the GSH:GSSG ratio, immune response will be profoundly affected.

Glutathione and the Nitric Oxide System

NO, an important factor in cell signalling, pathogen killing, ciliary beat function, and smooth muscle relaxation, is profoundly affected by GSH system function. In the extracellular compartment, GSH combines with NO to form s-nitrosoglutathione (GSNO). In healthy systems, GSNO is easily cleaved and is not only an important reservoir of GSH, but also an important reservoir of NO. GSH also appears to bear a relationship to the expression of iNOS [26-31]. NO in turn affects expression of gamma-glutamylcysteine synthetase, the rate-limiting enzyme for GSH synthesis, apparently to counteract NO cytotoxicity [32-35].

The Effects of Glutathione Transport Dysfunction in Cystic Fibrosis

In order to more fully discuss the effects of glutathione transport dysfunction in cystic fibrosis, two levels of analysis must take place. First, we must understand the consequences of CFTR mutation on total levels and redox ratios of glutathione in three compartments:

- CF cells whose primary means of effluxing GSH is the CFTR;
- CF cells that have other anion efflux channels redundant to the CFTR;
- The extracellular milieu in CF.

Second, since glutathione transport dysfunction has not been, generally speaking, a topic of research in cystic fibrosis, we must investigate what medical science knows about the effects of GSH deficiency in these three compartments in disease conditions other than CF for insights into what we might expect in CF as a result of this dysfunction.

Glutathione in the Three Compartments in CF

Research on glutathione status in CF is very new. Only a few research findings can be referenced. Nevertheless, what currently exists provides a basis for partial understanding.

In CF cells whose primary means of GSH efflux is the CFTR, such as bronchial epithelial cells, normal total levels of glutathione (GSH+GSSG) have been found [36]. (Indeed, it may be very difficult for such cells to suffer depletion of GSH, which may have ramifications for appropriate apoptosis in these cells.) However, there is currently no research concerning the GSH:GSSG ratio in these CF cells.

Second, in CF cells that possess redundant anion efflux channels to the CFTR (RACP cells, meaning Redundant Anion Channel Present), in particular the MRP family of channels (and GS-X pumps more broadly), depletion of total levels of glutathione has been found. Cells with such characteristics would include hepatocytes, leukocytes, erythrocytes, and lymphocytes, among others. Tirouvanziam found substantially lower levels of GSH in sputum neutrophils from CF patients compared to GSH levels in blood neutrophils, which also correlated with cell death rates [37]. Lands and colleagues found that total glutathione levels of the peripheral blood lymphocytes of CF persons were, in general, depressed [38]. Again, no studies of GSH:GSSG ratio have been conducted for this compartment. However, upregulation of MRP1 in CF erythrocytes has been noted [39].

Third, more plentiful research is available on glutathione status in the extracellular milieu in CF, especially in the lung ELF, but also in blood plasma. A noted previously, Brian Day and colleagues found a 50% reduction in lung epithelial lining fluid (ELF) GSH levels in uninfected CFTR knockout mice [10], and Finder et al. found a 49% reduction of GSH in in bronchoalveolar lavage fluid from CF patients [11]. Roum et al. found a profound deficit of GSH in CF lung ELF, with levels dropping to 5-10% of normal. Roum and colleagues also investigated GSH:GSSG ratios in CF lung ELF, and also found a large decrease, from a norm of over 9:1 in healthy persons to approximately 3:1 in CF patients [40]. In blood plasma, Brown et al. found a 50% decrease in total GSH, which was replicated by Roum et al. in a later study [41]. Roum et al. also found decreased GSH:GSSG ratio in CF blood plasma [40].

Emphasizing that transport of GSH is the issue, not synthesis or any other aspect of the glutathione system, studies have found normal synthesis of GSH in CF, and normal or even elevated levels of glutathione peroxidase, glutathione reductase, γ-glutamyl transpeptidase, and γ-glutamylcysteine transferase [42,43,17,44,45].

Glutathione Deficiency and Pathophysiology

The clearest way to demonstrate the importance of a properly functioning GSH system is to detail what scientific research tells us about the effects of GSH deficiency, even when studies have not been conducted concerning CF per se. We will discuss three main categories of known effects of GSH deficiency: impaired antioxidant capability, decreased mucolysis, and abnormal immune response, including decreased nitric oxide production and availability.

A) Impaired Antioxidant Capability

When a key antioxidant such as GSH is deficient in the extracellular compartment and in RACP cells, direct damage from oxidants increases greatly. In addition, glutathione deficiency in leukocytes (a type of RACP cell) has been shown to cause increased release of hydrogen peroxide [46]. Oxidant damage to lung epithelial cells from a diminished extracellular antioxidant screen reduces lung function, causing fibrosis and permitting greater adhesion of bacteria [20,21,47-49]. When GSH is deficient, other antioxidants may be consumed in higher-than-normal amounts to handle the increased oxidant burden. Thus, GSH deficiency is often accompanied by lower levels of alpha-tocopherol and ascorbate, and decreased activity of glutathione peroxidase, catalase, and superoxide dismutase, all of which are reversible when GSH level is normalized [50]. New research also points to the direct role of GSH in neutralizing HOCl, one of the deadliest oxidants to be found in the respiratory milieu, with the reaction being 2GSH + HOCl GSSG + H2O + HCl [51].

GSH deficiency also causes oxidant damage to the liver [52-62] and pancreas [63-65], resulting in impaired function of these organs, including reduced bile flow [54,59,61,66], and is associated with the onset of diabetes mellitus [67-73], rheumatoid arthritis [74], peripheral nerve damage [75], and myocardial injury [76]. GSH deficiency results in intestinal mucosal injury and chronic inflammation of the gut [77-82], decreased absorption of nutrients such as calcium [83], and general cachexia and growth retardation [84-87]. GSH deficiency also causes greater lipid peroxidation, which, in turn, causes cell damage [88-94]. (As peroxidation of arachidonic acid yields especially damaging metabolites, it is noteworthy that CF persons have been found to have threefold more arachidonic acid and threefold less DHA in the cell membrane than normal persons [95], and that the cytotoxicity of arachidonic acid is enhanced by GSH depletion [96]. The metabolism of arachidonic acid also entails the production of free radicals by virtue of the lipooxygenase and cyclooxygenase pathways, further increasing oxidant burden. For example, 8-isoprostane in breath condensate of CF persons is elevated three-fold above normal controls [97].

Loss of GSH antioxidant capability in the extracellular milieu has secondary effects, as well. One such effect is oxidant-derived inactivation of the anti-protease system [98-100]. Such inactivation produces its own cascade of harmful effects due to unbound neutrophil elastase (NE). In the lung, these include, as Barbero notes in a review of the scientific literature, "cleavage of fibronectin, lung elastin, immunoglobulins and immune complexes, complement receptors in neutrophils, and other receptors on T-cells and B-cells. Furthermore, NE inhibits ciliary beating and stimulates mucus production from goblet cells and facilitates P. aeruginosa adherence. Finally, by cleaving receptors for interleukin (IL)-1 and IL-2 or the T cell antigen receptor, it may hypothetically inhibit message transmission and immune recognition. Thus, besides destruction, [free NE] may lead to acquired immune suppression" [101]. GSH depletion has also been linked to increased levels of collagenase [102].

Other secondary effects of the loss of GSH antioxidant protection in the extracellular milieu include degradation of lung surfactant, both via oxidant damage and through the inability of the body to maintain appropriate levels of phosphatidycholine under conditions of GSH deficiency [03-105]. This in turn may be related to the linkage between GSH depletion and reduced lung surface tension [106]. S-glutathiolation protection of vulnerable proteins will also be reduced. Though it is intriguing to note that GSH depletion also leads to free radical-induced respiratory muscle fatigue, which contributes to respiratory failure in patients with lung disease [107], and that more generalized skeletal muscle fatigue also results from GSH depletion [108], since muscle cells are generally non-RACP cells, it is not clear whether these findings would be pertinent to the case of CF. However, it is relevant to the CF case to note that GSH depletion, by increasing airway inflammation, has been hypothesized to lead to the development of asthma [109]. When GSH in the ELF is deficient, the body decreases enzymatic activity transforming GSSG back into GSH, and instead further oxidizes GSSG into chloramines, long-lived oxidants capable of profound injury to the lung [110,111]. (For illustration, chloramines are the agent of lung damage when ammonia and bleach are mixed.) Oxidation products also serve to inhibit the enzymatic activities of glutathione reductase, essential in recycling of GSSG into GSH [112,113], and we would expect this inhibition in RACP cells. Oxidation appears to decrease gamma-glutamylcysteine transferase (g-GCT) activity, as well [114], and this would affect both RACP and non-RACP cells. These secondary effects, by damaging the integrity of lung tissue, increasing epithelial permeability, and further disrupting the GSH antioxidant system, allow for increased adhesion of pathogens [115]. Regulation of neutrophil adhesion is also affected by GSH depletion [116]. GSH depletion also causes oxidation of protein thiols, protein denaturation and aggregation, increases in insoluble proteins [117], all of which can serve to initiate stress responses in cells, such as induction of heat shock protein 70 (HSP70) [118,119] and stress-activated protein kinases [120], as well as disruption of other types of cell signalling [121], repair processes [122], protein synthesis [123-125], and even mitochondrial energy production [126]. GSH depletion also causes other cell structure alterations, including increased DNA damage [127], loss of junctional and cytoskeletal integrity [128,129], and abnormal cellular bodies [130-132]. We would hypothesize that these cellular effects would be seen in the RACP cells of CF patients.

It should be noted that glutathione deficiency in the ELF has been associated not only with cystic fibrosis, but also with such pulmonary diseases as acute respiratory distress syndrome (ARDS) [133], chronic obstructive pulmonary disease (COPD) [20], idiopathic interstitial pneumonia (IIP) [134], idiopathic pulmonary fibrosis (IPF--of non-smokers) [135], idiopathic respiratory distress syndrome (IRDS) [106], and diffuse fibrosing alveolitis (DFA) [136] A deficiency has also been found in the lungs of HIV-positive patients [137,138].

B) Impaired Ability to Maintain Proper Mucus Viscosity

Extracellular GSH deficiency impairs maintenance of proper mucus viscosity, as GSH facilitates cleavage of disulfide bonds in mucus [139]. Increased viscoelasticity of mucus further inhibits ciliary beating, and also allows for increased opportunity for bacterial colonization of the lung. [140-144]. Interestingly, GSH depletion has also been shown to provoke mucin secretion by tracheal epithelial cells [145], and increased NFkappaB due to GSH deficiency stimulates mucus oversecretion by epithelial cells in the presence of Pseudomonas aeruginosa [146]. However, since these are not RACP cells, these observations are only interesting if it is the case that despite their normal levels of total glutathione, CF epithelial cells have a significantly decreased GSH:GSSG ratio. Given the high amount of oxidant stress in CF, in part due to chronic and progressive extracellular GSH deficit caused by the CFTR mutation, this alteration might occur. If so, then it is also interesting to note that GSH deficit also precludes IFN-gamma inhibition of Na+ and fluid absorption [147,148], and perhaps NO regulation of ENaC, as well [149,150]. As noted above, oxidative stress due to GSH depletion leads to an increase in free NE, which also stimulates mucus secretion [151].

C) Abnormal Immune Response

Though GSH is well known for its antioxidant properties, and somewhat less well known for its role in maintaining proper mucus viscosity, it is not as widely known for the key role it plays in immune system regulation. Because RACP cells include leukocytes and lymphocytes, the literature in this area should be pertinent to the case of CF. The following discussion is not comprehensive, but rather serves to outline the broad parameters of the topic.

First, as noted in the introduction, the redox status of GSH is the primary mechanism by which this regulation takes place. GSH deficiency in immune system cells (which are RACP cells) triggers inflammation, and chronic GSH deficiency in these cells leads to chronic and exaggerated inflammation. Cellular GSH deficiency is related directly to increased transcription of NFkappaB [152-159]. NFkappaB codes for the inflammatory cytokines, and a deficit of either the water soluble or fat soluble antioxidants increases NFkappaB activity, which is a critical early event in the pathogenesis of many lung diseases [160]. This mechanism is demonstrated in HIV-infected macrophages, wherein there is increased activity of NFkappaB due to decreased GSH synthesis. Consequently, there is a progressive increase of inflammatory cytokines as the disease progresses (and as GSH continues to be diminished). Increasing the redox potential of infected macrophages correlates with a decrease in inflammatory cytokines, as well as a decrease in HIV replication [161-163]. The concept of cellular redox potential is particularly germane to immune cell function due to its influence on NFkappaB activity. Diseases that have a chronic inflammatory component, whether affecting a single organ (e.g., hepatitis), or as systemic inflammation (as in AIDS), will manifest GSH deficiency either in the affected organ or systemically, respectively. These deficits can occur due to insufficient GSH synthesis or transport, or consumption in pathological oxidative reactions that outpaces replenishment.

Accordingly, the cytokine profile of GSH deficiency includes elevated levels of AP-1 [155,156,158,159], TNF-alpha and its by-products [154,164-167], IL-1-induced MCP-1 [155,168], and IL-8 [158,164,169]. GSH also appears to exert some regulation over HIF-1alpha [157], regulates chemokine receptor expression [170], and appears to increase levels of IL-1a [171]. This cytokine profile leads to increased recruitment of neutrophils and macrophages [172,173], and, in general such a profile would produce chronic inflammation even in the absence of pathogen challenge.

However, under conditions of chronic GSH deficiency in RACP cells and in the extracellular milieu, the inflammation is for naught. GSH deficiency in neutrophils and macrophages decreases effectiveness of bactericidal action of these cells. There are several reasons for this: first, GSH deficiency in such cells produces premature apoptosis, both because GSH depletion is a necessary step in apoptosis, perhaps because GSH depletion is associated with the activation of sphingomyelinases [174], and because GSH deficiency allows for greater oxidant damage to these cells [46,175-186]. Second, GSH deficiency causes neutrophils to suffer microtubule damage, impaired release of lysosomal enzymes, depressed leukotaxis, and in general, decreased phagocytosis [46,187-189]. Third, premature apoptosis in a context of enhanced recruitment of neutrophils by cytokines causes increased spillage of toxic compounds and DNA into the extracellular milieu [190]. Such spillage promotes increased viscosity of secretions, increased oxidant and elastase burden, the establishment of a positive feedback loop to IL-8 production and further neutrophil recruitment, and, in general, an increased opportunity for pathogenic lung colonization [190]. Fourth, GSH appears to regulate the oxidative burst of neutrophils, with GSH deficiency leading to decreased burst activity [191]. The interplay of GSH and NO in bactericidal action will be discussed in a separate section below.

The immune response also becomes abnormal under conditions of chronic GSH deficiency because of an alteration of Th1/Th2 response. Depletion of GSH in antigen-presenting cells (APC, also a RACP cell) decreases interferon-gamma (IFN-gamma) and enhances Th2-associated humoral immunity responses at the expense of cell mediated immune response [147,192,193]. This alters the ability of APC to function normally, in part because GSH reduction of disulfide bonds is necessary for proteolysis of the antigen [147]. This interference of signalling between the APC and the T cells prevents proper T cell response [147,194,195]. Other cell signalling involving T cells may also be adversely affected [196]. As noted previously, IFN-gamma signalling is dysregulated by GSH depletion [148]. Extreme depletion of GSH in APC as well as in T cells has been shown to diminish both T cell proliferation and IL-12 production, as well as increasing apoptosis of T cells [147,195,197-207]. B cell and fibroblast proliferation also appears related to intracellular GSH level [208,209]. Activation and cytolytic activity of T cells and B cells is decreased with GSH depletion [193,210-214]. Again, this appears to be the result of cell structure abnormalities due to GSH depletion [215]. Movement towards a Th2 response has been associated with a negative outcome in many diseases [216-219].

D) Decreased Nitric Oxide Production and Availability

In the extracellular compartment, GSH deficiency will result in less extracellular GSNO, an important source of NO. In RACP cells (and perhaps non-RACP cells if depressed intracellular GSH:GSSG ratios were present in them), a variety of noteworthy consequences result. GSH deficiency has been shown to decrease iNOS expression and decrease levels of S-nitrosoglutathione (GSNO), which two phenomena may be interrelated [26-31]. NO and GSH appear to regulate cell energy metabolism [220,221], and NO stimulates enhanced expression of gamma-glutamylcysteine synthetase, the rate-limiting enzyme for GSH synthesis, apparently to counteract NO cytotoxicity [32-35]. GSNO is not only a reservoir of readily accessible NO, it is also a reservoir of easily accessible GSH, which becomes important under conditions in which cells become depleted of GSH through cytoprotective activities. Indeed, there appears to be a balance between GSH and GSNO, which under conditions of GSH depletion, favors cleavage of GSNO [222]. The balance appears to determine whether NO will be cytotoxic or cytoprotective [223-225]. Depletion of GSH markedly increases cell susceptibility to the harmful effects of peroxynitrite (ONOO-), leading to cytostasis and apoptosis [226-233]. In addition, under conditions of GSH depletion and resulting lower levels of GSNO (which is formed both intracellularly and extracellularly) and oxygen radical release from inflammatory cells, NO is readily transformed into nitrites and nitrates [234,235]. ONOO- has also been shown to inactivate glutathione reductase [113]. As NO is important in bactericidal action, lowered levels of NO significantly depress such action, leading to increased infection with organisms such as Pseudomonas aeruginosa [149]. GSH depletion reduces smooth muscle relaxation in response to NO, producing in the lung a tendency towards generalized bronchoconstriction [236,237]. NO also appears to regulate both the CFTR channel and a non-CFTR Cl- channel, and a decrease in NO leads to a decrease in conductance [238,239]. NO also appears to regulate ENaC sodium absorption via cGMP, with decreased NO leading to loss of the signal to downregulate sodium absorption [149,150]. Trans-epithelial potential difference, being regulated in part by sodium absorption, is thus seen to be regulated by iNOS, with decreased iNOS leading to increased potential difference [149]. Last, ciliary beat function is regulated by NO, with depletion of NO leading to impaired ciliary function [150].

CLINICAL TRIALS OF GSH USE IN CF PATIENTS

If GSH transport plays a role in the pathophysiology of cystic fibrosis, then it is natural to ask whether rectification of this problem might provide therapeutic benefit to CF patients. There are various approaches that have been discussed in the literature:

Reinstatement of Cellular Glutathione Transport. One approach, advocated by the research team that includes Henry Forman and John Tomich, is to create a synthetic peptide that will create a channel in the cell membrane allowing glutathione efflux [240]. Though at least several years away from clinical trials, reinstatement of transport in this manner would arguably have great therapeutic significance.

Increased Synthesis of GSH Through Cysteine Donors. As noted previously, cysteine is the rate-limiting component of GSH synthesis in the body. The use of cysteine donors, such as n-acetylcysteine (NAC) or special whey powders (e.g., Immunocal), will boost synthesis of GSH. Such an approach should not be overlooked, but increased synthesis will not solve the transport difficulties caused by CF mutation. The use of cysteine donors may well be complementary, however, to other approaches that tackle the transport problem more directly.

Exogenous Augmentation of GSH. Provision of GSH to the extracellular milieu could be therapeutic in CF. First, increasing the total level of glutathione and the redox ratio in the extracellular compartments of interest, expecially the lung, would decrease oxidant damage and also promote proper mucus viscosity. Second, ample extracellular GSH can rectify any chronic GSH deficit in RACP cells, with immune system cells of most interest here. Such rectification could help dampen the chronic exuberant inflammation characteristic of CF, as well as increase the efficacy of pathogen clearance. GSH augmentation has usually taken place in one of three ways: intravenous administration, oral administration, and aerosolized administration. Given that CF patients would have to use GSH on a daily basis as a maintenance therapy, the usefulness of IV administration is highly questionable. However, both oral administration and aerosolized glutathione deserve a more detailed discussion.

Oral Administration of GSH. There have been no clinical trials of oral glutathione in CF patients. We urge such trials, as alleviation of aspects of gastrointestinal symptoms in CF, as well as thinning of lung mucus, have been reported anecdotally by CF patients with use of oral glutathione. Some have argued that uptake of intact GSH by transporters in the human jejunum, though present, as noted previously, is not very effective. However, such studies have not considered long term use by a patient group with such a unique pathology involving cellular efflux of glutathione.

Aerosol Administration of GSH. There have been ten in vivo trials of aerosolized glutathione, with three of those trials focussing on CF patients [241-250]. In the first CF trial, whose principal investigator was James Roum, unbuffered GSH was administered for three days, b.i.d., each dose being 600 mg, to 7 CF patients [247]. Roum found the treatment well tolerated, and also that superoxide anion release by ELF inflammatory cells was significantly reduced. In the second trial, whose PI was Matthias Griese, 17 CF patients received buffered GSH (pH 7.0) over a 14 day period, with the maximum dose being 450 mg t.i.d [249]. Griese found restoration of normal levels of total glutathione in the ELF, with ELF total glutathione still doubled over baseline levels after twelve hours. Though inhalation was immediately followed by a transient drop in FEV1, this was spontaneously reversed in less than one hour, and the treatment was well tolerated. By the end of the trial, peak expiratory flow, FEV1, and FVC had all increased significantly by 6-7%. However, number of neutrophils, total protein, fraction of carbonyls and reduced thiols, and lipid peroxide content of BAL fluid remained unchanged. The third trial was controlled, with 10 CF patients on treatment and 9 on placebo with the PI being Clark Bishop [250]. Dosage was 66 mg/kg/day, divided into 4 doses given every 3-4 waking hours apart of buffered glutathione (pH approximately 6.0). Bishop also found the treatment to be well tolerated, and found peak flow to be significantly increased, and in an ancillary compliant analysis found cough to be signficantly decreased. FEF25-75 tended toward significant improvement, as well.

Other Approaches. Other approaches include aerosol administration of GSNO, which provides not only NO, but GSH as well to the lung compartment [251]. Complements to glutathione-centered approaches include support of a healthy glutathione system, which demands appropriate levels of riboflavin, selenium, magnesium, ascorbate, and E. Still other approaches include coaxing the expression of MRP-type channels at the apical surface of lung epithelia, through the use of agents such as colchicine [252]. These channels would then provide natural glutathione efflux.

Conclusion

Cystic fibrosis is, among other things, the first identified glutathione transport disease. Though cystic fibrosis is certainly multi-factorial, the pathophysiology of this disease appears to be linked, at least in part, to CFTR mutation-derived glutathione transport dysfunction. This new perspective on cystic fibrosis suggests possible therapeutic interventions that might offer significant amelioration of symptoms. In three small scale clinical trials of aerosolized glutathione in CF patients no adverse events were noted, and in two of the three trials, significant improvement in one or more measures of lung function were found even with as little as two weeks use. This encouraging beginning deserves follow-up, with large scale, multi-center clinical trials, examining not only aerosolized glutathione, but oral glutathione as well. Such a small and inexpensive intervention may well turn out to make a large difference in the lives of CF patients.

References

[1] Skach, W. R. *Cystic fibrosis: methods and protocols*. Humana Press; Totowa, NJ 2002.

[2] Boucher, R. C. New concepts of the pathogenesis of cystic fibrosis lung disease. *Eur. Respir. J. Jan 23(1)*:146-158; 2004.

[3] Roomans, G. M. Pharmacological approaches to correcting the ion transport defect in cystic fibrosis. *Am. J. Respir. Med. 2(5)*:H13-31; 2003.

[4] Coakley, R. D.; Grubb, B. R.; Paradiso, A. M.; Gatzu, J. T.; Johnson, L. G.; Kreda, S. M.; O'Neal, W. K.; Boucher, R. C. Abnormal surface liquids p++ regulation by cultured cystic fibrosis bronchial epithelium. *Proc. Natl. Acad. Sc. USA. Dec 23, 100(26)*:16083-16088; 2003.

[5] McShane, D.; Davies, J. C.; Davies, M. G.; Bush, A.; Geddes, D. M.; Alton, E. W. Airway surface p++ in subjects with cystic fibrosis. JOURNAL?

[6] Linsdell P and JW Hanrahan, "Glutathione Permeability of CFTR," *Am. J. Physiol. - Cell Physiol. 44(1)*: C323-C326, 1998 July.

[7] Gao L, Kim KJ, Yankaskas JR, Forman HJ, "Abnormal glutathione transport in cystic fibrosis airway epithelia," *Am J Physiol Lung Cell Mol Physiol* 1999 Jul;277(1):L113-8.

[8] Kogan I, Ramjeesingh M, Kidd J, Li C, Wang Y, Bear CE, "Characterization of glutathione permeability through the CFTR channel pore," *Ped Pulmonol* 2002 Oct; 24:189-90.

[9] Kogan I, Ramjessingh M, Li C, Kidd JF, Wang Y, Leslie EM, Cole SPC, Bear CE, "CFTR directly mediates nucleotide-regulated glutathione flux," *EMBO*, 2003 May 1; 22(9):1981-9.

[10] Velsor LW, van Heeckeren A, Day BJ, "Antioxidant imbalance in the lungs of cystic fibrosis transmembrane conductance regulator protein mutant mice," *Am J Physiol Lung Cell Mol Physiol* 2001 Jul;281(1):L31-8

[11] Finder, J. D.; Engman, C. L.; Kagan, V. E.; Tyurina, Y. Y. Brondoalveolar lavage fluid from patients with cystic fibrosis have diminished levels of reduced glututione. *Ped. Pulm. Supplement 25*; A158; 239; 2003.

[12] Meister, A. Glutathione metabolism. *Methods Enzymol 251*:3-7; 1995.

[13] Buhl R et al., "Augmentation of the Antioxidant Screen of the Epithelial Surface of the Lower Respiratory Tract by Aerosol Administration of Glutathione," *Proc. Natl. Acad. Sci. USA 87*:4063-67, 1990 June.

[14] Iantomasi T et al., "Glutathione transport system in human small intestine epithelial cells," *Biochim. Biophys. Acta 1330(2)*: 274-83, 1997 December 4.

[15] Hunjan MK and DF Evered, "Absorption of glutathione from the gastro-intestinal tract," *Biochim. Biophys. Acta 815(2)*: 184-8, 1985 May 14.

[16] Favilli F et al., "Effect of orally administered glutathione on glutathione levels in some organs of rats: role of specific transporters," *Br. J. Nutr. 78(2)*: 293-300, 1997 August.

[17] Hagen TM et al., "Bioavailability of dietary glutathione: effect on plasma concentration," *Am. J. Physiol. 259 (4 Pt 1)*: G524-9, 1990 October.

[18] Vina, J.; Bannister, J. V.; Bannister, W. H. *Glutathione: metabolism and physiological functions*. CRC Press: Boca Raton, FL; 1990.

[19] Pietarinen-Runtti P, Lakari E, Raivio KO, Kinnula VL, "Expression of antioxidant enzymes in human inflammatory cells," *Am J Physiol Cell Physiol* 2000 Jan; 278(1):C118-25.

[20] Rahman I, MacNee W, "Lung glutathione and oxidative stress: implications in cigarette smoke-induced airway disease," *Am J Physiol* 1999, 277 (Lung Cell Molecular Physiol 21): L1067-L1088.

[21] Kelly FJ, "Glutathione: in defence of the lung," *Food Chem Toxicol* 1999 Sep-oct; 37(9-10):963-6.

[22] Cantin A. M.; North S. L.; Hubbard R. C.; Crystal R. G.; "Normal alveolar epithelial lining fluid contains high levels of glutathione," *J Appl Physiol* 1987, 63:152-157.

[23] Klatt, P.; Lamas, S. Regulation of protein function by S-glutathiolation in response to oxidative and nitrosative stress. *Eur. J. Biochem.* Aug 267(16):4928-4944; 2000.

[24] Noszal B, Visky D, Kraszni M, "Population, acid-base, and redox properties of N-acetylcysteine conformers," *J Med Chem 43(11)*:2176-82, 2000 Jun 1

[25] Ziment I, "Acetylcysteine: a drug that is much more than a mucokinetic," *Biomed Pharmacother 42(8)*:513-9, 1988.

[26] Chen G, Wang SH, Warner TD, "Regulation of iNOS mRNA levels in endothelial cells by glutathione, a double-edged sword," *Free Radic Res* 2000 Mar;32(3):223-34

[27] Kang KW, Pak YM, Kim ND, "Diethylmaleate and buthionine sulfoximine, glutathione-depleting agents, differentially inhibit expression of inducible nitric oxide synthase in endotoxemic mice," *Nitric Oxide* 1999 Jun;3(3):265-271.

[28] Vos TA, Goor H, Tuyt L, Jager-Krikken A, Leuvenink R, Kuipers F, Jansen PL, Moashage H, "Expression of inducible nitric oxide synthase in endotoxemic rat hepatocytes is dependent on the cellular glutathione status," *Hepatology* 1999 Feb;29(2):421-426.

[29] Wang F, Wang LY, Wright D, Parmely MJ, "Redox imbalance differentially inhibits lipopolysaccharide-induced macrophage activation in the mouse liver," *Infect Immun* 1999 Oct;67(10):5409-5416.

[30] Davidson CA, Kaminski PM, Wolin MS, "NO elicits prolonged relaxation of bovine pulmonary arteries via endogenous peroynitrite generation," *Am J Physiol* 1997 Aug;273(2 Pt 1):L437-444.

[31] Singh SP et al., "The chemistry of the S-nitrosoglutathione/glutathione system," *Proc. Natl. Acad. Sci., USA, 93*:14428-14433, 1996 December.

[32] Moellering D, McAndrew J, Patel RP, Cornwell T, Lincoln T, Cao X, Messina JL, Forman HJ, Jo HJ, Darleyusmar VM, "Nitric oxide-dependent induction of glutathione synthesis through increased expression of gamma-glutamylcysteine synthetase," *Archives of Biochemistry and Biophysics* 1998 Oct 1;358(1):74-82.

[33] Li H, Marshall ZM, Whorton AR, "Stimulation of cystine uptake by nitric oxide:regulation of endothelial cell glutathione levels," *Am J Physiol* 1999 Apr;276(4 Pt 1):C803-11.

[34] Kuo PC, Abe KY, Schroeder RA, "Interleukin-1-induced nitric oxide production modulates glutathione synthesis in cultured rat hepatocytes," *Am J Physiol* 1996 Sep;271(3 Pt 1):C851-862.

[35] Levonene AL, Laasko J, Vaskonen T, Mervaala E, Karppanen H, Lapatto R, "Down-regulation of renal glutathione synthesis by systemic nitric oxide synthesis inhibition in spontaneously hypertensive rats," *Biochem Pharmacol* 2000 Feb 15;59(4):441-443.

[36] Gao L, Kim KJ, Yankaskas JR, Forman HJ, "Abnormal glutathione transport in cystic fibrosis airway epithelia," *Am J Physiol Lung Cell Mol Physiol* 1999 Jul;277(1):L113-118.

[37] Tirouvanziam RM, Tjioe I, Moss RB, Parks DR, Herzenberg LA, Wine JJ, "Multiparameter study of CF blood and lung leukocytes using 3-laser, 11-color cytometry," *Ped Pulmonol* 2001 Oct; 22:271-272.

[38] Lands LC, Grey V, Smountas AA, Kramer VG, McKenna D, "Lymphocyte glutathione levels in children with cystic fibrosis," *Chest* 1999 Jul;116(1):201-205.

[39] Abraham EH, Sterling KM, Kim RJH, Parker HW, Boyle WE, "Expression of CFTR and of DF508 CFTR in the reb blood cell membrane," abstract presented at the 13th *Annual European Cystic Fibrosis Conference*, June 2000, Stockholm, Sweden, abstract 14.

[40] Roum JH, Buhl R, McElvaney NG, Borok Z, Crystal RG, "Systemic deficiency of glutathione in cystic fibrosis," *J Appl Physiol* 1993 Dec;75(6):2419-2424.

[41] Brown RK, Wyatt H, Price JF, Kelly FJ, "Pulmonary dysfunction in cystic fibrosis is associated with oxidative stress," *Eur Respir J* 1996;9:334-339.

[42] Hagiwara K, Naito K, Kurokawa Y, Ichikawa T, "Kidney injury induced by lipid peroxide produced by vitamin E deficiency and GSH depletion in rats," *J Nutr Sci Vitaminol (Tokyo)* 1991 Feb; 37(1):99-107.

[43] Tabary O, Escotte S, Couetil JP, Hubert D, Dusser D, Puchelle E, Jacquot J, "Genistein inhibits constitutive and inducible NFkappaB activation and decreases IL-8 production by human cystic fibrosis bronchial gland cells," *Am J Pathol* 1999 Aug;155(2):473-481.

[44] Wong CH et al., "Cough Induced by Low pH," *Respiratory Medicine. 93(1)*:58-61, 1999 January.

[45] Jurima-Romet M and PN Shek, "Lung Uptake of Liposome-entrapped Glutathione After Intratracheal Administration," *J. Pharm. Pharmacol. 43*:6-10, 1991.

[46] Boxer LA, Oliver JM, Speilberg SP, Allen JM, Schulman JD, "Protection of Granulocytes by Vitamin E in Glutathione Synthetase Deficiency," *New Engl J Med* 1979 Oct 25;301(17): 901-905.

[47] Rahman Q, Abidi P, Afaq F, Schiffmann D, Mossman BT, Kamp DW, Athar M, "Glutathione redox system in oxidative lung injury," *Crit Rev Toxicol* 1999 Nov; 29(6):543-568.

[48] Smith LJ, Anderson J, "Oxygen-induced lung damage. Relationship to lung mitochondrial glutathione levels," *Am Rev Respir Dis* 1992 Dec; 146(6):1452-1457.

[49] Abidi P, Afaq F, Arif JM, Lohani M, Rahman Q, "Chrysolite-mediated imbalance in the glutathione redox system in the development of pilmonary injury," *Toxicol Lett* 1999 May 20;106(1):31-39.

[50] Thanislass J, Raveendran M, Devaraj H, "Buthionine sulfoximine-induced glutathione depletion. Its effect on antioxidants, lipid peroxidation and calcium homeostasis in the lung," *Biochem Pharmacol* 1995 Jul 17; 50(2):229-234.

[51] Forman HJ, Gao L, Broughman J, Iwamoto T, Venglarik CJ, Tomich JM, "Glutathione Transpoet and Impaired Antioxidant Function in Cystic Fibrosis," symposium session S16.4 presented at the Fourteenth Annual North American Cystic Fibrosis Conference, Baltimore, Maryland, November 9-12, 2000.

[52] Lauterburg BH, and ME Velez, "Glutathione deficiency in alcoholics: risk factor for paracetamol hepatotoxicity," *Gut 29(9)*:1153-1157, 1988 Sep.

[53] Fernandez-Checa JC et al., "Mitochondrial glutathione depletion in alcoholic liver disease," *Alcohol 10(6)*:469-475.

[54] Purucker E et al., "Glutathione status in liver and plasma during development of biliary cirrhosis after bile duct ligation," *Res Exp Med (Berlin) 198(4)*:167-174, 1998 Dec.

[55] Loguercio C et al., "Effect of liver cirrhosis and age on the glutathione concentration in the plasma, erythrocytes, and gastric mucosa of man," *Free Radic Biol Med 20(3)*:483-488, 1996.

[56] Barbaro G, Di Lorenzo G, Soldini M, Bellomo G, Belloni G, Grisorio B, Barbarini G, "Vagal system impairment in human immunodeficiency virus-positive patients with chronic hepatitis C: does hepatic glutathione deficiency have a pathogenic role?," *Sand J Gastroenterol* 1997 Dec; 32(12):1261-1256.

[57] Nath RG, Ocando JE, Richie JP Jr, Chung FL, "Effect of glutathione depletion on exocyclic adduct levels in the liver DNA of F344 rats," *Chem Res Toxicol* 1997 Nov;10(11):1250-1253.

[58] Sokol RJ, Taylor SF, Devereaux MW, Khandwala R, Sondheimer NJ, Shikes RH, Mierau G, "Hepatic oxidant injury and glutathione depletion during total parenteral nutrition in weanling rats," *Am J Physiol* 1996 Apr;270(4 Pt 1):G691-700.

[59] Ankrah NA, Dunyo SK, Nyarko AK, Appiah-Opong R, Ofsuhene M, "Biliary excretion in persons with low blood glutathione," *East Afr Med J* 1998 Apr;75(4):204-207.

[60] Wang X, Kanel GC, DeLeve LD, "Support of sinusoidal endothelial cell glutathione prevents hepatic veno-occlusive disease in the rat," *Hepatology* 2000 Feb;31(2):428-434.

[61] Bouchard G, Yousef IM, Barriault C, Tuchweber B, "Role of glutathione and oxidative stress in phalloidin-induced cholestasis," *J Heptaol* 2000 Apr; 32(4):550-560.

[62] Kobayashi T, Robinson MK, Robinson V, DeRosa E, Wilmore DW, Jacobs DO, "Glutathione depletion alters hepatocellular high-energy phosphate metabolism," *J Surg Res* 1993 Mar;54(3):189-195.

[63] Demols A, Van Laethem JL, Quertinmont E, Legros F, Louis H, LeMoine O, Deviere J, "N-acetylcysteine decreases severity of acute pancreatitits in mice," *Pancreas* 2000 Mar; 20(2):161-169.

[64] Gomez-Cambronero L, Camps B,de La Asuncion JG, Cerda M, Pellin A, Pallardo FV, Calvete J, Sweiry JH, Mann GE, Vina J, Sastre J, "Pentoxifylline ameliorates cerulein-induced pancreatitits in rats: role of glutathione and nitric oxide," *J Pharmacol Exp Ther* 2000 May 1;293(2):670-676.

[65] Wallig MA, "Xenobiotic metabolism, oxidant stress and chronic pancreatitis: focus on glutathione," *Digestion* 1998;59 Suppl 4:13-24.

[66] Paulusma CC, van Geer MA, Evers R, Heijn M, Ottenhoff R, Borst P, Oude Elferink RP, "Canalicular multispecific organic anion transporter/multidrug resistance protein 2 mediates low-affinity transport of reduced glutathione," *Biochem J* 1999 Mar 1;338(Pt 2):393-401.

[67] Ho E, Chen G, Bray TM, "Supplementation of N-acetylcysteine inhibits NFkappaB activation and protects against alloxan-induced diabetes in CD-1 mice," *FASEB J* 1999 Oct; 13(13):1845-1854.

[68] Vijayalingam S, Parthiban A, Shanmugasundaram KR, Mohan V, "Abnormal antioxidant status in impaired glucose tolerance and non-insulin-dependent diabetes mellitus," *Diabet Med* 1996 Aug; 13(8):715-719.

[69] Papadopoulos MC, Koumenis IL, Dugan LL, Giffard RG, "Vulnerability to glucose deprivation injury correlates with glutathione levels in astrocytes," *Brain Res* 1997 Feb 14;748(1-2):151-156.

[70] Ciuchi E, Odetti P, Prando R, "The effect of acute glutathione treatment on sorbitol level in erythrocytes from diabetic patients," *Diabetes Metb* 1997 Feb;23(1):58-60.

[71] Ankrah NA, Appiah-Opong R, "Toxicity of low levels of methylglyoxal: depletion of blood glutathione and adverse effect on glucose tolerance in mice," *Toxicol Lett* 1999 Sep 20;109(1-2):61-67.

[72] Domninguez C, Ruiz E, Gussinye M, Carrascosa A, "Oxidative stress at onset and in early stages of type 1 diabetes in children and adolescents," *Diabetes Care* 1998 Oct;21(10):1736-1742.

[73] Paolisso G et al., "Plasma GSH/GSSG affects glucose homeostasis in healthy subjects and non-insulin dependent diabetics," *Am J Physiol 262(3 Pt. 1)*: E435-40, 1992 Sep.

[74] Agha AM, El-Khatib AS, Al-Zuhair H, "Modulation of oxidant status by meloxicam in experimentally induced arthritis," *Pharmacol Res* 1999 Oct;40(4):385-392.

[75] Raya A, Gallego J, Bosch-Morell F, Roma J, Romero FJ, "Phenytoin-induced glutathione depletion in rat peripheral nerve," *Free Radic Biol Med* 1995 Nov;19(5):665-567.

[76] Lee KJ, Andrejuk T, Dziuban SW Jr, Goldfarb RD, "Deleterious effects of buthionine sulfoximine on cardiac function during continuous endotoxemia," *Proc Soc Exp Biol Med* 1995 Jun;209(2):178-184.

[77] Ardite E, Sanas M, Panes J, Romero FJ, Pique JM, Fernandez-Checa JC, "Replenishment of glutathione levels improves mucosal function in experimental acute colitis," *Lab Invest* 2000 May;80(5):735-744.

[78] Goldin E, Ardite E, Elizalde JI, Odriozola A, Panes J, Pique JM, Fernanadez-Checa JC, "Gastric mucosal damage in experimental diabetes in rats: role of endogenous glutathione," *Gastroenterology* 1997 Mar;112(3):855-863.

[79] Yoshikawa T, Minamiyama Y, Ichikawa H, Takahashi S, Naito Y, Kondo M, "Role of lipid peroxidation and antioxidants in gastric mucosal injury induced by hypoxanthine-xanthine oxidase system in rats," *Free Radic Biol Med* 1997;23(2):243-250.

[80] Sido B, Hack V, Hochlehnert A, Lipps H, Herfarth C, Droge W, "Impairment of intestinal glutathione synthesis in patients with inflammatory bowel disease," *Gut* 1998 Apr;42(4):485-492.

[81] Miralles-Barrachina O, Savoye G, Belmonte-Zalar L, Hochain P, Ducrotte P, Hecketsweiler B, Lerebours E, Dechelotte P, "Low levels of glutathione in endoscopic biopsies of patients with Crohn's colitis: the role of malnutrition," *Clin Nutr* 1999 Oct;18(5):313-317.

[82] Bengmark S and Heppsson B, "Gastrointestinal surface protection and mucosa reconditioning," *J. Parenter Enteral Nutr 19(5)*:410-5, 1995 Sep-Oct.

[83] Tolosa de Talamini N, Marchionatti A, Baudino V, Alisio A, "Glutathione plays a role in the chick intestinal calcium absorption," *Comp Biochem Physiol A Physiol* 1996 Oct;115(2):127-132.

[84] Ushmorov A, Hack V, Droge W, "Differential reconstitution of mitochondrial respiratory chain activity and plasma redox state by cysteine and ornithine in a model of cancer cachexia," *Cancer Res* 1999 Jul 15;59(14):3527-3534.

[85] Liberman MW, Wiseman AL, Shi ZZ, Carter BZ, Barrios R, Ou CN, Chevez-Barrios P, Wang Y, Habib GM, Goodman JC, Huang SL, Lebovitz RM, Matzuk MM, "Growth retardation and cysteine deficiency in gamma-glutamyl transpeptidase-deficient mice," *Proc Natl Acad Sci USA* 1996 Jul 23;93(15):7923-7926.

[86] Droge W, "Cysteine and glutathione in catabolic conditions and immunological dysfunction," *Curr Opin Clin Nutr Metab Care*, 1999 May;2(3):227-233.

[87] Golden MH, "Oedematous malnutrition," *Br Med Bull* 1998;54(2):433-444.

[88] Scholz RW et al., "Mechanism of Interaction of Vitamin E and Glutathione in the Protection against Lipid Peroxidation," *Annals of the New York Academy of Sciences, 570*:514-517, 1989.

[89] Higuchi, Y, Matsukawa S, "Glutathione depletion induces giant DNA and high-molecular-weight DNA fragmentation associated with apoptosis through lipid peroxidation and protein kinase C activation in C6 glioma cells," *Arch Biochem Biphys* 1999 Mar; 1;363(1):33-42

[90] Scholz RW, Reddy PV, Wynn MK, Graham KS, Liken AD, Gumpricht E, Reddy CC, "Glutathione-dependent factors and inhibition of rat liver microsomal lipid peroxidation," *Free Radic Biol Med* 1997; 23(5):815-28

[91] Thanislass J, Raveendran M, Devaraj H, "Buthionine sulfoximine-induced glutathione depletion. Its effect on antioxidants, lipid peroxidation and calcium homeostasis in the lung," *Biochem Pharmacol* 1995 Jul 17; 50(2):229-34

[92] Hagiwara K, Naito K, Kurokawa Y, Ichikawa T, "Kidney injury induced by lipid peroxide produced by vitamin E deficiency and GSH depletion in rats," *J Nutr Sci Vitaminol (Tokyo)* 1991 Feb; 37(1):99-107

[93] Angelini P, Cirelli F, Quarticelli A, Chicco D, Vendemiale G, Altomare E, "Administration of glutatione and lipid peroxidation induced during fasting," *Boll Soc Ital Biol Sper* 1990 Nov; 66(11):1097-1104

[94] Rosenblat M, Aviram M, "Macrophage glutathione content and glutathione peroxidase activity are inversely related to cell-mediated oxidation of LDL: in vitro and in vivo studies," *Free Radic Biol Med* 1998 Jan 15;24(2):305-317.

[95] Freedman SD, Katz MH, Parker EM, Laposata M, Urman MY, Alvarez JG, "A membrane lipid imbalance plays a role in the phenotypic expression of cystic fibrosis in cftr (-/-) mice," *Proc Natl Acad Sci USA* 1999 Nov 23; 96(24):13995-4000.

[96] Chen Q, Galleano M, Cederbaum AI, "Cytotoxicity and apoptosis produced by arachidonic acid in Hep G2 cells overexpressing human cytochrome P4502E1," *J Biol Chem* 1997 Jun 6;272(23):14532-14541.

[97] Montuschi P, Karitonov SA, Ciabattoni G, Corradi M, van Rensen L, Geddes DM, Hodson ME, Barnes PJ, "Exhaled 8-isoprostane as a new non-invasive biomarker of oxidative stress in cystic fibrosis," *Thorax*, 2000, 55(3):205-209.

[98] Buhl R et al, "Oxidant-Protease Interaction in the Lung: Prospects for Antioxidant Therapy," *Chest*, 110(6): 267S-272S, 1996 December supplement.

[99] Gillissen A, Birrer P, McElvaney NG, Buhl R, Vogelmeier C, Hoyt RF Jr, Hubbard RC, Crystal RG, "Recombinant secretory leukoprotease inhibitor augments gluathione levels in lung epithelial lining fluid," *J Appl Physiol* 1993 Aug;75(2):825-32

[100] Vogelmeier C, Biedermann T, Maier K, Mazur G, Behr J, Krombach F, Buhl R, "Comparative loss of activity of recombinant sefretory leukoprotease inhibitor and alpha 1-protease inhibitor caused by different forms of oxidative streaa," *Eur Respir J* 1997 Sep;10(9):2114-9

[101] Barbero, GJ, "Therapeutic Approaches to Cystic Fibrosis," *Bulletin of the World Health Organization, 72(3)*: 341-352, 1994.

[102] Brenneisen P. Briviba K, Wlaschek M, Wenk J, Scharffetter-Kochanel K, "Hydrogen peroxide (H2O2) increases the steady-state mRNA levels of collagenase/MMP-1 in human dermal fibroblasts," *Free Radic Biol Med* 1997;22(3):515-524.

[103] Jain A et al., "Ascorbic acid prevents oxidative stress in glutathione deficient mice: effects on lung type 2 cell lamellar bodies, lung surfactant, and skeletal muscle," *Proc. Natl. Acad. Sci. USA 89(11)*:5093-7, 1992 June.

[104] Jain A, Mehta T, Auld PA, Rodrigues J, Ward RF, Schwartz MK, Martensson J, "Glutathione metabolism in newborns: evidence for glutathione deficiency in plasma, bronchoalveolar lavage fluid, and lymphocytes in prematures," *Pediatr Pulmonol* 1995 Sep;20(3):160-156.

[105] Madesh M, Benard O, Balasubramanian KA, "Glutathione modulates lipid composition of human colon derived HT-29 cells," *Int J Biochem Cell Biol* 1998 Dec;30(12):1345-1352.

[106] Boda D, Nemeth I, Pinter S, "Surface tension, glutathione contenet and redox ratio of the tracheal aspirate fluid of premature infants with IRDS," *Biol Neonate* 1998 Oct;74(4):281-288.

[107] Supinski G, "Free radical induced respiratory muscle dysfunction," *Mol Cell Biochem* 1998 Feb;179(1-2):99-110.

[108] Bounous G, Molson J, "Competition for glutathione precursors between the immune system and the skeletal muscle: pathogenesis of chronic fatigue syndrome," *Med Hypotheses* 1999 Oct;53(4):347-349.

[109] Shaheen SO, Sterne JA, Songhurst CE, Burney PG, "Frequent paracetamol use and asthma in adults," *Thorax* 2000 Apr;55(4):266-270.

[110] Ogino T et al., "Neutrophil Antioxidant Capacity During the Respiratory Burst -- Loss of Glutathione Induced by Chloramines," *Free Radical Biology and Medicine 23(3)*: 445-452, 1997.

[111] Bilzer M and BH Lauterberg, "Gutathione metabolism in activated human neutrophils: stimulation of glutathione synthesis and consumption of glutathione by reactive oxygen species," *Eur. J. Clin. Investigation 21(3)*: 316-322, 1991 June.

[112] Remiao F, Carmo H, Carvalho FD, Bastos ML, "Inhibition of glutathione reductase by isoproterenol oxidation products," *J Enzyme Inhib* 2000;15(1):47-61.

[113] Barker JE, Heales SJ, Cassidy A, Bolanos JP, Land JM, Clark JB, "Depletion of brain glutathione results in a decrease of glutathione reductase activity; an enzyme susceptible to oxidative damage," *Brain Res* 1996 Apr 15;16(1-2):118-122.

[114] van Klaveren RJ, Hoet PH, Pype JL, Demedis M, Nemery B, "Increase in gamma-glutamyltransferase by glutathione depletion in rat type II pneumocytes," *Free Radic Biol Med* 1997;22(3):525-534.

[115] Li XY, Donaldson K, Rahman I, MacNee W, "An investigation of the role of glutathione in increased epithelial permeability induced by cigarette smoke in vivo and in vitro," *Am J Respir Crit Care Med* 1994 Jun;149(6):1518-1525.

[116] Kokura S, Wolf RE, Yoshikawa T, Granger DN, AW TY, "Molecular mechanisms of neutrophil-endothelial cell adhesion induced by redox imbalance," *Cric Res* 1999 Mar 19;84(5):516-524.

[117] Freeman ML, Huntley SA, Meredith MJ, Senisterra GA, Lepock J, "Destabilization and denaturation of cellular protein by glutathione depletion," *Cell Stress Chaperones* 1997 Sep;2(3):191-198.

[118] Calabreses V, Testa G, Ravagna A, Bates TE, Guiffrida Stella AM, "HSP70 induction in the brain following ethanol administration in the rat: regulation by glutathione redox state," *Biochem Biophys Res Commun* 2000 Mar 16;269(2):397-400.

[119] Liu H, Lightfoot R, Stevens JL, "Activation of heat shock factor by alkylating agents is triggered by glutathione depletion and oxidation of protein thiols," *J Biol Chem* 1996 Mar 1;271(9):4805-4812.

[120] Wilhelm D, Bender K, Knebel A, Angel P, "The level of intracellular glutathione is a key regulator for the induction of stress-activated signal transduction pathways including Jun N-terminal protein kinases and p38 kinase by alkylating agents," *Mol Cell Biol* 1997 Aug ; 17(8):4792-4800

[121] Kirlin WG, Cai J, Thompson SA, Diaz D, Kavanagh TJ, Jones DP, "Glutathione redox potential in response to differentiation and enzyme inducers," *Free Radic Biol Med* 1999 Dec;27(11-12):1208-18

[122] Lertratanangkoon K, Savaraj N, Scimeca JM, Thomas ML, "Glutathione depletion-induced thymidylate insufficiency for DNA repair synthesis," *Biochem Biophys Res Commun* 1997 May 19;234(2):470-475.

[123] Asensi M, Garcia-Espana A, Pallardo FV, Vina J, Esrrela JM, "Effect of nonprotein thiols on protein synthesis in isolated rat hepatocytes," *Experientia* 1996 Feb 15;52(2):111-114.

[124] Fussell JC, Kelly FJ, "Effects of deamethasone on lung protein turnover," *Biochem J 273(Pt 1)*:93-7. 1991 Jan 1.

[125] Murthy MR, "Protein synthesis in growing-rat tissues. II. Polyribosome cocentration of brain and liver as a function of age," *Biochim Biophys Acta 119(3)*:599-613, 1966 Jun 22.

[126] Thanislass J, Raveendran M, Sivasithamparam N, Devaraj H, "Effect of chronic glutathione deficiency on rat lung mitochondrial function," *Pulm Pharmacol* 1996 Apr;9(2):119-122.

[127] Rojas E, Valverde M, Kala SV, Kala G, Lieberman MW, "Accumulation of DNA damage in the organs of mice deficient in gamma-glutamyltranspeptidase," *Mutat Res* 2000 Feb 14;447(2):305-316.

[128] Gilmont RR, Dardano A, Young M, Engle JS, Adamson BS, Smith DJ Jr, Rees RS, "Effects of glutathione depletion on oxidant-induced endothelial cell injury," *J Surg Res* 1998 Nov;80(1):62-68.

[129] Fiorentini, C, Falzano L, Rivabene R, Fabbri A, Malorni W, "N-acetylcysteine protects epithelial cells against the antioxidant imbalance due to Clostridium difficile toxins," *FEBS Lett* 1999 Jun 18;453(1-2):124-128.

[130] Kamei H, "Cystine starvation induces reversible large-body formation from nuclear bodies in T24 cells," *Exp Cell Res* 1997 Nov 25;237(1):207-216.

[131] Zuelke KA, Jones DP, Perreault SD, "Glutathione oxidation is associated with altered microtubule function and disrupted fertilization in mature hamster oocytes," *Biol Reprod* 1997 Dec;57(6):1413-1439.

[132] Jain A, Martensson J, Mehta T, Krauss AN, Auld PM, Meister A, "Ascorbic acid prevents oxidative stress in glutathione-deficient mice: Effects on lung type 2 lamellar bodies, lung surfactant, and skeletal muscle," *Proc Natl Acad Sc USA*, 1992 June :89: 5093-5097.

[133] Moss M, Guidot DM, Wong-Lambertina M, Ten Hoor T, Perez RL, Brown LA, "The effects of chronic alcohol abuse on pulmonary glutathione homeostasis," *Am J Respir Crit Care Med* 2000 Feb 1;161(2 Pt 1):414-419

[134] Kitamura, S, "The 74th annual meeting president lecture: Pathogenesis and therapy of acute lung injury," *Kekkaku* 1999 Sep; 74(9):693-697.

[135] Rahman I, Skwarska E, Henry M, Davis M, O'Connor CM, FitzGerald MX, Greening A, MacNee, W, "Systemic and pulmonary oxidative stress in idiopathic pulmonary fibrosis," *Free Rad Biol Med* 1999 Jul;27(1-2):60-8

[136] Behr J, Degenkolb B, Maier K, Braun B, Beinert T, Krombach F, Vogelmeier C, Fruhmann G, "Increased oxidation of extracellular glutathione by bronchoalveolar inflammatory cells in diffuse fibrosing alveolitis," *Eur Respir J* 1995 Aug; 8(8):1286-1292.

[137] Staal FJT, Ela SW, Roederer M, Anderson MT, Herzenberg LA, "Glutathione deficiency and human immunodeficiency virus infection," *Lancet* 1992; 339:909-912.

[138] Pacht ER, Diaz P, Clanton T, Hart J, Gadek JE, "Alveolar glutathione fluid decreases in asymptomatic HIV-seropositive subjects over time," *Chest* 1997 Sep;112(3):785-788.

[139] Smith CV, Jones DP, Guenther TM, Lash, LH, Lauterberg BH, "Compartmentation of Glutathione: Implications for the Study of Toxicity and Disease," *Toxic and Appl Pharmacol 140*, 1-12, 1996.

[140] Houtmeyers E, Gosselink R, Gayan-Ramirez G, Decramer M, "Regulation of mucociliary clearance in health and disease," *Eur Respir J* 1999 May; 13(5):1177-1188.

[141] King M, Rubin BK, "Mucus-controlling agents: past and present," *Respir Care Clin N Am* 1999 Dec; 5(4):575-94

[142] Houtmeyers E, Gosselink R, Gayan-Ramirez G, Decramer M, "Effects of drugs on mucus clearance," *Eur Respir J* 1999 Aug;14(2):452-67

[143] Connolly MA, "Mucolytics and the critically ill patient: help or hindrance?" *AACN Clin Issues* 1995 May; 6(2):307-15

[144] Clarke SW, "Rationale of airway clearance," *Eur Respir J Suppl* 1989 Jul; 7:599s-603s.

[145] Jiang N, Dreher KL, Dye JA, Li Y, Richards JH, Martin LD, Adler KB, "Residual oil fly ash induces cytotoxicity and mucin secretion by guinea pig tracheal epithelial cells via an oxidant-mediated mechanism," *Toxicol Appl Pharmacol* 2000 Mar 15;163(3):221-230.

[146] Li JD, Feng W, Gallup M, Kim JH, Gum J, Kim Y, Basbaum C, "Activation of NF-kappaB via a Src-dependent Ras-MAPK-pp90rsk pathway is required for Pseudomonas aerugionosa-induced mucin overproduction in epithelial cells," *Proc Natl Acad Sci USA*, 1998, 95(10):5718-5723.

[147] Peterson JD, Herzenberg LA, Vasquez K, Waltenbaugh C, "Glutathione levels in antigen-presenting cells modulate Th1 versus Th2 response patterns," *PNAS* 1998 March 17;95(6):3071-3076.

[148] Galietta LJV, Folli C, Marchetti C, Romano L, Carpani D, Conese M, Zegarra-Moran O, "Modification of transepithelial ion transport in human cultured bronchial epithelial cells by interferon-gamma," *Am J Physiol - Lung Cell Mol Physiol* 2000 Jun;278(6):L1186-1194.

[149] Kelley TJ, Drumm ML, "Inducible nitric oxide synthase expression is reduced in cystic fibrosis murine and human airway epithelial cell lines," *J Clin Invest*, 1998 Sep;102(6):1200-1207.

[150] Mayer B, Pfeiffer S, Schrammel A, Koesling D, Schmidt K, Brunner F, "A new pathway of nitric oxide cylclic GMP signalling involving s-nitrosoglutathione," *J Biol Chem* 1998 Feb 6;273(6):3264-3270.

[151] Fischer B, Voynow J, "Neutrophil elastase induces MUC5AC messenger RNA expression by an oxidant-dependent mechanism," *Chest* 2000 May;117(5 Suppl 1):317S-320S.

[152] Cho S, Urata Y, Ilada T, Goto S, Yamaguchi M, Sumikawa K, Kondo T, "Glutathione downregulates the Phosphorylation of I kappa-B: Autoloop Regulation of the NF-kappa B-Mediated Expression of NF-kappa B Subunits by TNF-alpha in Mouse Vascular Endothelial Cells," *Biochemical and Biophysical Research Communications* 253(1):104-108, 1998.

[153] Droge W et al., "Modulation of Lymphocyte Functions and Immune Responses by Cysteine and Cysteine Derivatives," *The American Journal of Medicine 91(3C)*: 140-143, 1991 September 30.

[154] Sen CK, Khanna S, Reznick AZ, Roy S, Packer L, "Glutathione regulation of tumor necrosis factor-alpha-induced NF-kappa B activation in skeletal muscle-derived L6 cells," *Biochem Biophys Res Commun* 1997 Aug 28;237(3):645-9

[155] Desai A, Huang X, Warren JS, "Intracellular glutathione redox status modulates MCP-1 expression in pulmonary granulomatous vasculitis," *Lab Invest* 1999 Jul;79(7):837-47

[156] Luo Y, Hattori A, Munoz J, Qin ZH, Roth GS, "Intrastriatal dopamine injection induces apoptosis through oxidation-involved activation of transcription factors AP-1 and NF-kappaB in rats," *Mol Pharmacol* 1999 Aug;56(2):254-64

[157] Haddad JJ, Olver RE, Land SC, "Antioxidant/pro-oxidant equilibrium regulates HIF-1alpha and NF-kappaB redox sensitivity: evidence for inhibition by glutathione oxidation in alveolar epithelial cells," *J Biol Chem* 2000 May 4

[158] Tanaka C, Kamata H, Takeshita H, Yagisawa H, Hirata H, "Redox regulation of lipopolysaccharide (LPS)-induced interleukin-8 (IL-8) gene expression mediated by NF kappa B and AP-1 in human astrocytoma U373 cells," *Biochem Biophys Res Commun* 1997 Mar 17;232(2):568-73

[159] Rahman I, MacNee W, "Regulation of redox glutathione levels and gene transcription in lung inflammation: therapeutic approaches," *Free Radic Biol Med 28(9)*:1405-20, 2000 May 1

[160] Christman JW, Sadikot RT, Blackwell TS, "The role of nuclear factor-kappa B in pulmonary diseases," *Chest,* 2000, 117(5):1482-1487.

[161] Roederer M, Staal FJ, Osada H, Herzenberg LA, Herzenberg LA, "CD4 and CD8 T cells with high intracellular glutathione levels are selectively lost as the HIV infection progresses," *Int Immunol*, 1991 Sep; 3(9):933-7

[162] Garaci E, Palamara AT, Cirolo MR, D'Agostini C, del-Latif MS, Aquaro S, Lafavia E, Rotilio G, "Intracellular GSH content and HIV replication in human macrophages," *J Leukoc Biol*, 1997 Jul;62(1):54-9

[163] Palamara AT, Perno CF, Aquaro S, Bue MC, Dini L, Garaci E, "Glutathione inhibits HIV replication by acting at the late stages of the virus life cycle," *AIDS Res Hum Retroviruses*, 1996 Nov 1;12(16):1537-1541.

[164] Gosset P. Wallaert B, Tonnel AB, Fourneau C, "Thiol regulation of the production of TNF-alpha, IL-6 and IL-8 by human alveolar macrophages," *Eur Respir J* 1999 Jul;14(1):98-105

[165] Hashimoto S, Gon Y, Matsumoto K, Takeshita I, Asai Y, Asai Y, Machino T, Horie T, "Regulation by intracellular glutathione of TNF-alpha-induced p38 MAP kinase activation and RANTES production by human pulmonary vascular endothelial cells," *Allergy* 2000 May;55(5):463-9

[166] Yamauchi N, Watanabe N, Kuriyama H, Neda H, Maeda M, Himeno T, Tsuji Y, Niitsu Y, "Suppressive effects of intracellular glutathione on hydroxyl radical production induced by tumor necrosis factor," *Int J Cancer* 1990 Nov 15;46(5):884-888.

[167] Peristeris P, Clark BD, Gatti S, Faggioani R, Mantovani A, Mengozzi M, Orencole SF, Sironi M, Ghezzi P, "N-acetylcysteine and glutathione as inhibitors of tumor necrosis factor production," *Cell Immunol* 1992 Apr;140(2):390-399.

[168] Rovin BH, Dickerson JA, Tan LC, Fassler J, "Modulation of IL-1-induced chemokine expression in human mesangial cells through alterations in redox status," *Cytokine* 1997 Mar;9(3):178-186.

[169] Pena LR et al., "Treatment with glutathione precursor decreases cytokine activity," *J. Parenter. Enteral. Nutr. 23(1)*:1-6, 1999 January-February.

[170] Saccani A, Saccani S, Orlando S, Sironi M, Bernasconi S, Ghezzi P, Mantovani A, Sica A, "Redox regulation of chemokine receptor expression," *Proc Natl Acad Sci USA*, 2000 Mar 14;97(6):2761-2766.

[171] Morita A, Grewe M, Grether-Beck S, Olaizola-Horn S, Krutmann J, "Induction of proinflammatory cytokines in human epidermal carcinoma cells by in vitro ultraviolet A1 irradiation," *Photochem Photobiol* 1997 Apr;65(4):630-535

[172] Lombard-Gillooly K, Hubbard AK, "Modulation of silica-induced lung injury by reducing lung non-protein sulfhydryls with buthionine sulfoximine," *Toxicol Lett* 1993 Mar;66(3):305-15

[173] Cuzzocrea S, Constantino G, Zingarelli B, Mazzon E, Macali A, Caputi AP, "The protective role of endogenous gluathione in carrageenan-induced pleurisy in the rat," *Eur J Pharmacol* 1999 May 14;372(2):187-97.

[174] Liu B, Hannun YA, "Inhibition of neutral magnesium-dependent sphingomyelinase by glutathione," *J Biol Chem* 1997 Jun 27;272(26):16281-15287.

[175] Watson RW, Rotstein OD, Nathens AB, Dackiw AP, Marshall JC, "Thiol-mediated redox regulation of neutrophil apoptosis," *Surgery* 1996 Aug;120(2):150-157.

[176] Nakatani T, Tawaramoto M, Opare Kennedy D, Kojima A, Matsui-Yuasa I, "Apoptosis induced by chelation of intracellular zinc is associated with depletion of cellular reduced glutathione level in rat hepatocytes," *Chem Biol Interact* 2000 Mar 15;125(3):151-63

[177] Coppola S, Ghibelli L, "GSH extrusion and the mitochondrial pathway of apoptotic signalling," *Biochem Soc Trans* 2000 Feb;28(2):56-61

[178] Colell A, Garcia-Ruiz C, Miranda M, Ardite E, Mari M, Morales A, Corrales F, Kaplowitz N, Fernandez-Checa JC, "Selective glutathione depletion of mitochondria by ethanol sensitizes hepatocytes to tumor necrosis factor," *Gastroenterology* 1998 Dec;115(6):1541-51

[179] Nicole A, Santiard-Baron D, Ceballos-Picot I, "Direct evidence for glutathione as mediator of apoptosis in neuronal cells," *Biomed Pharmacother* 1998;52(9):349-55

[180] Rosenfeld ME, "Inflammation, lipids, and free radicals: lessons learned from te atherogenic process," *Semin Reprod Endrocrinol* 1998;16(4):249-61

[181] Hardwick SJ, Carpenter KL, Allen EA, Mitchinson MJ, "Glutathione (GSH) and the toxicity of oxidised low-density lipoprotein to human monocyte-macrophages," *Free Radic Res* 1999 Jan;30(1):11-9

[182] Aoshiba K, Yasui S, Nishimura K, Nagai A, "Thiol depletion induces apoptosis in cultured lung fibroblasts," *Am J Respir Cell Mol Biol* 1999 Jul;21(1):54-64

[183] Vahrmeijer AL, van Dierendonck JH, Schutrups J, van de Velde CJ, Mulder GJ, "Effect of glutathione depletion on inhibition of cell cycle progression and induction of apoptosis by mephalan (L-phenylalanine mustard) in human colorectal cancer cells," *Biochem Pharmacol* 1999 Aug 15;58(4):655-64

[184] Yang CF, Shen HM, Ong, CN, "Ebselen induces apoptosis in HepG(2) cells through rapid depletion of intracellular thiols," *Arch Biochem Biophys* 2000 Feb 15;374(2):142-52

[185] Li Y, Maher P, Schubert D, "A role for 12-lipoxygenase in nerve cell death caused by glutathione depletion," *Neuron* 1997 Aug;19(2):453-63.

[186] Iwata S et al., "Adult T cell leukemia (ATL)-derived factor/human thioredoxin prevents apoptosis of lymphoid cells induced by L-cystine and glutathione depletion: possible involvement of thiol-mediated redox regulation in apoptosis caused by pro-oxidant state," *J. Immunol.* 158(7):3108-17, 1997 April.

[187] Wedner HJ et al., "Inhibition of human polymorphonuclear leukocyte function by 2-cyclohexene-1-one: A role for glutathione in cell activation," *J. Clin. Invest. 68(2)*:535-43, 1981 August

[188] Aziz AS et al., "Effects of selenium on polymorphonuclear leukocyte function in goats," *Am. J. Vet. Res., 45(9)*:1715-8, 1984 September.

[189] Voetman AA, Loos JA, Roos, D, "Changes in the Levels of Glutathione in Phagocytosing Human Neutrophils," *Blood* 1980 May;55(5):741-747.

[190] Tirouvanziam R, "CFTR, glutathione, and neutrophil function," 1999 Nov, http://63.193.197.190/Subsets/tirouv/index.htm

[191] Atalay M, Marnila P, Lilius, EM, Hanninen O, Sen OK, "Glutathione-dependent modulation of exhausting exercise-induced changes in neutrophil function of rats," *Eur J Appl Physiol* 1996;74(4):342-7.

[192] ven der Meide PH, de Labie MC, Botman CA, van Bennekom WP, Olsson T, Aten J, Weening JJ, "Mercuric chloride down-regulates T cell interferon-gamma production in brown Norway but not in Lewis rats; role of glutathione, *Eur J Immunol* 1993 Mar;23(3):675-81

[193] Smyth MJ, "Glutathione modulates activation-dependent proliferation of human peripheral blood lymphocyte populations without regulating their activated function," *J Immunol* 1991 Mar 15;146(6):1921-1927.

[194] Nathens AB, Rotstein OD, Dackiw AP, Gorczynski R, "The glutathione depleting agent diethylmaleate pronolong renal allograft survival," *J Surg Res* 1998 Jun;77(1):75-9

[195] Robinson MK, Rodrick ML, Jacobs DO, Rounds JD, Collins KH, Saporoschetz IB, Mannick JA, Wilmore DW, "Glutathione depletion in rats impairs T-cell and macrophage immune function," *Arch Surg* 1993 Jan;128(1):29-34

[196] Ginn-Pease ME, Whisler RL, "Optimal NF kappa B mediated transcriptional responses to Jurkat T cells exposed to oxidative stress are dependent on intracellular glutthione and costimulatory signals," *Biochem Biophys Res Commun* 1996 Sep 24;226(3):695-702

[197] Aukrust P. Svardal AM, Muller F, Lunden B, Nordoy I, Froland SS, "Markedly distrubed glutathione reodx status in CD45RA+CD4+ lymphocytes in human immunodeficiency virus type 1 infection is associated with selective depletion of this lymphocyte subset," *Blood* 1996 Oct 1;88(7):2626-33

[198] Shenker BJ, Guo TL, O I, Shapiro IM, "Induction of apoptosis in human T-cells by methyl mercury: temporal relationship between mitochondiral dysfunction and loss of reductive reserve," *Toxicol Appl Pharmacol* 1999 May 15;157(1):23-35

[199] Herzenberg LA, De Rosa SC, Dubs JG, Roederer M, Anderson MT, Ela SW, Deresinski SC, Herzenberg LA, "Glutathione deficiency is asociated with impaired survival in HIV disease," *Proc Natl Acad Sci USA* 1997 Mar 4;94(5):1967-1972.

[200] Hamilos DL, Zelarney P, Mascari JJ, "Lymphocyte proliferation in glutathione-depleted lymphocytes: direct relationship between glutathione availability ant he proliferative response," *Immunopharmacology* 1989 Nov-Dec;18(3):223-35

[201] Gringhius SI, Leow A, Papendrecht-Van Der Voort EA, Remans PH, Breedveld FC, Verweij CL, "Displacement of linker for activation of T cells from the plasma

membrane due to redox balance alterations results in hyporesponsiveness of synovial fluid T lymphocytes in rheumatoid arthritis," *J Immunol* 2000 Feb 15;164(4):2170-2179.

[202] Aidoo A, Lyn-Cook LE, Morris SM, Kodell RL, Casciano DA, "Comparative study of intracellular glutathione content in rat lymphocyte cultures treated with 2-mercaptoethanol and interleukin-2," *Cell Biol Toxicol* 1991 Jul;7(3):215-27

[203] Gmunder H, Roth S, Eck HP, Gallas H, Mihm S, Droge W, "Interleukin-2 mRNA expression, lymphokine production and DNA synthesis in glutathione-depleted rats," *Cell Immunol* 1990 Oct 15;130(2):520-8

[204] Ting CC, Wang J, Hargrove ME, "Reversal of multiple-site tumor cell-induced immunosuppression by specific cytokines and pharmacological agents," *Immunopharmacology* 1995 Aug;30(2):119-30

[205] Hyde H, Brothwick NJ, Janossy G, Salmon M, Akbar AN, "Upregulation of intracellular glutathione by fibroblast-derived factor(s): enhanced survival of activated T cells in the presence of low Bcl-2," *Blood* 1997 Apr 1;89(7):2453-2460.

[206] Messina JP, Lawrence DA, "Cell cycle progression of glutathione-depleted human peripheral blood mononuclear cells is inhibited at S phase," *J Immunol* 1989 Sep 15;143(6):1974-81.

[207] Fidelus RK and MF Tsan, "Glutathione and lymphocyte activation: a function of ageing and auto-immune disease," *Immunology* 61(4):503-8, 1987 August.

[208] Jeannin P, Delneste Y, Lecoanet-Henchoz S, Gauchat JF, Life P, Homes D, Bonnefoy JY, "Thiols decrease human interleukin (IL) 4 production and IL-4-induced immunoglobulin synthesis," *J Exp Med* 1995 Dec 1;182(6):1785-92

[209] Rigacci S, Iantomasi T, Marraccini P, Berti A, Vincenzini MT, Ramponi G, "Evidence for glutathione involvement in platelet-derived growth-factor-mediated signal," *Biochem J* 1997 Jun 15;324(Pt 3):791-6

[210] Romero DL, Mounho BJ, Lauer FT, Born JL, Burchiel SW, "Depletion of glutathione by benzo(a)pyrene metabolites, ionomycin, thatpsigargin, and phorbol myristate in human peripheral blood mononuclear cells," *Toxicol Appl Pharmacol* 1997 May;144(1):62-9

[211] Liang SM, Liang CM, Hargrove ME, Ting CC, "Regulation by glutathione of the effect of lymphokines on differentiation of primary activated lymphocytes. Influence of glutathione on cytotoxic activity of CD3-AK-.," *J Immunol* 1991 Mar 15;146(6):1909-13

[212] Gmunder H, Droge W, "Differential effects of glutathione depletion on T cell subsets," *Cell Immunol* 1991 Nov;138(1):229-37

[213] Ting CC, Hargrove HE, Liang SM, Liang CM, Sharrow SO, "Dichotomy of glutathione regulation of the activation of resting and preactivated lymphocytes," *Cell Immunol* 1992 Jun;142(1):40-53

[214] Gmunder H, Eck HP, Benninghoff B, Roth S, Droge W, "Macrophages regulate intracellular glutathione levels of lymphocytes. Evidence for an immunoregulatroy role of cysteine," *Cell Immunol* 1990 Aug;129(1):32-46.

[215] Hargrove ME, Wang J, Ting CC, "Regulation by glutathione of the activation and differentiation of IL-4-dependent activated killer cells," *Cell Immunol* 1993 Jul;149(2):433-43

[216] Sprietsma JE, "Zinc-controlled Th1/Th2 switch significantly determines development of disease," *Med Hypotheses* 1997 Jul;49(1):1-14

[217] Spriestma JE, "Cysteine, glutathione (GSH) and zinc and copper ions together are effective, natral, intracellular inhibitors of (AIDS) viruses," *Med Hypotheses* 1999 Jun;52(6):529-38

[218] Spriestma JE, "Modern diets and diseases: NO-zinc balance. Under Th1, zinc and nitorgen monoxide (NO) collectively protect against viruses, AIDS, autoimmunity, diabetes, allergies, asthma, infectious diseases, atherosclerosis and cancer," *Med Hypotheses* 1999 Jul;53(1):6-16

[219] Moser C, Johansen HK, Song Z, Hougen HP, Rygaard J, Hoiby N, "Chronic Pseudomonas aeruginosa lung infection is more severe in Th2 responding BALB/c mice compared to Th1 responding C3H/HeN mice," *APMIS* 1997 Nov;105(11):838-42

[220] Nishikawa M, Sato EF, Kashiba M, Kuroki T, Utsumi K, Inoue M, "Role of glutathione in nitric oxide-dependent regulation of energy metabolism in rat hepatoma cells," *Hepatology* 1998 Feb;27(2):422-426.

[221] Bolanos JP, Almeida A, Stewart V, Peuchen S, Land JM, Clark JB, Heales SJ, "Nitric oxide-mediated mitochondrial damage in the brain: mechanisms and implications for neurodegenerative diseases," *J Neurochem* 1997 Jun;68(6):2227-40.

[222] D'Emilia DM, Lipton SA, "Ratio of S-nitrosohomocyst(e)ine or other thiols determines neurotoxicity in rat cerebrocortical cultures," *Neuroscience Letters* 1999;265:103-106.

[223] Stefanelli C, Pignatti C, Tantani B, Stanic I, Bonavita F, Muscari C, Guarnieri C, Clo C, Caldarera CM, "Nitric oxide can function as either a killer molecule or an antiapoptotic effector in cardiomyocytes," *Biochim Biophys Acta* 1999 Jul 8;1450(3):406-13

[224] Rosenberg PA, Li Y, Ai S, Altiok N, Back SA, Volpe JJ, "Intracellular redox state determines whether nitric oxide is toxic or protective to rat oligodendrocytes in culture," *J Neurochem* 1999 Aug;73(2):476-84

[225] Chiueh CC, Rauhala P, "The redox pathway of S-nitrisoglutathione, glutathione and nitric oxide in cell to neuron communications," *Free Radic Res* 1999 Dec;31(6):641-50

[226] Boggs SE, McCormick TS, Lapetina EG, "Glutathione Levels Determine Apoptosis in Macrophages," *Biochem Biophys Res Commun* 1998 Jun 18;247(2):229-33

[227] Zhao ZH, Francis CE, Welch G, Loscalzo J, Ravid K, "Reduced glutathione prevents nitric oxide-induced apoptosis in vascular smooth muscle cells," *Biochimica er Biophysica Acta - Molecular Cell Research* 1997 Nov 27;1359(2):143-52

[228] Ju C, Yoon KN, Oh YK, Kim HC, Sin CY, Ryu JR, Ko KH, Kim WK, "Synergistic depletion of astrocytic glutathione by glucose deprivation and peroxynitrite: correlation with mitochondrial dysfunction and subsequent cell death," *J Neurochem* 2000 May;74(5):1989-98

[229] Callsen D, Brune B, "Role of mitogen-activated protein kinases in S-nitrosoglutathione-induced macrophage apoptosis," *Biochemistry* 1999 Feb 23;38(8):2279-86

[230] Lemaire G, Alvarez-Pachon FJ, Beuneu C, Lepoivre M, Petit JF, "Differential cytostatic effects of NO donors and NO producing cells," *Free Radic Biol Med* 1999 May;26(9-10):1274-83

[231] Romao PR, Fonseca SG, Hothersall JS, Noronha-Dutra AA, Ferreira SH, Cunha FQ, "Glutathione protects macrophages and Leishmania major against nitric oxide-mediated cytotoxicity," *Parasitology* 1999 Jun;118(Pt 6):559-66

[232] Aleryani S et al., "Superoxide-mediated decomposition of biological S-nitrosothiols," *J Biol Chem*, 273(11):601-5, 1998 March 13.

[233] Arnelle, DR and Stamler JS, "NO+, NO, and NO- donation by S-nitrosothiols: implications for regulation of physiological functions by S-nitrosylation and acceleration of disulfide formation," *Arch Biochem Biophys* 318(2):279-85, 1992 April 20.

[234] Jones KL, Bryan TW, Jinkins PA, Simpson KL, Grisham MB, Owens MW, Milligan SA, Markewitz BA, Robbins RA, "Superoxide released from neutrophils causes a reduction in nitric oxide gas," *AJP - Lung Cellular and Molecular Physiology* 1998 Dec;275(6):L1120-6

[235] Zavodnik IB, Lapshina EA, Rekawiecka K, Zavodnik LB, Barstosz G, Bryszewska M, "Membrane effects of nitrite-induced oxidation of human red blood cells," *Biochim Biophys Acta* 1999 Oct 15;1421(2):306-16

[236] Belvisi MG, Ward JK, Mitchell JA, Barnes PJ, "Nitric oxide as a neurotransmitter in human airways," *Arch Int Pharmacodyn Ther* 1995 Jan-Feb;329(1):97-110

[237] Gaston B et al., "Relaxation of Human Bronchial Smooth Muscle by S-Nitrosothiols in Vitro," *The Journal of pharmacology and experimental therapeutics. 268(2)*: 978-984, 1994 February.

[238] Kamosinska B, Radomski MW, Duszyk M, Radomski A, Man SF, "Nitric oxide activates chloride currents in human lung epithelial cells," *Am J Physiol* 1997 Jun;272(6 PT 1):L1098-104

[239] Dong YJ, Chao AC, Kouyama K, Hsu YP, Bocian RC, Moss RB, Gardner P, "Activation of CFTR chloride current by nitric oxide in human T lymphocytes," *EMBO J* 1995 Jun 15;14(12):2700-2707.

[240] Gao L, Broughman JR, Iwamoto T, Tomich JM, Venglarik CJ, Forman HJ. "Synthetic chloride channel restorese glutathione secretion in cystic fibrosis airway epithelia." *Am. J. Physiol. Lung Cell Mol. Physiol* 2001 July; 28(1):L24-30.

[241] Buhl R, Vogelmeier C, Critenden M, Hubbard RC, Hoyt RF Jr., Wilson, EM, Cantin AM, Crystal RG, "Augmentation of the glutathione in the fluid lining the epithelium of the lower respiratory tract by directly administering glutathione," *Proc. Natl. Acad. Sci. USA,* 1990 June, 87:4063-67

[242] Buhl R, Holroyd K, Borok Z, Roum J, Bokser A, Grimes G, Czerski D, Cantin A, Crystal RG, "Reversal of the glutathione deficiency in the lower respiratory tract of HIV-Seropositive individuals by glutathione aerosol therapy," *Clin. Res.*, 1990, 38(2): 596A

[243] Borok Z, Buhl R, Grimes GJ, Bokser AD, Hubbard RC, Holroyd KJ, Roum JH, Czerski DB, Cantin AM, Crystal RG, "Effect of Glutathione Aerosol on Oxidant-Antioxidant Imbalance in Idiopathic Pulmonary Fibrosis," *Lancet*, 1991 July 17, 338:215-6,

[244] Marrades RM, Roca J, Barbera JA, de Jover L, MacNee W, Rodriguez-Roisin R, "Nebulized Glutathione Induces Bronchoconstriction in Patients with Mild Asthma," *Am. J. Respir. Crit. Care Med.,* 1997, 156:425-30

[245] Bernorio S, Pecis M, Zucchi A, Guerra G, Migliorini V, Negri L, Corsano A, "Glutathione in Bronchial Hyperresponsiveness," *J. Aerosol Medicine 9(2)*:207-213, 1996

[246] Testa B, Mesolella M, Testa D, Giuliano A, Costa G, Maione F, Iaccarino F, "Glutathione in the upper respiratory tract," *Ann Otol Rhinol Laryngol* 1995;104:117-9

[247] Roum JH, Borok Z, McElvaney NG, Grimes GJ, Bokser AD, Buhl R, Crystal RG, "Glutathione aerosol suppresses lung epithelial surface inflammatory cell-derived oxidants in cystic fibrosis," *J Appl Physiol* 1999 Jul;87(1):438-43

[248] Bagnato GF, Gulli S, DePasquale R, Giacobbe O, Spatari G, Purello D'Ambrosio F. "Effect of inhaled glutathione on airway response to 'fog' challenge in asthmatic patients." *Respiration* 1999 Nov-Dec; 66(6):518-521.

[249] Griese M, ramakers J, Krasselt A, Starosta V, Van Konigsbruggen S, Fischer R, Ratjen F, Mullinger B, Huber RM, Maier K, Rietschel E, Scheuch G. "Improvement of alveolar glutathione, lung function, but not oxidative stress in cystic fibrosis." *Am. J. Respir. Crit. Care Med,* 2004 Jan 15 (e published ahead of publication).

[250] Bishop C, Hudson V, Hilton S, Saxey C, Dastrup T, Redding M, Bishop N, "Glutathione augmentation in cystic fibrosis." *Ped. Pulm.*, 2003 Supplement 25, A242;267.; forthcoming in Chest

[251] Snyder AH, McPherson ME, Hunt JF, Johnson M, Stumler JS, Gaston B. "Acute effects of aerosolized S-nitroglutathione in cystic fibrosis." *Am. J. Respir. Crit. Care Med,* 2002 April; 165(7):922-966.

[252] Sermet-Gaudelus I, Stoven V, Annereau JP, Witko-Sarsat V, Reinert P, Guyot M, Deschamps-Latscha B, Lallemand JY, Lenoir G. "Interest of colchicine for the treatment of cystic fibrosis patients. Preliminary report." *Mediators Inflamm.* 1999; *(1):13-5.

In: New Developments in Birth Defects Research
Editor: Nelson A. Gaslem, pp. 207-223

ISBN 1-60021-400-2

Chapter 8

GENES THAT MODULATE CYSTIC FIBROSIS DISEASE SEVERITY ARE ENCODED NEAR THE *CFTR* GENE ON 7Q31 – 7QTEL

Frauke Stanke and Burkhard Tümmler

Clinical Research Group, Department of Pediatrics, Medizinische Hochschule Hannover, D-60623 Hannover, Germany.

ABSTRACT

Cystic fibrosis (CF), the most common severe autosomal recessive trait among Caucasians, is caused by molecular lesions in the cystic fibrosis transmembrane conductance regulator gene (*CFTR*). The course of the multi-organ disease CF is highly variable suggesting the influence of environmental factors and/or modulating genes other than *CFTR* on the disease phenotype.

The gene causing Cystic fibrosis (CF) was uncovered in 1989.[1] Within the cystic fibrosis transmembrane conductance regulator (*CFTR*) gene, more than 1300 variants have been described so far.[2] The allelic heterogeneity of the *CFTR* gene has instigated many genotype-phenotype studies [3-5] which all demonstrate that except for the pancreatic status, course and severity of the multi-organ CF cannot be predicted on the basis of the *CFTR* mutation genotype. Moreover, the variability of CF disease has also been observed among unrelated patients carrying the same *CFTR* mutation genotype [6,7] and within CF sib pairs.[8] These observations have been accepted by the CF community to indicate the role of other factors than the *CFTR* gene in shaping the disease phenotype, and several studies have been launched to study the role of inherited modulators in CF.

In 1994, the European CF twin and sibling study has been initiated during an EU BIOMED symposium. More than 500 CF twin and sibling pairs from 158 CF clinics of 14 European countries were enrolled in the study in 1995-1996. Out of these, less than 40 families with F508del homozygous twins or sibs were selected to study inherited modulators of CF disease based on their extreme clinical phenotype. This chapter describes the rationale for selecting these pairs [9] and summarizes the findings on the candidate gene region on 7q31.3-7qtel [10] among this set of highly informative CF siblings.

Cystic fibrosis (CF), the most common severe autosomal recessive trait among Caucasians, is caused by molecular lesions in the cystic fibrosis transmembrane conductance regulator gene (*CFTR*). The course of the multi-organ disease CF is highly variable suggesting the influence of environmental factors and/or modulating genes other than *CFTR* on the disease phenotype. To evaluate the cause of CF disease variability, the *European CF twin and sibling study* collected data on two clinical parameters most sensitive for course and prognosis of CF for a cohort of more than 300 CF twin and sibling pairs. In order to analyze the effect of modulating genes on CF disease severity, F508del homozygous sibling pairs with extreme clinical phenotype as judged by nutritional status (weight as % of predicted weight for height) and pulmonary status (CF population centiles for FEV1%pred) were selected by a ranking algorithm. These highly concordant and highly discordant F508del homozygous sib pairs were typed at single nucleotide polymorphisms (SNPs) and short tandem repeat polymorphisms (STRPs) in the 24-cM *CFTR*-spanning region between D7S525 and D7S495. Allele frequencies differed significantly at D7S495 comparing concordant mildly affected, concordant severely affected and discordant sib pairs. A rare haplotype of two SNPs within the leptin gene promoter was found exclusively among the concordant mildly affected pairs. A retrospective genotype-phenotype analysis of 54 F508del homozygotes from the CF clinic in Hannover for whom longitudinal growth data were available suggests that the leptin-promoter-haplotypes found predominantly among the concordant mildly affected pairs predispose to an elevated growth gain during puberty. Furthermore, all concordant sib pairs shared the paternal F508del chromosome between *CFTR* and D7S495, whilst the cohort of discordant sib pairs inherited equal proportions of recombined and non-recombined paternal chromosomes. We conclude that disease manifestation in CF is modulated by loci in the partially imprinted region 3' of *CFTR* that determine stature, food intake and energy homeostasis, such as the Silver-Russel-Syndrome candidate gene region and *LEP*.

Introduction

The gene causing Cystic fibrosis (CF) was uncovered in 1989.[1] Within the cystic fibrosis transmembrane conductance regulator (*CFTR*) gene, more than 1300 variants have been described so far.[2] The allelic heterogeneity of the *CFTR* gene has instigated many genotype-phenotype studies [3-5] which all demonstrate that except for the pancreatic status, course and severity of the multi-organ CF cannot be predicted on the basis of the *CFTR* mutation genotype. Moreover, the variability of CF disease has also been observed among unrelated patients carrying the same *CFTR* mutation genotype [6,7] and within CF sib pairs.[8] These observations have been accepted by the CF community to indicate the role of other factors than the *CFTR* gene in shaping the disease phenotype, and several studies have been launched to study the role of inherited modulators in CF.

In 1994, the European CF twin and sibling study has been initiated during an EU BIOMED symposium. More than 500 CF twin and sibling pairs from 158 CF clinics of 14 European countries were enrolled in the study in 1995-1996. Out of these, less than 40 families with F508del homozygous twins or sibs were selected to study inherited modulators of CF disease based on their extreme clinical phenotype. This chapter describes the rationale for selecting these pairs [9] and summarizes the findings on the candidate gene region on 7q31.3-7qtel [10] among this set of highly informative CF siblings.

Selection of Informative Patient Pairs

It is reasonable to assume that the *CFTR* mutation genotype, environmental factors and inherited modulators will influence the outcome of CF disease. Hence, to study inherited modulators it is advantageous to select a set of patients where the role of confounding variables is minimized. To standardize the *CFTR* mutation genotype, only F508del homozygous sibs were selected for genotyping. As a consequence, the influence of the major disease causing gene is normalized for all individuals of the study population and the role of other factors – for instance, inherited modulators – is emphasized. Considering a sib pair that is characterized by a concordant phenotype, random environmental effects can be excluded as a cause of the disease manifestation. Again, the role of other influences of CF disease severity – such as inherited factors – is emphasized. Finally, the selection of extreme phenotypes is likely to increase the informativity of the sample [11-13] as the phenotypic contrast between mildly and severely affected patients can be utilized in a case-control design of an association study.

Quantitative Description of CF Disease Severity and Intrapair Discordance

CF is a multi-organ disease with a variety of symptoms. Two quantitative parameters which are most sensitive to course and prognosis of CF disease [14-17] were selected to define CF disease severity among the European CF twins and sibs: wfh% (= weight expressed as weight% predicted for height, reference data set published by Prader *et al.* [18]) and the FEV1%pred (reference data set published by Knudson *et al.* [19]) — derived CF population centiles, so-called FEVPerc (= CF centiles for FEV1%pred, defined using the reference data set by EUCFRegistry [9]). These two parameters, wfh% and FEVPerc, respectively, account for the severity of CF disease in the two major afflicted organ systems, the gastrointestinal and pulmonary tract. The parameter FEVPerc is corrected for the progression of lung disease with age in a CF population by describing CF population centiles for FEV1%pred. Please note that centiles for both, wfh% and FEVPerc, are age-independent within the CF patient population [9] and therefore, these parameters are appropriate measures of disease severity when patients are heterogeneous with respect to their age due to a cross-sectional study design.

To allow the assessment of CF disease severity using one quantitative parameter only, wfh% and FEVPerc were combined using a non-parametric approach as described in detail elsewhere.[9] Briefly, after all patients have been enrolled into the study, rank numbers were assigned to wfh% and FEVPerc values. In a x-y-plot of rank number for wfh% vs. rank number for FEVPerc (Figure 1a), the distance from origin defines the overall CF disease severity of a patient and the distance of two data points of a sib pair (= DELTA) defines the intrapair discordance of a sib pair. When 29 monozygous twin pairs and 12 dizygous twin pairs were compared in their intrapair difference in wfh%, their intrapair difference in FEVPerc and the composite parameter DELTA, discordance between these twin groups of different zygosity was comparable in wfh% (p = 0.48) and FEVPerc (p = 0.12) while monozygous twins were significantly more concordant in their composite parameter DELTA (p = 0.04). As higher concordance among monozygous compared to dizygous twins is generally accepted as an indication of inherited factors, the composite parameter appears to be more sensitive towards this inherited increment in CF disease than each of the individual parameters describing nutritional and pulmonary status.[9] For this reason, we conclude that the selection of candidates for an association study based on this composite parameter will increase the power to detect inherited modulators.

114 F508del homozygous patient pairs for whom wfh% and FEVPerc were available for both siblings in 1996 were ranked according to these composite parameters to define the groups concordant / mildly affected patient pairs (CON+), composed of two siblings with mild disease, concordant / severely affected patient pairs (CON-), comprised of two severely diseased siblings and discordant pairs (DIS) wherein one sibling is mildly affected and the other is severely affected.

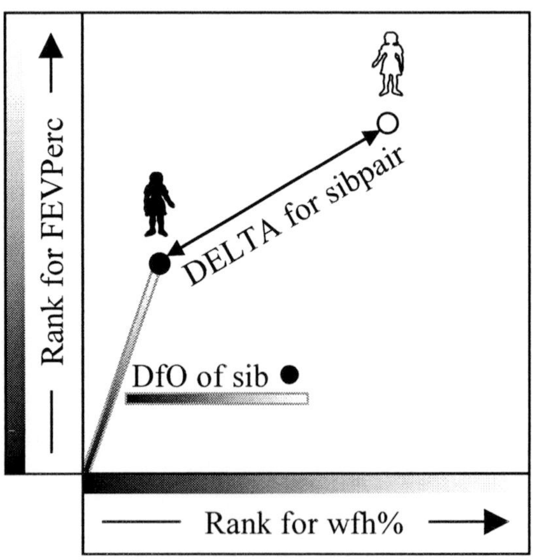

Figure 1. Definition of composite parameters for ranking CF twin and sibpairs according to their disease severity and intrapair discordance. Disease severity of a sib is judged via distance from origin (=DfO) within above diagram of rank for wfh% and rank for FEVPerc. The intrapair discordance is quantified by parameter DELTA depicting the distance of two data points, representative for one sib pair, within the same diagram. See Mekus *et al.* [9] for details.

To analyse inherited modulators on chromosome 7q, only dizygous pairs were considered. DNA could be obtained for 10 pairs ranked CON-, 11 pairs ranked CON+ and 13 pairs ranked DIS. Concordant and discordant patient pairs differed significantly in their discordance as represented by intrapair differences of wfh% and FEVPerc ($p < 0.001$, Mann-Whitney rank test [10]) and their disease severity as represented by intrapair sum of wfh% and FEVPerc ($p < 0.001$, Mann-Whitney rank test comparing CON+ and CON- pairs [10]).

The CFTR Gene Region: a Candidate for the Modulation of CF Disease Severity?

Among Caucasians, CF is the most frequent severe disease inherited in an autosomal recessive fashion. Based on the incidence, 1 out of 20-30 healthy Caucasians are expected to be carrier for one CF disease causing allele. It has been speculated that an advantage of the heterozygous carrier state has lead to this comparably high prevalence of CF-causing alleles in the general population.[20] Moreover, three frequent *CFTR* mutations – i.e. F508del, N1303K, and G542X – that have emerged by independent mutation events all occur on the same *CFTR* flanking SNP haplotype,[21-25] which points to an advantage transmitted by the genetic background on chromosomes carrying this haplotype.

To analyze whether the genetic background of the *CFTR* gene region has an impact on CF disease severity, 34 dizygous patient pairs were analyzed at several SNP and STRP loci within the *CFTR*-spanning region between D7S525 and D7S495 (see table 1 for details).

RESULTS

CFTR Intragenic and Flanking SNPs: MetH, XV2c, TUB20 and J3.11

Four marker loci near or within the *CFTR* gene have been studied on the F508del homozygous sib pairs (Table 1).[10] The SNPs MetH and J3.11 are localized in approximately 1 Mb distance 5' and 3' to the *CFTR* gene. Genotype-phenotype associations among F508del homozygotes with respect to loci within the *CFTR* linkage group have previously been suggested when an association of the J3.11 allele 2 with milder pulmonary disease [34] and an association of the MetH-J3.11 haplotype 2-1 with low weight [35] was reported. Furthermore, an association of allele 2 at marker locus CS.7 (located within a 40-kb distance 3'of XV2c) and postnatal female survival in the Czech population has been reported.[36]

As expected for F508del chromosomes, the F508del-typical archaic MetH-XV2c-TUB20-J3.11 haplotype 1-1-2-1 was most frequently observed among the European CF sib pairs (estimated to account for 60% of chromosomes among the CON+ pairs, respectively). Allele frequencies at these four marker loci were indistinguishable comparing CON+, CON- and DIS patient pair groups. However, all our CON+ sibs carried the allele 1 at XV2c and the mildest nine CON+ pairs were homozygous for allele 1 at MetH. Hence, published reports and the findings within this study agree with the hypothesis that a 'benign' phenotype is associated with the 'archaic' *CFTR* haplotype.[10]

Table 1. Markers analyzed on 7q31-7qtel.

Marker	Type(1)	Pos.[Mb](2)	Pos[cM](3)	Pos[cM](4)	Pos[cM](5)	Reference
D7S525	STRP	109.20	121.4	153.1	90.2	[26]
MetH	SNP	115.89	—	—	—	[27]
XV2c	SNP	116.52	—	—	—	[28]
TUB20	SNP	116.82	—	—	—	[21]
DHS1 (5)	SNP	116.89	—	—	—	[29]
DHS2 (5)	SNP	116.89	—	—	—	[29]
J3.11	SNP	117.41	—	—	—	[27]
D7S680	STRP	126.23	130.8	164.8	97.1	[26]
D7S514	STRP	126.58	130.2	163.8	97.1	[26]
D7S635	STRP	126.58	130.2	163.8	97.1	[26]
D7S2501	STRP	127.06	130.8	164.8	97.1	[26]
AFM16yc 9	STRP	127.11	—	—	—	[26]
D7S504	STRP	127.17	130.8	164.8	97.1	[26]
D7S1875	STRP	127.30	130.8	164.8	97.1	[26]
LEP1 (5)	SNP	127.43	—	—	—	[30-31]
LEP2 (5)	SNP	127.43	—	—	—	[30-31]
D7S461	STRP	127.90	—	—	—	[26]
D7S530	STRP	128.76	134.6	172.0	97.1	[26]
D7S649	STRP	130.27	136.1	173.5	98.7	[26]
D7S640	STRP	132.06	137.8	175.6	100.3	[26]
D7S500	STRP	134.52	140.6	179.9	101.9	[26]
D7S495	STRP	137.42	144.7	184.6	105.1	[26]

(1) STRP = short tandem repeat polymorphism (microsatellite); SNP = single nucleotide polymorphism

(2) position on physical map as given by UNISTS 05/2004 (XV2c, J3.11, D7S514, D7S2501, D7S504, D7S1875, D7S461, D7S649, D7S640, D7S500) and by relative position on NT_079596 [32]

(3) position on Marshfield sex-averaged genetic map.[33] Please note that the distance between D7S525 and D7S495 is 23.3 cM on the sex-averaged map, 31.5 cM on the female recombination map, but only 14,9 cM on the male recombination map.

(4) position on Marshfield female recombination map [33]

(5) position on Marshfield male recombination map [33]

(6) These SNPs refer to: DHS1: AC000061:72957 C/T and DHS2: AC000061:73211C/T, both within DHS at *CFTR*4572+15.6 kb; LEP2: *LEP*-2548G/A and *LEP*-2549C/A; LEP1: *LEP*-1387G/A (see appendix for details)

Discordant Sib Pairs Trace Inherited Modulators Encoded in Trans

Mild pulmonary disease has previously been correlated with the allele 2 at J3.11.[34] In our CF twin and sibling cohort, we did not see an association of J3.11 genotype with pulmonary disease severity. This might be due to a difference in age distribution of the respective patient panels: we have selected siblings with extreme clinical phenotypes from a patient cohort aged 6–38 years (mean: 18 years), while Santis and co-workers [34] investigated adult patients (range: 18–40 years). Effects that manifest later in life might not be detected within our cohort. However, we observed that genotypes at J3.11 segregated with the intrapair discordance in the lung function parameter FEVPerc. Among our discordant pairs, we observed a higher intra-pair difference in FEVPerc for pairs homozygous for allele 1 at J3.11 compared with sib pairs heterozygous at J3.11 ($p = 0.05$, Mann-Whitney rank test).[10] This finding cannot be exclusively explained by sequences encoded in linkage disequilibrium to J3.11 as two siblings of any CF patient pair must have inherited the same genetic information starting at F508del up to any recombination breakpoint that has been observed only 3' to J3.11 among the CF twin and sibling pairs. Thus, inherited modulators causing the intrapair discordance of F508del homozygous sib pairs must be encoded elsewhere in the genome where the siblings do not obligatorily carry the same alleles. Near J3.11, few genes have been annotated and the only gene with a well-defined function for pulmonary disease is the *CFTR* gene itself. We hypothesize that the trans-acting factors differentially interact with allelic variants of regulatory sequences in the 3'region of *CFTR*. Plausible candidates are the conserved non-coding sequences [37] and/or DNAse hypersensitive sites.[38] Recently, two functional SNPs within the DNAse hypersensitive site DHS 4572+15.6 kb were described.[29] We have tested 51 F508del homozygous dizygous patient pairs for variants at these two polymorphisms. Only two haplotypes were observed among the 102 F508del chromosomes, the frequent haplotype being present on 93% of F508del-chromosomes. The rare DHS-haplotype was observed on seven F508del alleles only, whereby the phenotype of the corresponding pair was ranked discordant in five cases.

Modulation of CF Disease Severity by QTLs for Growth and Stature at 7q31.3 - 7qtel

The three highly informative microsatellite markers D7S525, D7S514 and D7S495 were typed for the 34 F508del homozygous sibling pairs (Table 1).[10] At D7S495, localized in a 21-cM distance 3'to *CFTR*, the allele distributions were significantly different between the clinically different patient pair cohorts ($P=0.01$ for the comparison of CON– and CON+ allele distributions, and $P=0.03$ for the comparison of CON– and DIS allele distributions). Strikingly, allele 10 at D7S495 was observed on a third of the F508del chromosomes of the 11 mildly affected patient pairs, but did not occur among the ten severely affected patient pairs (Figure 2).[10] This finding implies a skewed distribution of functional polymorphisms of this chromosome 7q segment in the phenotypically different sib-pairs.

Obesity related traits have been mapped to several markers located between *CFTR* and 7qtel in different populations (Figure 3a) as genomewide scans have identified quantitative trait loci for stature near D7S635, near D7S649 and in a region between D7S649 and D7S438.[39-42]

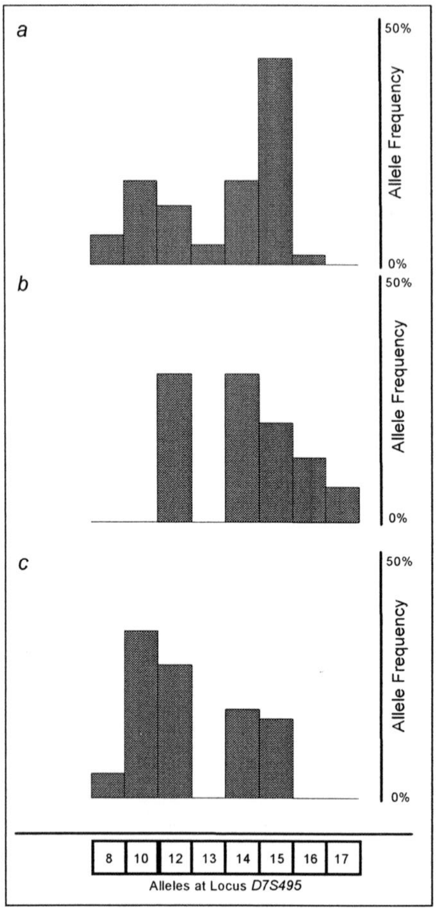

Figure 2. Allelic association among CF twin and sib pairs at D7S495. Allele distribution at D7S495 among DIS (Figure 2a; 26 chromosomes), CON- (Figure 2b; 20 chromosomes) and CON+ (Figure 2c; 22 chromosomes) F508del homozygous patient pairs. Comparison of CON-/CON+: 0.02; comparison of CON-/DIS: p=0.04 after Bonferroni-Correction for multiple testing as previously described.[10] Alleles at $(CA)_n$ repeat locus D7S495 are given as *arbitrary repeat units*. The actual physical sizes are: *8*: 150 bp; *10:* 154 bp; *12:* 158 bp; *13:* 160 bp; *14:* 162 bp; *15:* 164 bp; *16:* 166 bp; *17:* 168 bp.

A Rare LEP Promoter Haplotype is Observed Among Mildly Affected Patient Pairs

The human homologue of the murine obesity gene *LEP* has a pivotal role in energy homeostasis and the regulation of long-term energy balance,[43] immunomodulation [44] and reproduction.[45] To analyze *LEP* as a candidate gene for modulation of disease severity, two SNPs with high polymorphism information content as judged by published allele frequencies for the non-CF population [30-31] were selected for genotyping. These SNPs, LEP1 and LEP2, are both localized within the promoter of the *LEP* gene within a 1 kb distance. Among CON– and DIS pairs, only the LEP1-LEP2 haplotypes 1-1 and 2-2 were observed. The recombined LEP1-LEP2 haplotype 2-1 was exclusively observed in concordant/mildly affected patient pairs: among the informative meioses, every fifth CON+ chromosome carried the LEP1-LEP2 haplotype 2-1. In contrast, among CON- pairs, the LEP1-LEP2 haplotype 2-2 was observed on four out of five chromosomes among the informative meiosis. [10]

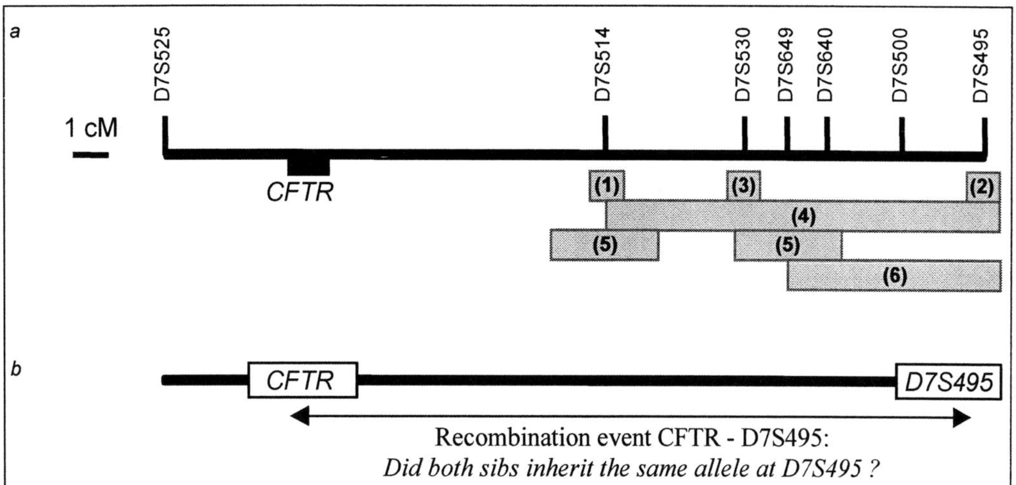

		CON- and CON+	DIS	
maternal chromosomes	yes	10	7	p = 0.275
	no	11	6	
paternal chromosomes	yes	21	5	p = 0.00007
	no	0	8	

Figure 3. Modulation of growth and stature in region 7q31-7qtel. Modulation of growth and stature on 7q31-7qtel observed for the non-CF population (3a) and for F508del homozygous CF patients (3b).[10] Please note that recombination events on maternal chromosomes have been detected in F508del homozygous sibpairs irrespective of their intra-pair discordance while recombination events on paternal chromosomes were exclusively observed among discordant sib pairs (p = 0.00007).[10] — Numbers in grey boxes below the genetic map in 3a correspond to literature data on: variation of (1) extremity skinfolds and (2) of waist circumference in Mexican-Americans;[39] (3) response to a very-low-calorie diet in a Finnish population of morbidly obese woman;[40] (4) candidate gene region for growth retardation by maternal isodisomy 7 and/or Silver Russel Syndrome;[47] (5) and (6) QTL for stature.[41-42]

As leptin was reported to be the permissive factor for puberty [45] and pubertal growth is known to be different in CF children compared to the non-CF population,[46] we have analyzed longitudinal growth data on 54 F508del homozygotes from the Hannover CF clinic for whom DNA was available for *LEP* genotyping. For reference, the growth curves of a non-CF population [18] were evaluated to predict the pubertal gain of body height for the respective pre-pubertal height centiles. All patients carrying the LEP1-LEP2 haplotype 2-1 (observed in six individuals) gained at least as much height during puberty compared to non-CF children with equal pre-pubertal height centiles whereas the same applies to only half of the patients homozygous for the LEP1-LEP2 haplotype 2-2 (observed in a total of 16 patients). This preliminary evaluation of the Hannover data set suggests that the leptin-promoter-haplotypes found predominantly among the concordant mildly affected pairs predispose to an elevated growth gain during puberty.

Analysis of Recombination Events Among Discordant Pairs Reveal a Parent-of-Origin Effect

By definition for this autosomal recessive disease, two F508del homozygous siblings have inherited the same genetic material at the *CFTR* locus and adjacent sequences localized 5' and 3' to *CFTR*. Absolute linkage disequilibrium is only disrupted if a recombination event has occurred during meiosis in the last generation. After typing the F508del homozygous sib pairs, we noticed that different D7S495 alleles were inherited from parent to offspring in 19 out 34 families. To analyze these recombination events, we have typed additional microsatellite markers located between *CFTR* and D7S495 (Table 1). Single recombination events were seen in all three phenotypic groups; however, recombination events on both F508del chromosomes were only observed among discordant patients in five of the 13 pairs. Maternal chromosomes recombined with similar rates in the different patient-pair cohorts.[10] In contrast, recombination frequencies were different on concordant and discordant paternal chromosomes (Figure 3b, P=0.00007, Fisher's exact test).[10] No recombination was observed on concordant paternal chromosomes.

This finding can be translated as a parent-of-origin effect: apparently, phenotypic concordance among CF sibs can be attributed to shared paternal sequences, while it does not have consequences whether or not two siblings have inherited the same genes from their mother. Interestingly, the region D7S686-7qtel was described as a candidate region for growth retardation by maternal isodisomy 7 and Silver-Russel-Syndrome (Figure 3a).[47] A paternally expressed gene that modulates growth in humans might explain why recombination events on the maternal chromosome were observed in all three phenotypic groups, while recombinations on the paternal allele were detected only among the discordant pairs: All concordant pairs shared the paternal allele between *CFTR* and D7S495 including the imprinted and non-imprinted genes controlling growth and stature implying a paramount effect of this chromosomal region on the impairment of growth in CF. The shared 28-cM segment of paternal chromosomes in concordant pairs contains more than 100 annotated genes, at least a dozen of which can be reasonably associated with growth and development. Hence, in contrast to the highly significant association of a single locus with the manifestation of a meconium ileus in CF,[48] in our case no singular candidate gene could be a priori hypothesized that accounts for the observed segregation of shared paternal chromosomes with concordance in clinical phenotype. Among the candidate genes for the modulation of growth and stature on chromosome 7q, the paternally expressed gene *MEST/PEG1*, encoded near D7S649 (Figure 3a), was named as a candidate for the Silver-Russel-Syndrome.[49-50] We have checked whether the recombination breakpoints on the paternal chromosome map 5' to *MEST/PEG*. However, we could identify a recombination breakpoint 5' to *MEST/PEG1* only in one out of eight cases, while in four out of eight cases the recombination breakpoint was located 3' to *MEST/PEG1*.[10] As this genomic region contains a cluster of imprinted genes besides *MEST/PEG1*,[51] we conclude that at least in some cases a paternally imprinted gene other than *MEST/PEG1* modulates the intra-pair discordance among our F508del homozygotes.

DISCUSSION

Heterozygote Advantage Mediated by Genes Encoded in the CFTR Linkage Group?

In a cohort of F508del homozygous twins and siblings selected for extreme clinical phenotypes, we have found evidence in regions 5' and 3'to, but not within, the major disease-causing gene itself for the existence of CF modulating genes. We conclude that functional polymorphisms in *LEP*, paternally imprinted loci such as *MEST/PEG1*, the stature QTLs and probably some further genes that hitchhike with F508del-*CFTR* in affected family members significantly shape the clinical manifestation of CF. The advantage or disadvantage of the apparently asymptomatic heterozygous CF carriers, however, is confined to the region that still is in linkage disequilibrium with *CFTR*. Based on assumptions of mutation rate of STRPs and of the demographic history of the European population, the age of the F508del mutation has been estimated from F508del-*CFTR* marker haplotypes to be 500–2,000 generations old.[52] Consequently, only genes with a genetic distance of 1 cM or less from *CFTR* are still in linkage disequilibrium on F508del-*CFTR* chromosomes. Hence, besides *CFTR* itself less than ten genes, including *CAV1, CAV2, MET , WNT2, GASZ* and *CORTBP2* [32] can modulate the fitness of F508del heterozygotes compared with the general population, as described by Dahl *et al.* [53] for non-smoking F508del carriers. In contrast, for affected F508del homozygotes the major modifier genes on chromosome 7q31-7qtel are co-inherited with F508del-*CFTR* in CF families, but are already in linkage equilibrium in the present-day F508del carrier population.

Detecting Modulators Encoded in Trans by Typing Discordant Pairs

In an association study using a classical case-control-design, the contrast between mildly and severely affected patients is employed to detect inherited modulators. For a study composed of affected sibpairs, the comparison of allele distributions between concordant mildly affected and concordant severely affected patient pairs points towards inherited modulators encoded close to the markers typed, as demonstrated within this chapter for the role of growth and stature modulating genes in CF. While in principle, the same contrast might be recognized by comparing the mildly and the severely affected patient of a discordant pair, observations at the *CFTR* gene region delineate another mechanism that provides an attractive opportunity to map disease modulating factors: near the *CFTR* gene region, two CF sibs must have inherited the same information from their parents together with their disease-causing lesion. Association of a discordant phenotype with J3.11 genotypes (Mekus *et al.* [10] and this chapter) thus points towards the consequences of inherited modulators that are encoded elsewhere in the genome. In this case, the interaction of transcription factors encoded in trans with regulatory elements localized in close proximity to the marker tested is a most obvious underlying mechanism, but for other genes scenarios such as interaction between ligand and receptor are equally valid and can be recognized through an allelic imbalance observed by comparing the discordant pairs to the concordant phenotypes. For the described association of J3.11 genotypes with the intrapair discordance in lung function,[10] all variants within known or still unrecognized regulatory elements of the *CFTR* gene and the corresponding transcription factors are plausible candidates. Fine mapping of SNPs within the respective regions [54] such as the two functional SNPs within the DNAseI hypersensitive site at +15.6kb 3‘ to the *CFTR* gene [29] that might define rare haplotypes among discordant pairs (this chapter) will resolve the extent to which haplotypes at the 3' end to *CFTR* have an impact on the manifestation of CF disease severity.

Genes that Modulate of Growth and Stature in Humans are Modulators of CF

The analysis of CF sib pairs at the *CFTR* gene region has demonstrated that gene(s) localized 3' to the *CFTR* gene determine the severity of CF disease. This is evident through the marked allelic association at D7S495, by the observation that a rare *LEP* promoter haplotype was observed exclusively among concordant mildly affected patient pairs, and by the finding that recombination events 3' to *CFTR* on paternal chromosomes were observed among discordant pairs but absent from concordant pairs (Mekus *et al.* [10] and this chapter). The molecular entities determining growth and stature among humans [41-42, 55] and causing Silver-Russel-Syndrome mediated by maternal uniparental disomy of chromosome 7q31-7qter [47] are still unknown. Furthermore, it is unknown whether the QTL for stature that has been reproducibly mapped to 7q31-7qtel [41-42, 55] is identical to the locus causing Silver-Russel-Syndrome or whether these are separate entities that map to the same chromosomal location by chance. In that respect, refined mapping of the recombination breakpoints on paternal chromosomes among the concordant CF sib pairs, thereby defining the region containing the modulator of CF disease severity encoded 3' to *CFTR*, might assist in delimiting the candidate gene region for modulation of growth and stature among humans.

Mapping CF Modulating Genes

The analysis of genes that modulate the CF phenotype using a candidate gene approach is widely used (reviewed by Drumm [56] and Merlo & Boyle [57]). Most studies rely on genotyping results for one candidate gene locus of a group of CF patients, and clinical parameters are compared between patient groups carrying different genotypes at the candidate gene locus. This approach is problematic with respect to a correction for multiple testing when many clinical variables are considered and/or the initially analyzed cohort is subdivided based on dichotomous variables, and as a consequence the same genotype data is analyzed multiple times. An alternative approach to circumvent this bias is the a-priory definition of patient groups, and following use of the phenotypic contrast between them to compare genotype and/or allele frequencies at candidate gene loci [9, 58]. Using this more robust design, the relative impact of candidate genes on the CF phenotype can be estimated if the same patient group is typed at multiple candidate gene loci. Furthermore, a duplication of the reported association in a second sample can be used to confirm an initial finding if the definition of phenotype and the clinical characteristics are similar in both data sets used for the association study. Future strategies for therapeutic intervention could be directed at those reliable modulators that have a high impact on CF disease manifestation.

Acknowledgements

The European CF Twin and Sibling Study was initiated in 1994 under the umbrella of the EU BIOMED II program. We are indebted to patients, parents and members of the European Cystic Fibrosis Twin and Sibling Study Consortium for their ongoing support.

This work was funded by the Deutsche Forschungsgemeinschaft (SFB280 Projekt A13) and by the European Union (QLG1-CT-2001-01005). Initial funding of the Clinical Research Group "Molecular Pathology of Cystic Fibrosis" by the Deutsche Forschungsgemeinschaft is gratefully acknowledged. This study was also supported in part by grants provided grants provided by the Mukoviszidose e.V. and by the Deutsche Fördergemeinschaft für Mukoviszidoseförderung e.V..

Appendix

Genotyping

All marker were typed based on PCR-based methods.[10] Microsatellites were analyzed by direct blotting electrophoresis of PCR product amplified with one biotinylated primer and subsequent chemoluminescence detection. All SNPs were assayed by PCR-RFLP whereby the alleles were named according to the standard nomenclature [59] with "1" denoting the uncut allele and "2" denoting the cut allele. Primer sequences for PCR amplification of markers D7S525, D7S680, D7S514, D7S635, D7S2501, AFM16yC9, D7S504, D7S1875, D7S461, D7S530, D7S649, D7S640, D7S500, D7S495 were taken from internet resources. Analysis for SNP markers MetH, XV2c, TUB20, and J3.11 was carried out as described by Horn *et al.*,[27] Rosenbloom *et al.*,[28] Dörk *et al.* [21] and Horn *et al.*,[27] respectively. LEP1 targets two nucleotide exchanges at positions –2548 and –2549 of the LEP promoter [30-31] which both destroy a *Hha*I site (primers used for amplification: 5'-ATTTCCTGTAATTTTCCCGTGAGAA-3' and 5'-AGTGGTCCTGAGGTGACGTACATC-3') and LEP2 detects –1387G/A (primers used for amplification: 5'-GGTGGGCATCACAGTACTACCG-3' and 5'-TCGTTTGTAGTTCCCCGCTTTAC-3'). The two SNPs within the DHS at 4572+15.6kb [29] were targeted with *BspH*I (for DHS1 = AC000061:72957C/T) and *Age*I (for DHS2=AC000061:73211C/T) upon amplification of a 384 bp product using primers 5'-GTACACCACTACGCCCAGGT-3' and 5'-TAAAGGGCATTCAGGACACC-3'.

References

[1] Rommens JM, Iannuzzi MC, Kerem BS, Drumm ML, Melmer G, Dean M et al. Identification of the cystic fibrosis gene: chromosome walking and jumping. *Science* 1989;245:1059–1065.

[2] The Cystic Fibrosis Analysis Consortium. Cystic fibrosis mutation database. Avaliable at: http://www.genet.sickkids.on.ca/cftr

[3] Koch C, Cuppens H, Rainisio M, Madessani U, Harms H, Hodson M et al. European Epidemiologic Registry of Cystic Fibrosis (ERCF): comparison of major disease manifestations between patients with different classes of mutations. *Pediatr Pulmonol* 2001;31:1-12.

[4] Zielenski J. Genotype and phenotype in cystic fibrosis. Respiration 2000; 67:117-33.

[5] Rowntree RK, Harris A. The phenotypic consequences of CFTR mutations. *Ann Hum Genet* 2003;67:471-85.

[6] Johannsen HK, Nir M, Hʊiby N, Koch C, Schwartz M. Severity of cystic fibrosis in patients homozygous and heterozygous for ΔF508 mutation. *Lancet* 1991;337:631–634.

[7] Lester LA, Kraut J, Lloyd-Still J, Karrison T, Mott C, Billstrand C et al. ΔF508 genotype does not predict disease severity in an ethnically diverse cystic fibrosis population. *Pediatrics* 1994;93:114–118.

[8] Santis G, Osborne L, Knight RA, Hodson ME. Independent genetic determinants of pancreatic and pulmonary status in cystic fibrosis. *Lancet* 1990;336:1081-1084.

[9] Mekus F, Ballmann M, Bronsveld I, Bijman J, Veeze H, Tümmler B. Categories of deltaF508 homozygous cystic fibrosis twin and sibling pairs with distinct phenotypic characteristics. *Twin Res* 2000;3:277–293.

[10] Mekus F, Laabs U, Veeze H, Tümmler B. Genes in the vicinity of CFTR modulate the cystic fibrosis phenotype in highly concordant or discordant F508del homozygous sib pairs. *Hum Genet* 2003;112:1-11.

[11] Eaves L, Meyer J. Locating human quantitative trait loci: guidelines for the selection of sibling pairs for genotyping. *Behav Genet* 1994;24:443–455.

[12] Risch N, Zhang H. Extreme discordant sib pairs for mapping quantitative trait loci in humans. *Science* 1995;268:1584–1589.

[13] Dolan CV, Boomsma DI. Optimal selection of sib pairs from random samples for linkage analysis of a QTL using the EDAC test. *Behav Genet* 1998;28:197–206.

[14] Corey M, Farewell V. Determinants of mortality from cystic fibrosis in Canada, 1970–1989. *Am J Epidemiol* 1996;143:1007–1017.

[15] Corey M, Edwards L, Levison H, Knowles M. Longitudinal analysis of pulmonary function decline in patients with cystic fibrosis. *J Pediatr* 1997;131:809–814.

[16] Lai HC, Corey M, FitzSimmons S, Kosorok MR, Farrell PM. Comparison of growth status of patients with cystic fibrosis between the United States and Canada. *Am J Clin Nutr* 1999;69:531–538.

[17] Sharma R, Florea VG, Bolger AP, Doehner W, Florea ND, Coats AJ et al. Wasting as an independent predictor of mortality in patients with cystic fibrosis. *Thorax* 2001;56:746–750.

[18] Prader A, Largo RH, Molinari L, Issler C. Physical growth of Swiss children from birth to 20 years of age. First Zurich longitudinal study of growth and development. *Helv Pediatr Acta Suppl* 1989;52:1-125.

[19] Knudson RJ, Lebowitz MD, Holberg CJ, Burrows B. Changes in the normal maximal expiratory flow volume curve with growth and ageing. *Am Rev Respir Dis* 1983;127:725-734.

[20] Romeo G, Devoto M, Galietta LJV. Why is the cystic fibrosis gene so frequent? *Hum Genet* 1989;94:1–5.

[21] Dörk T, Neumann T, Wulbrand U, Wulf B, Kälin N, Maass G et al. Intra- and extragenic marker haplotypes of *CFTR* mutations in cystic fibrosis families. *Hum Genet* 1992;88:417–425.

[22] Sereth H, Shoshani T, Bashan N, Kerem BS. Extended haplotype analysis of cystic fibrosis mutations and its implications for the selective advantage hypothesis. *Hum Genet* 1993;92:289–295.

[23] Morral N, Dörk T, Llevadot R, Dziadek V, Mercier B, Ferec C et al. Haplotype analysis of 94 cystic fibrosis mutations with seven polymorphic *CFTR* DNA markers. *Hum Mutat* 1996;8:149–159.

[24] Cuppens H, Teng H, Raeymaekers P, De Boeck C, Cassiman JJ. *CFTR* haplotype backgrounds on normal and mutant *CFTR* genes. *Hum Mol Genet* 1994;3:607–614.

[25] Morral N, Dörk T, Llevadot R, Dziadek V, Mercier B, Ferec C et al. Haplotype analysis of 94 cystic fibrosis mutations with seven polymorphic *CFTR* DNA markers. *Hum Mutat* 1996;8:149–159.

[26] Dib C, Faure S, Fizames C, Samson D, Drouot N, Vignal A et al. A comprehensive genetic map of the human genome based on 5264 microsatellites. *Nature* 1996;380:152–154.

[27] Horn GT, Richards B, Wright G, Landes GM, Klinger KW. Analysis and detection of genetic polymorphisms near the cystic fibrosis and Huntington's disease loci. *Cytogenet Cell Genet* 1989;51:1015.

[28] Rosenbloom CL, Kerem BS, Rommens JM, Tsui LC, Wainwright B, Williamson R et al. DNA amplification for detection of the XV2c polymorphism linked to cystic fibrosis. *Nucleic Acids Res* 1989;17:7117.

[29] Rowntree R, Harris A. DNA polymorphisms in potential regulatory elements of the CFTR gene alter transcription factor binding. *Hum Genet* 2002;111:66-74.

[30] Mammes O, Betoulle D, Aubert R, Giraud V, Tuzet S, Petiet A et al. Novel polymorphism in the 5'region of the *LEP* gene. Association with leptin levels and response to low-calorie diet in human obesity. *Diabetes* 1998;47:487–489.

[31] Li WD, Reed DR, Lee JH, Xu W, Kilker RL, Sodam BR et al. Sequence variants in the 5'flanking region of the leptin gene are associated with obesity in woman. *Ann Hum Genet* 1999;63:227–234.

[32] The National Center for Biotechnology Information. Human genome resources at NCBI. Available at: http://www.ncbi.nlm.nih.gov/

[33] The Marshfield center for medical genetics. Genetic maps. Available at: http://research.marshfieldclinic.org/genetics/

[34] Santis G, Osborne L, Knight RA, Ramsay M, Williamson R, Hodson ME. Cystic fibrosis haplotype association and the Delta F508 mutation in adult British CF patients. *Hum Genet* 1990;85:424–425.

[35] Wulbrand U, Dörk T, Tümmler B, Krawczak M. Genetic determinants in cystic fibrosis. *Lancet* 1991;337:623.

[36] Macek M Jr, Macek M Sr, Krebsova A, Nash E, Hamosh A, Reis A et al. Possible association of the allele status of the CS.7/*Hha*I polymorphism 5'of the *CFTR* gene with postnatal female survival. *Hum Genet* 1997;99:565–572.

[37] VISTA Genome Browser. Available at: http://pipeline.lbl.gov/

[38] Nuthall HN, Moulin DS, Huxley C, Harris A. Analysis of DNAse hypersensitive sites at the 3'end of the cystic fibrosis transmembrane regulator gene (*CFTR*). *Biochem J* 1999;341:601– 611.

[39] Duggirala R, Sern MP, Mitchell BD, Reinhart LJ, Shipman PA, Uresandi OC et al. Quantitative variation in obesity-related traits and insulin precursors linked to the *OB* gene region on human chromosome 7. *Am J Hum Genet* 1996;59:694–703.

[40] Oksanen L, Öhman M, Heiman M, Kainulainen K, Kaprio J, Mustajoki P et al. Markers for the gene *OB* and serum leptin levels in human morbid obesity. *Hum Genet* 1997;99:559–564.

[41] Hirschhorn J N, Lindgren C M, Daly MJ, Kirby A, Schaffner SF, Burtt NP et al. Genomewide linkage analysis of stature in multiple populations reveals several regions with evidence of linkage to adult height. *Am J Hum Genet* 2001;69:106–116.

[42] Perola M, Ohman M, Hiekkalinna T, Leppavuori J, Pajukanta P, Wessman M et al. Quantitative-trait-locus analysis of body-mass index and of stature, by combined analysis of genome scans of five Finnish study groups. *Am J Hum Genet* 2001;69:117–123.

[43] Woods SC, Seeley RJ, Porte D Jr, Schwartz MW. Signals that regulate food intake and energy homeostasis. *Science* 1998;280:1378–1382.

[44] Lord GM, Matarese G, Howard JK, Baker RJ, Bloom SR, Lechler RI. Leptin modulates the T-cell immune response and reverses starvation-induced immunosuppression. *Nature* 1998;394:897–901.

[45] Baldelli R, Dieguez C, Casanueva F. The role of leptin in reproduction: experimental and clinical aspects. *Ann Med* 2002;34:5-18.

[46] Byard PJ (1994) The adolescent growth spurt in children with cystic fibrosis. *Ann Hum Biol* 1994;21:229-40.

[47] Hannuila K, Lipsanen-Nymawn M, Kontiokari T, Kere J. A narrow segment of maternal uniparental disomy of chromosome 7q31-qter in Silver-Russel-Syndrome delimits a candidate gene region. *Am J Hum Genet* 2001;68:247–253.

[48] Zielenski J, Corey M, Rozmahel R, Markiewicz D, Aznarez I, Casals T et al. Detection of a cystic fibrosis modifier locus for meconium ileus on human chromosome 19q13. *Nat Genet* 1999;22:128–129.

[49] Kobayashi S, Kohda T, Miyoshi N, Kuroiwa Y, Aisaka K, Tsutsumi O et al. Human *PEG1/MEST*, an imprinted gene on chromosome 7. *Hum Mol Genet* 1997;6:781– 786.

[50] Hayashida S, Yamasaki K, Asada Y, Soeda E, Niikawa N, Kishino T. Construction of a physical and transcript map flanking the imprinted *MEST/PEG1* region at 7q32. *Genomics* 2000;66: 221–225.

[51] Blagitko N, Schultz U, Schinzel AA, Ropers HH, Kalscheuer VM. Gamma2-COP, a novel imprinted gene on chromosome 7q32, defines a new imprinting cluster in the human genome. *Hum Mol Genet* 1999;8:2387–2396.

[52] Wiuf C. Do delta F508 heterozygotes have a selective advantage? *Genet Res* 2001;78:41–47.

[53] Dahl M, Tybjaerg-Hansen A, Wittrup HH, Lange P, Nordestgaard BG. Cystic fibrosis DeltaF508 heterozygotes, smoking, and reproduction: studies of 9141 individuals from a general population sample. *Genomics* 1998;50:89–96.

[54] Phylactides M, Rowntree R, Nuthall I, Ussery D, Wheeler A, Harris A. Evaluation of potential regulatory elements identified as DNAseI hypersensitive sites in the CFTR gene. *Eur J Biochem* 2002;269: 533-559.

[55] Wu X, Cooper RS, Boerwinkle E, Turner ST, Hunt S, Myers R et al. Combined analysis of genomewide scans for adult height: results from the NHLBI family blood pressure program. *Europ J Hum Genet* 2003;11:271-274.

[56] Drumm M. Modifier genes and variation in cystic fibrosis. Respir Res 2001;2:125-128.

[57] Merlo CA, Boyle MP. Modifier genes in cystic fibrosis lung disease. *J Lab Clin Med* 2003;141:237-241.

[58] Knowles MR, Konstan M, Schluchter M, Handler A, Bucur C, Pace R et al. Multi-center study of gene modifiers for CF lung disease. *Pediatric Pulmonology* 2003;S25:99-100.

[59] European Working Group on Cystic Fibrosis Genetics. Gradient of distribution in Europe of the major CF mutation and of its associated haplotype. *Hum Genet* 1990;85:436–445.

INDEX

A

B

C

D

E

F

I

J

K

L

M

N

O

P

Q

R

S

T

U

V